Glaucoma Medical Therapy

Ophthalmology Monographs

A series published by Oxford University Press in cooperation with the American Academy of Ophthalmology

Series Editor: Richard K. Parrish, II, MD, Bascom Palmer Eye Institute

American Academy of Ophthalmology Clinical Education Secretariat:
Louis B. Cantor, MD, Indiana University School of Medicine
Gregory L. Skuta, MD, Dean A. McGee Eye Institute

GLAUCOMA MEDICAL THERAPY

Principles and Management,
Second Edition

Edited by

PETER A. NETLAND, MD, PhD

Published by Oxford University Press
In cooperation with
The American Academy of Ophthalmology

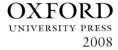

OXFORD
UNIVERSITY PRESS
2008

OXFORD
UNIVERSITY PRESS

Oxford University Press, Inc., publishes works that further
Oxford University's objective of excellence
in research, scholarship, and education.

Oxford   New York
Auckland   Cape Town   Dar es Salaam   Hong Kong   Karachi
Kuala Lumpur   Madrid   Melbourne   Mexico City   Nairobi
New Delhi   Shanghai   Taipei   Toronto

With offices in
Argentina   Austria   Brazil   Chile   Czech Republic   France   Greece
Guatemala   Hungary   Italy   Japan Poland   Portugal   Singapore
South Korea   Switzerland   Thailand   Turkey   Ukraine   Vietnam

Published by Oxford University Press, Inc.
198 Madison Avenue, New York, New York 10016
www.oup.com

Oxford is a registered trademark of Oxford University Press

Library of Congress Cataloging-in-Publication Data
Glaucoma medical therapy : principles and management / edited by Peter A. Netland.—2nd ed.
    p. ; cm. — (Ophthalmology monographs ; 13)
Includes bibliographical references and index.
ISBN 978-0-19-532850-9
1. Glaucoma—Chemotherapy.   I. Netland, Peter A.   II. American Academy
of Ophthalmology.   III. Series.
[DNLM: 1. Glaucoma—drug therapy.   2. Intraocular Pressure—drug effects.
W1 OP372L v.13 2007 / WW 290 G550152 2007]
RE871.G554 2007
617.7'41061—dc22   2007013167

9 8 7 6 5 4 3 2 1

Printed in China
on acid-free paper

Legal Notice

The American Academy of Ophthalmology provides the opportunity for material to be presented for educational purposes only. The material represents the approach, ideas, statement, or opinion of the author, not necessarily the only or best method or procedure in every case, nor the position of the Academy. Unless specifically stated otherwise, the opinions expressed and statements made by various authors in this monograph reflect the author's observations and do not imply endorsement by the Academy. The material is not intended to replace a physician's own judgment or give specific advice for case management. The Academy does not endorse any of the products or companies, if any, mentioned in this monograph.

Some material on recent developments may include information on drug or device applications that are not considered community standard, that reflect indications not included in approved FDA labeling, or that are approved for use only in restricted research settings. This information is provided as education only so that physicians may be aware of alternative methods of the practice of medicine, and should not be considered endorsement, promotion, or in any way encouragement to use such applications. The FDA has stated that it is the responsibility of the physician to determine the FDA status of each drug or device he or she wishes to use in clinical practice, and to use these products with appropriate patient consent and in compliance with applicable law.

The Academy and Oxford University Press (OUP) do not make any warranties as to the accuracy, adequacy, or completeness of any material presented here, which is provided on an "as is" basis. The Academy and OUP are not liable to anyone for any errors, inaccuracies, or omissions obtained here. The Academy specifically disclaims any and all liability for injury or other damages of any kind for any and all claims that may arise out of the use of any practice, technique, or drug described in any material by any author, whether such claims are asserted by a physician or any other person.

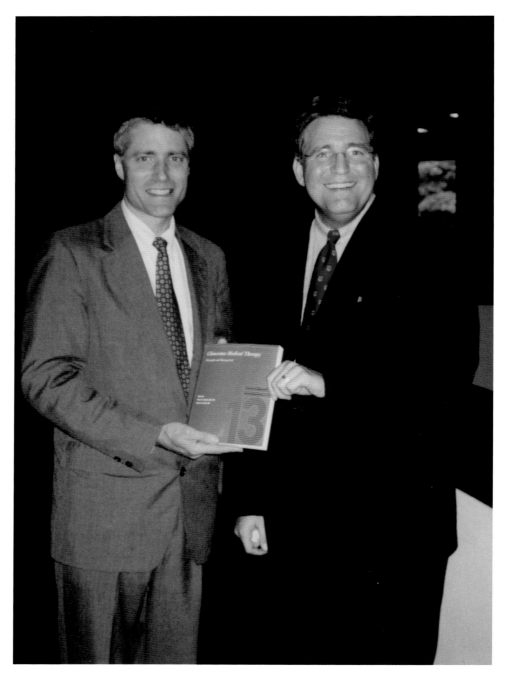

Peter A. Netland, MD, PhD (*left*), and Robert C. Allen, MD (*right*), Memphis, Tennessee, 2000.

Preface

*I*n the latter part of the nineteenth century, effective medical treatment for glaucoma was championed by physicians who had studied under Albrecht von Graefe. In 1876, Ludwig Laqueur, a professor in Strasbourg, France, recommended the use of an extract of the calabar bean, the seed of an African vine that is a source of physostigmine. At about the same time, Adolf Weber, a practicing ophthalmologist in Darmstadt, Germany, advocated the use of an extract of jaborandi, a South American shrub that contains pilocarpine. Although these drugs did not treat the underlying cause of glaucoma, they successfully controlled intraocular pressure in many patients. Miosis-inducing parasympathomimetic drugs remained the mainstay of medical therapy for glaucoma for the next 75 years, until the introduction of oral acetazolamide and topical epinephrine in the 1950s, followed by topical ophthalmic beta blockers in the 1970s.

In recent years, a large number of drugs have been developed for the treatment of glaucoma. With the increasing choices of alternative medications, miotic drugs, acetazolamide, and epinephrine are now less frequently used to treat chronic glaucoma. Prostaglandin analogs, topical carbonic anhydrase inhibitors, and adrenergic agonists have played an increasingly important role in the medical therapy of glaucoma. While naturally available substances provided the earliest glaucoma medications, new drugs are now developed through computational and synthetic chemical techniques. Currently available glaucoma medications have been approved for clinical use based upon their ability to lower intraocular pressure, although medications are being considered with other primary mechanisms of action that are thought to be potentially beneficial in glaucoma therapy. The clinical use of drugs for glaucoma therapy has evolved, adapting with the advent of each new drug.

Clinicians need to understand, synthesize, and use data about medications that have specific benefits and risks for their glaucoma patients.

An ideal drug would have no side effects, would be effortless to administer, would cost nothing, and would be 100% effective in controlling or eliminating the problem. Currently, the ideal drug for glaucoma does not exist. Nonetheless, investigators continually strive to improve glaucoma medical therapy, which will likely continue to improve in the future. New experimental and clinical investigations are promising and may open new therapeutic targets for treatment of glaucoma in the future. The focus of this book is the current art and science of clinically available drugs for medical therapy of glaucoma. The contributors have attempted to provide evidence-based information about the topic, while providing perspective from clinical experience.

This is a peer-reviewed, edited, multiauthor book, with chapters contributed by individuals with expertise in the medical therapy of glaucoma. The book is intended to provide information about glaucoma medical therapy for practicing ophthalmologists and ophthalmologists in training. Other practitioners who have clinical contact with glaucoma patients also may find the content of this monograph valuable. The material in this book on the medical management of glaucoma complements the surgical orientation of the second edition of *Glaucoma Surgery: Principles and Techniques*, edited by Robert N. Weinreb, MD, and Richard P. Mills, MD, and published by the American Academy of Ophthalmology and Oxford University Press.

In the second edition of this book, all chapters have been thoroughly revised and updated, and new chapters regarding fixed-combination drugs and medical treatment in pregnancy and pediatric patients have been added. Some chapters have required addition of extensive new material because of the changes in medical therapy of glaucoma since the publication of the first edition of the book in 1999. In 2005, Robert C. Allen, MD, co-editor for the first edition, succumbed to the complications of uveal melanoma. He was an esteemed clinical colleague and investigator, prolific academic, respected department chair, devoted family man, and cherished friend.

The contributors to this edition of *Glaucoma Medical Therapy* have dedicated their efforts to the memory of Dr. Robert C. Allen (1950–2005).

Peter A. Netland, MD, PhD

Educational Objectives

The educational objectives of this monograph are to

- Identify the different categories of drugs and combinations of drugs used to treat glaucoma
- Outline the treatment regimens employed with specific medications
- Describe the side effects and contraindications of specific medications
- Demonstrate how different drugs may be used either alone or in combination to achieve the desired therapeutic effect
- Provide updated information on medications and their role in glaucoma therapy
- Familiarize the reader with the effect of systemic medications on intraocular pressure
- Explain the use of osmotic drugs in the management of angle-closure glaucoma and secondary glaucomas
- Educate the reader on the use of medications in specific types of glaucoma, such as pediatric, pigmentary, corticosteroid-induced, and neovascular glaucoma
- Encourage the reader to monitor patient compliance with recommended regimens and offer suggestions to improve compliance
- Define maximum tolerable medical therapy
- Analyze the use of medications in conjunction with laser or filtration surgery

Acknowledgments

This book was a team effort, and I am indebted to the contributors to this monograph for giving so generously of their time and expertise. I am also grateful to the reviewers for this book, who, despite their anonymity, provided important peer review of this material. The Foundation of the American Academy of Ophthalmology and the Clinical Education Staff provided skilled assistance for the first edition of this book, particularly Pearl C. Vapnek, managing editor of the Ophthalmology Monographs series. In developing the first edition, help and encouragement were afforded by the Ophthalmology Monographs Committee, including Drs. H.S. Eustis, A. Capone, W.W. Culbertson, J.C. Fleming, C.L. Karp, B.G. Haik, and M.A. Johnstone. Clinical Education Secretaries provided valuable guidance for the first and second editions, including Drs. T.A. Weingeist, M.A. Kass, T. Liesegang, and G.L. Skuta. Dr. Richard K. Parrish, II, the series editor, has provided important oversight for the monograph series, including the second edition of this book. I am especially thankful for the expert assistance of Mary E. Smith, MPH, RDMS, project manager for the book at the University of Tennessee. The team at Oxford University Press provided excellent publishing support for the second edition, including editorial assistant Nicholas C. Liu, production editor Brian Desmond, marketing manager John Hercel, and sales manager Marnie Vandenberg. I am especially indebted to Catharine Carlin, editor at Oxford University Press, for her support and encouragement throughout the development of the second edition of this book.

I am most grateful for the memory of my co-editor for the first edition of *Glaucoma Medical Therapy*, Dr. Robert C. Allen. Book coauthors usually have a unique bond, but our relationship surpassed even that closeness. I will miss Bob's advice, support, and friendship.

Contents

Contributors

Robert C. Allen, MD (deceased)
Department of Ophthalmology
Medical College of Virginia
Richmond, Virginia

R. Rand Allingham, MD
Department of Ophthalmology
Duke University Medical Center
Durham, North Carolina

Yaniv Barkana, MD
Department of Ophthalmology
Assaf Harofe Medical Centre
Beer Yaacov, Zerifin, Israel

Carl B. Camras, MD
Department of Ophthalmology
   and Visual Sciences
University of Nebraska Medical
   Center
Omaha, Nebraska

Pouya N. Dayani, MD
Department of Ophthalmology
   and Visual Sciences
Washington University School
   of Medicine
St. Louis, Missouri

Robert D. Fechtner, MD
Institute of Ophthalmology and
   Visual Science
University of Medicine and Dentistry
   of New Jersey
Newark, New Jersey

B'Ann True Gabelt, MS
Department of Ophthalmology
   and Visual Sciences
University of Wisconsin
Madison, Wisconsin

Lisa S. Gamell, MD
Department of Ophthalmology
Beth Israel Medical Center
New York, New York

Thomas W. Hejkal, MD, PhD
Department of Ophthalmology
   and Visual Sciences
University of Nebraska Medical Center
Omaha, Nebraska

Eve J. Higginbotham, MD
Department of Ophthalmology
Emory School of Medicine
Morehouse School of Medicine
Atlanta, Georgia

Nauman R. Imami, MD
Henry Ford Medical Center
Detroit, Michigan

Malik Y. Kahook, MD
UPMC Eye Center
University of Pittsburgh School
    of Medicine
Pittsburgh, Pennsylvania

Elliott M. Kanner, MD, PhD
Hamilton Eye Institute
University of Tennessee Health
    Science Center
Memphis, Tennessee

Michael A. Kass, MD
Department of Ophthalmology
    and Visual Sciences
Washington University School
    of Medicine
St. Louis, Missouri

Paul L. Kaufman, MD
Department of Ophthalmology
    and Visual Sciences
University of Wisconsin
Madison, Wisconsin

Albert S. Khouri, MD
Institute of Ophthalmology and
    Visual Science
University of Medicine and Dentistry
    of New Jersey
Newark, New Jersey

Allan E. Kolker, MD
St. Louis, Missouri

Paul J. Lama, MD
Institute of Ophthalmology and
    Visual Science
University of Medicine and Dentistry
    of New Jersey
Newark, New Jersey

Simon K. Law, MD, PharmD
Jules Stein Eye Institute
University of California, Los Angeles
Los Angeles, California

David A. Lee, MD, MS, MBA
Jules Stein Eye Institute
University of California, Los Angeles
Los Angeles, California

Jeffrey M. Liebmann, MD
Manhattan Eye, Ear and
    Throat Hospital
New York University Medical Center
New York, New York

Felipe A. Medeiros, MD
Hamilton Glaucoma Center
University of California, San Diego
La Jolla, California

Peter A. Netland, MD, PhD
Hamilton Eye Institute
University of Tennessee Health
    Science Center
Memphis, Tennessee

Tony Realini, MD
West Virginia University Eye Institute
Morgantown, West Virginia

Robert Ritch, MD
New York Eye and Ear Infirmary
New York, New York

Howard I. Savage, MD
Wilmer Institute
Johns Hopkins University
Baltimore, Maryland

Joel S. Schuman, MD
UPMC Eye Center
University of Pittsburgh School
    of Medicine
Pittsburgh, Pennsylvania

Robert N. Weinreb, MD
Hamilton Glaucoma Center
University of California, San Diego
La Jolla, California

Glaucoma Medical Therapy

Ocular Pharmacology

SIMON K. LAW AND DAVID A. LEE

Ocular medications have an important role in the treatment of glaucoma. Medications are usually considered the first line of treatment for glaucoma, and in most glaucoma patients medications alone can control their disease. Glaucoma medications lower intraocular pressure (IOP) by either reducing aqueous production or increasing aqueous outflow through either the conventional or the unconventional pathways. Frequently, multiple glaucoma medications are used in combination to adequately lower IOP. A clear understanding of the pharmacokinetics of these medications is important to knowing several details:

1. Whether the drug itself or a metabolite is responsible for the therapeutic effect
2. The optimal route of drug administration
3. The optimal dosage regimen
4. The relationship between drug concentrations in tissues and their pharmacologic or toxicologic response

Pharmacokinetics is the study of the time-course changes of drug concentrations and their metabolites in tissues. It involves the determination of the rates of four processes: absorption, distribution, metabolism, and excretion.[1] Biopharmaceutics is the study of the effects of drug formulation on the pharmacologic and therapeutic activity.[2] It deals with the relationships between the drug response and the drug's physical state, salt form, particle size, crystalline structure, surface area, dosage form, adjuvants, or preservatives present in the formulation. Pharmacokinetic and biopharmaceutic data are important for making informed judgments on drugs and their formulations—judgments that may allow the proper selection of an appropriate

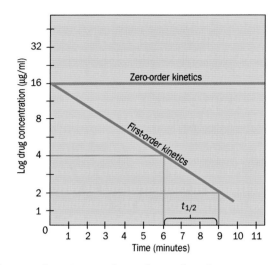

Figure 1.2. Pharmacokinetics: semilogarithmic plot of concentration versus time.

adequate mixing of drug with the precorneal tear film and the residence time of drug in the precorneal area.[4]

A relatively stagnant precorneal tear film layer has a thickness of about 7–9 μm and is composed of mucin, water, and oil.[10] Eyelid blinking facilitates the mixing of the drug with the precorneal tear film. A gradient of drug concentration between the precorneal tear film and the cornea and bulbar conjunctival epithelia acts as a driving force for passive drug diffusion into the cornea and conjunctiva.[7] The lag time is the time between the instillation of drug and its appearance in aqueous, which reflects the rate of drug diffusion across the cornea.

The amount of drug penetrating the eye is linearly related to its concentration in the tears, unless the drug interacts or binds with other molecules present in the cornea or the cornea becomes saturated because of limited drug solubility. The rate of drug concentration decline in the tears is proportional to the amount of drug remaining in the tears at the time and approximates first-order kinetics. This rate of decline depends on the rate of dilution by fresh tears and the drainage rate of tears into the cul-de-sac.[11,12]

In normal humans, the basal rate of tear flow is approximately 1 μL/min, and the physiologic turnover rate is approximately 10% to 15% per minute, which decreases with age. Basal tear flow is usually lower in patients with keratoconjunctivitis sicca and slightly higher in contact lens wearers.[13] The half-life of the exponential decline of fluorescence in the precorneal tear film in normal humans, as measured by fluorophotometry, varies between 2 and 20 minutes. This variability also applies to other substances. The loss rate constant for fluorescein varies depending on the amount of tearing. Reflex tearing caused by stinging from instillation of an irritating drug produces a higher loss rate. Lid closure and local or general anesthesia can decrease the tear flow rate. Physical, psychological, and emotional factors can increase tearing.

Blinking movements force part of the instilled volume through the puncta into the nasolacrimal duct. Each blink eliminates 2 μL of fluid from the cul-de-sac.[4] Aside from elimination by drainage through the nasolacrimal route, evaporation of tears, and deposition of drug on lid margins, drug may be bound to proteins in tears and metabolized by enzymes in tears and tissue.[14] These processes tend to limit the amount of drug entering the eye. As a result of limited residence time in the precorneal area imposed by these factors, but mainly because of rapid drainage, only a small fraction of the dose (1% to 10%) reaches the internal structures. This fraction may be increased by prolonging the residence time at the absorptive surfaces and enhancing the penetration rate through the corneal epithelium, by making the molecule more lipophilic. Transcorneal movement can be increased by changing the barrier properties of the corneal epithelium, by applying an anesthetic, by preservatives in topical medications, or after damaging the epithelium. Conversion of epinephrine to its dipivalyl ester derivative increases its lipophilicity and serves as a prodrug to increase penetration through the epithelium.

The distribution of drugs within the eye depends on many factors. The eye is relatively isolated from the systemic circulation by the blood–retina, blood–vitreous, and blood–aqueous barriers. These barriers comprise the tight junctions between the capillary endothelial cells in the retina and iris, between the nonpigmented ciliary epithelial cells, and between the retinal pigment epithelial cells.[15] These tight junctions exclude large molecules such as plasma proteins from entering the eye from the blood circulation, but allow many smaller molecules (molecular weight <500 daltons) and drugs to pass. The blood–aqueous barrier is evidenced by the low concentration of proteins in the aqueous and the failure of intravenously injected fluorescein to enter the aqueous unless the eye is inflamed. Many drugs in the blood circulation are unable to enter the eye because of these blood–ocular barriers.

The fraction of a topical drug that is absorbed by the eye can enter the systemic blood circulation by at least two pathways:

1. Along with the bulk flow of aqueous by way of the conventional outflow pathways of trabecular meshwork, Schlemm's canal, aqueous collecting channels, and episcleral venous plexus
2. By being absorbed into the blood vessels of the uvea, choroid, and retina

A drug in the aqueous that leaves through the uveoscleral outflow pathway through the iris base and ciliary body may be reabsorbed into the choroidal vessels from the suprachoroidal space.

Drug loss from the precorneal area limits the time available for absorption into the eye. The time to peak drug levels in the eye is determined by the residence time in the precorneal area.[16] Most drugs delivered topically to the eye exhibit similar apparent times to peak concentrations in aqueous as the drug drains out of the cul-de-sac within the first 5 minutes. The time it takes for most drugs to reach their peak concentrations in the aqueous is within a rather narrow range of 20–60 minutes.[17] Within the cornea, drug may diffuse laterally to the limbus and enter the eye at the iris root. Drugs may also be absorbed from the cul-de-sac across the conjunctiva and enter the eye through the sclera. The sclera poses less of a barrier to hydrophilic drugs than does the cornea, but both are comparable for lipophilic drugs.[8]

The main route of drug entry into the anterior chamber is through the cornea. Drugs in the aqueous equilibrate with drugs in the tissues in contact with that fluid. Drugs are not distributed uniformly within the eye; molecules may selectively concentrate in certain parts. Most drugs are eliminated from the anterior chamber by bulk flow of aqueous. Normally, turnover of aqueous in human eyes is rapid, with a half-life of approximately 52 minutes.[5] In the case of drugs that decrease the formation of aqueous, their effects on the turnover of aqueous may alter the drug elimination rate to favor a longer duration of action.

The distribution of drugs by diffusion from the anterior chamber to the tissues of the posterior segment is hindered by physical barriers, such as the iris, lens, and ciliary body, as well as by the bulk flow of aqueous anteriorly through the pupil. Most topically applied ophthalmic drugs can reach therapeutic concentrations in the anterior segment tissues but not in the posterior segment tissues. There are significant challenges to the delivery of drugs to the retina by topical administration due to these barriers. Therefore, the most commonly used route of administration to deliver drugs to the retina and vitreous is by intravitreal injection. Also, drug concentrations in the posterior segment of the eye can be measured by obtaining tissue samples, such as vitreous or retinal biopsy specimens. Ultimately, the drug enters various cells and acts on enzymes or receptors. Drug molecules may be bound to proteins or pigment and are unable to act until freed from these binding sites.

The relationship between iris color and ocular drug effects was reported as early as 1929.[18] Topically applied mydriatic drugs had a slower onset of action in dark-pigmented irides compared with light-pigmented irides. Onset and duration of drug action after topical application were correlated with the retention of drug in the melanin-containing iris. Binding of the drugs by melanin is a very important factor in the control of drug action in the ocular compartments. Many liposoluble drugs are bound by melanin and slowly released later. Ocular drug response may vary from individual to individual depending on the degree of melanin pigmentation of the iris.

After a drug has been applied, it can be metabolized by enzymes in the tears, adnexa, and ocular tissues.[19] A broad range of active enzymes have been reported in eye tissues, including esterases, oxidoreductases, lysosomal enzymes, peptidases, glucuronide and sulfate transferases, glutathione-conjugating enzymes, catechol O-methyltransferase, monoamine oxidase, and corticosteroid beta-hydroxylase. Esterase activity in the cornea is involved in the conversion of ester prodrugs, such as dipivalylepinephrine, to their parent compounds. Cholinesterase inhibitors may interfere with prodrug ester hydrolysis in the eye and modify the drug effect.[20]

Stereochemical factors may affect drug penetration, metabolism, and receptor interaction. Chiral molecules possess an asymmetric carbon atom in the structure and exist in two enantiomeric forms, dextro (*d*) and levo (*l*), which rotate polarized light in opposite directions.[21] Well-known chiral molecules are amino acids and the catecholamines epinephrine and norepinephrine. The equal mixture of the two enantiomers is called a *racemate*. One of the stereoisomers is generally preferred by the enzyme, the transporter, or the receptor. Naturally occurring *l*-epinephrine or *l*-norepinephrine is physiologically more active than the unnatural *d*-isomer.[22]

Occasionally, drugs containing chiral centers are available as racemates even though the therapeutic benefit may be derived primarily from one isomer. The less active isomer may compete with a more active isomer for an enzyme, a transport system, or the receptor. The metabolic disposition of the racemic drug may appear highly complex because the ratio of the molecular species, *d/l*, can change in an unpredictable way. In body fluids, one isomer may be converted to another isomer, leading to a racemization of the drug. Occasionally, the "inactive" isomer may exhibit toxicity. The possible differences in behavior between isomers and racemates should be kept in mind when new medications are investigated clinically.

1.2 AQUEOUS HUMOR DYNAMICS

Aqueous humor is formed by the ciliary processes, flows from the posterior chamber through the pupil into the anterior chamber, and exits via the trabecular route at the angle and the uveoscleral route. It is being continuously formed and drained. The ciliary processes consist of about 80 processes, each of which contains a large number of fenestrated capillaries in a core of stroma. The surface of the ciliary process is covered by a double layer of epithelium: the outer pigmented and the inner nonpigmented layers. The apical surfaces of these two layers face each other and are joined by tight junctions. The epithelium double layer protrudes into the posterior chamber, providing a large surface area for aqueous secretion.

1.2.1 *Theories of Production.* The aqueous humor is produced by three processes: simple perfusion, ultrafiltration, and active secretion. Diffusion of solutes across cell membranes occurs down a concentration gradient. Substances with high lipid-solubility coefficients penetrate easily through biologic membranes. Ultrafiltration refers to a pressure-dependent movement along a pressure gradient. Diffusion and ultrafiltration are passive requiring no active cellular participation. They are responsible for the formation of the "reservoir" of the plasma ultrafiltrate in the stroma, from which the posterior chamber aqueous humor is derived by means of active secretion. In active secretion, energy from hydrolysis of adenosine triphosphate (ATP) is used to secrete substances against a concentration gradient. Sodium is transported into the posterior chamber, resulting in water movement from the stromal pool into the posterior chamber.[23]

The identity of the precise ion or ions transported is not known, but sodium, chloride, and bicarbonate are involved. The enzymes sodium-potassium–activated adenosine triphosphatase (Na^+,K^+-ATPase) and carbonic anhydrase (CA), abundantly present in the nonpigmented epithelium, are intimately involved in the process of active secretion. Na^+,K^+-ATPase provides the energy for the metabolic pump that transports sodium into the posterior chamber, while CA catalyzes reaction of $CO_2 + H_2O$ to $H^+ + HCO_3^-$. HCO_3^- is essential for the active secretion of aqueous humor.

Inhibition of calcium causes a reduction of the nonpigmented epithelium intracellular HCO_3^- available for transport with Na^+ from the cytosol of the nonpigmented epithelium to the aqueous, required to maintain electroneutrality. A reduction of H^+ decreases H^+–Na^+ exchange and, again, the availability of intracellular Na^+ for transport into the intercellular channel. In addition, a reduction in the intracellular pH inhibits Na^+,K^+-ATPase.[23]

1.2.2 *Rate of Production*. In human, the rate of aqueous humor turn over is approximately 1% to 1.5% of the anterior chamber volume per minute. The rate of aqueous humor formation is approximately 2.5 μL/min. It is affected by a variety of factors, including the integrity of the blood–aqueous barrier, blood flow to the ciliary body, and neurohumoral regulation of vascular tissue and the ciliary epithelium. Aqueous formation varies diurnally and drops during sleep.

1.2.3 *Aqueous Outflow*. Aqueous humor outflow consist of pressure-dependent and pressure-independent pathways. The pressure-dependent outflow refers to the trabecular meshwork–Schlemm's canal–venous system, while the pressure-independent outflow refers to any nontrabecular outflow and is also called uveoscleral outflow.

The trabecular meshwork is divided into three layers: uveal, corneoscleral, and juxtacanalicular. The juxtacancalicular meshwork is adjacent to the Schlemm's canal and is thought to be the major site of outflow resistance. Aqueous moves both across and between the endothelial cells lining the inner wall of Schlemm's canal. A complex system of channels connects Schlemm's canal to the episcleral veins, which subsequently drain into the anterior ciliary and superior ophthalmic veins.

In the uveoscleral pathway, the predominant route appears to be the aqueous passage from the anterior chamber into the ciliary muscle, and then into the supraciliary and suprachoroidal spaces. The fluid then exits the eye through the intact sclera or along the nerves and the vessels that penetrate it. The reasons for the pressure independence of this pathway are not entirely clear but might be consequent to the complex nature of the pressure and resistance relationships between the various fluid compartments within the soft intraocular tissues along the route.[23,24]

1.3 TEAR FILM DYNAMICS

The cul-de-sac compartment is the space into which topical eye medications are instilled. The human cul-de-sac has a volume of about 7 μL, which can expand momentarily and variably to 30 μL. That fraction of an instilled drop that is in excess of the cul-de-sac volume drains into the nasolacrimal duct within 15 seconds after instillation or is lost by overflow onto the cheek with forceful blinking. A normal blink eliminates about 2 μL of fluid from the cul-de-sac.[4]

The volume of eye drops delivered from commercial product containers is typically in the 25- to 35-μL range but can be as high as 75 μL. Currently, the practical lower limit of drop volume deliverable from commercial containers is 20–25 μL without further modification of the container's tip. For optimal ocular bioavailability, the drop size should be 20 μL or less.[25,26]

Instillation of multiple drops at one time, in the belief that it will increase ocular bioavailability, achieves little more than increasing the possibility for delivering a large systemic dose of the drug, which could result in a higher incidence of side effects or toxicity. If a drop of one medication is followed closely by a drop of another medication or of saline solution, a substantial washout occurs, with a concomitant lessening of the effect.[27] A 30-second interval between drops results in a 45% washout loss of drug effect, whereas a 2-minute interval results in only 17% loss of effect. After a 5-minute interval, a second drop will cause almost no washout effect on the first drop.

In the normal, nonirritated eye, the tear turnover rate averages 16% per minute. Instillation of the average drop stimulates lacrimation to increase the turnover rate to 30% per minute. The washout effect of this spontaneous tear flow results in almost complete disappearance of an instilled drug from the cul-de-sac within 5 minutes. At least 80% of eye-drop–applied drug leaves by lacrimal drainage and not by entering the eye. In general, drugs are readily absorbed across the highly vascularized nasopharyngeal mucosa into the systemic circulation.

Nasolacrimal occlusion may decrease the systemic absorption, increase the ocular penetration of topically applied ophthalmic drugs, and improve the therapeutic index.[27–29] Nasolacrimal occlusion may allow a reduction in the dosage and frequency of administration of various glaucoma drugs. The benefit of nasolacrimal occlusion should be determined individually for each patient. The patient must be trained to perform punctal occlusion properly, or its benefit may not be realized. Simple eyelid closure, so that the lacrimal pump system is not activated, may also reduce nasolacrimal drainage of topical medication.

1.4 DRUG FORMULATION

Ophthalmic drugs are formulated to bring the active drugs into contact with the eye surface to allow for absorption. Extension of corneal contact time may result in increased drug penetration and a higher intraocular drug level. The most common formulations for ophthalmic drug delivery are solutions and suspensions. In addition to the active drug, ophthalmic solutions or suspensions contain other ingredients to control various characteristics of the formulation, such as the buffering and pH, osmolality and tonicity, viscosity, and antimicrobial preservation. Although these ingredients are listed as inactive, they can affect the permeability of the drug across the ocular surface barrier and alter the therapeutic effectiveness of the drug.

1.4.1 *Solution Versus Suspension.* Ophthalmic solutions are the most commonly used ocular drug delivery systems and are the least expensive to formulate.[7] All of the ingredients are completely dissolved, so there is only minimal interference with vision. Drugs in solution are immediately available for absorption. However, the aqueous solution dosage form can be considered only for drugs with sufficient aqueous solubility to prevent them from precipitating under adverse storage conditions. In some cases, one or more cosolvents may be added to the formulation to facilitate dissolution or maintain the drug in solution.

Ophthalmic suspensions are sterile preparations of drug with low water solubility dispersed in a liquid vehicle. They are formulations mainly for certain salts of corticosteroids, for example, prednisolone acetate and fluorometholone acetate. The drug is present in a micronized form, generally <10 μm in diameter.[30] The aqueous phase of the suspension is saturated with the drug. Different salts of the same drug can vary in water solubility, so a salt may be obtained that renders an otherwise-soluble drug insoluble. The small drug particles of a suspension presumably remain in the cul-de-sac longer than an aqueous solution and can prolong the drug's availability, although there are no reported data to prove this phenomenon.[30] The drug delivery from a suspension is characterized by two consecutive phases. The first phase is a rapid delivery of the dissolved drug. The second is a slower but more prolonged delivery from the dissolution of the retained particles.[31]

The surface area accessible for drug dissolution and the ocular bioavailability from topically applied suspensions are correlated with particle size.[32] As particle size decreases, the more rapid dissolution rate of the drug particle in the tear film may result in higher bioavailability. However, a suspension of very small particle sizes can drain from the cul-de-sac without prolonging the availability of the drug. Owing to the particle sedimentation property, adequate shaking of the suspension is required before use to obtain accurate dosing. Particle size influences the rate of settling of the suspension of the drug particles upon shaking the container. Generally, suspensions of larger particle sizes have a faster rate of settling and a lower rate of resuspension upon shaking. In addition, larger particles can lead to increased ocular irritation, with enhanced tearing and drug loss by drainage. To minimize potential irritation, particle size should be <10 μm.[33] However, the 10-μm limit may not be clear-cut, because other factors, such as concentration, density, and shape, may contribute to the comfort threshold and retention in the cul-de-sac.[30]

1.4.2 *Buffering and pH*. The pH of an ophthalmic formulation is important to achieve the optimal condition of chemical and physical stability for the formulation, the solubility of the active ingredient as well as the adjuvant ingredients (e.g., preservatives and any viscosity-improving polymers), and the comfort of the ophthalmic formulation.[34]

Most ophthalmic drugs, being weak acids or bases, are present in solutions as both the nonionized (nondissociated) and the ionized (dissociated) species. The drug may by itself provide the necessary buffering action if its pK_a is in the appropriate range. The degree of ionization of a drug in solution is determined by the pK_a of the drug and the pH of the solution. A pH that favors a higher proportion of the nonionized species could result in a higher transcorneal permeability.[35] The normal tear pH given in the literature ranges from 7.0 to 7.4, depending on different methods of measurement.[36] The in vivo pH of the formulation depends on the solution pH and the tear pH. The pH of the tears may modify the final in vivo pH of the drug and, subsequently, the drug's effectiveness.[37] On the other hand, the pH of the tears, which have their own buffer system, may be temporarily altered by the ophthalmic drops and subsequently elicit reflex tearing. This can cause excessive washout of the drug, which interferes with absorption.

1.4.3 *Osmolality and Tonicity*. Tear osmolality varies between 302 and 318 mOsm/kg with the eyelids open, increasing by 1.43 mOsm/kg during the day, and varies between 288 and 293 mOsm/kg after prolonged eyelid closure.[34] There are significant individual variations in the tonicity of normal human tears. To avoid irritation, ophthalmic formulations intended for topical instillation should be approximately isotonic with the tears. The eye can tolerate a considerable range of tonicity between 266 and 445 mOsm/kg before any pain or discomfort is detected.[38] Also, the tears can adjust the tonicity of the topically applied solutions by osmosis. Increased tonicity of topical drops is immediately diluted by the tears. Because ophthalmic drugs listed in the *Physicians' Desk Reference* do not exceed 5% of an active compound, they are within the acceptable range of tonicity between 220 and 640 mOsm/kg. Excessive ranges of tonicity can elicit reflex tearing. Examples are a few ophthalmic solutions, such as pilocarpine 8% and 10%, phenylephrine 10%, and sulfacetamide 10%, that cause a strong burning and stinging sensation upon instillation.[39]

The tonicity of ophthalmic products is generally adjusted to physiologically compatible values by using sodium chloride. In cases where a precipitating effect of sodium chloride may reduce the solubility of the drug or other ingredients, the nonionizing substance mannitol may be used.

1.4.4 *Viscosity.* Increasing the viscosity of a topically applied ocular formulation is expected to reduce drainage, increase the residence time in the conjunctival sac, and thus lead to enhanced intraocular penetration and therapeutic effect. Improvement in ocular drug delivery is observed over the viscosity range from 1 to 15 cp (centipoise), and it is suggested that the optimal viscosity should be 12–15 cp.[40] Further increases in viscosity above this level do not appear to proportionally increase the drug concentration in aqueous. Formulations with higher viscosity cause ocular surface irritation, resulting in reflex blinking, lacrimation, and increased drainage of the applied formulation. Higher viscosity may also have the effect of inhibiting product–tear mixing accompanied by optical surface distortion, which produces visual disturbance for the patient. Formulations with viscosity of 30 cp or higher impart a sticky feel to the formulation, making it uncomfortable to use.

The most commonly used agents for increasing viscosity include polyvinyl alcohol (PVA) and derivatives of methylcellulose. The viscosities of solutions containing 1.4% PVA and 0.5% hydroxypropyl methylcellulose, which are the concentrations usually used in ophthalmic products, are about 10 and 20 cp or less, respectively.[34]

1.4.5 *Preservatives.* Ophthalmic drug delivery systems packaged in a multiple-dose container must contain a suitable mixture of substances to prevent the growth of microorganisms or to destroy any that are accidentally introduced when the container is open during use. Common preservatives in ophthalmic preparations are quaternary cationic surfactants such as benzalkonium chloride and benzododecium bromide; mercurials such as thimerosal, chlorobutanol, and parahydroxy benzoates; and aromatic alcohols. It has been shown that preservatives used in ophthalmic solutions can be toxic to the ocular surface following topical administration and can enhance the corneal permeability of various drugs.[41]

Benzalkonium chloride is the most commonly used preservative in ophthalmic preparations. As a surfactant, benzalkonium chloride can increase the solubility of drugs that are hydrophilic and exert their bactericidal effect by emulsification of the bacterial cell walls. Ocular damage from these agents is most likely due to emulsification of the cell membrane lipids.[42] Adverse reactions are not uncommon with this preservative. Although most of the side effects are reversible, irreversible cytopathologies can also be seen. The compound is known to cause edema, desquamation, punctate keratitis, and papillary conjunctivitis.[43] Benzalkonium chloride binds to soft contact lenses and tends to concentrate in the contact lens. Parallel use of soft contact lens and vehicles containing benzalkonium chloride can result in severe but reversible and temporary epithelial keratitis without significant endothelial damage.

Another preservative used only with brimonidine tartrate is Purite, which is a stabilized oxychloro complex that has oxidative properties and is different from benzalkonium chloride. Purite may be better tolerated in eyes sensitive to benzalkonium chloride.

Adverse ocular side effects attributed to the organomercurials are less common. Hypersensitivity to the organomercurials appears to be the most dramatic side effect incurred with these agents and is estimated to occur in about 10% to 50% of patients. Hyperemia, edema, and blepharoconjunctivitis may result.[43]

1.4.6 *Drug Delivery by Prodrugs.* The main route of entry of topically applied drugs into the anterior chamber is through the cornea. One way to increase the penetration of the corneal epithelium is by increasing the lipophilicity of the drug. Dipivefrin (Propine), latanoprost (Xalatan), travoprost (Travatan), and nepafenac (Nevanac) are examples of prodrugs developed for this purpose. The ester group in these compounds increases their lipophilicity and enhances corneal permeability. These prodrugs are then converted into the active drugs, the acidic forms, by the esterase enzymes in the cornea. Prodrugs allow increased penetration into the anterior chamber and may reduce local and systemic side effects by decreasing the concentration of drug required.

1.5 NEW DRUG DELIVERY VEHICLES

To deliver ophthalmic drugs into contact with the eye surface to permit absorption, detailed formulation requirements have to be satisfied in terms of pH, osmolality, tonicity, and viscosity to achieve chemical and physical stability, solubility, and comfort for the patient. New vehicles are under investigation to further prolong the corneal contact time. Currently, solutions and suspensions remain the most commonly used vehicles for ophthalmic drug delivery.

1.5.1 *Emulsions.* Emulsions are traditionally defined as two-phase systems in which one liquid is dispersed throughout another liquid in the form of small droplets. The development of the specialized submicrometer emulsion has created new interest in this delivery system. The emulsion is characterized by the droplet size of the oily phase in the range of 0.1–0.3 μm. The nonionic surfactants used in stabilizing this emulsion are nonirritating. Emulsions have the advantage of allowing the delivery of lipid-soluble drugs in an aqueous-like form. By formulation of the drug in an emulsion, the drug can be protected from susceptible oxidation or hydrolysis. Animal studies have demonstrated improved performance of some ophthalmic drugs formulated in a specialized submicrometer emulsion.[44] The increased ocular retention time probably explained the improved bioavailability and enhanced effectiveness. Specialized submicrometer emulsions also demonstrated a reduction of ocular irritation, although the mechanism is currently unknown.

1.5.2 *Gels.* Gels are single continuous or multiphase semisolid systems. Drug release from a gel occurs by diffusion and erosion of the gel surface. Because gels can also be degraded by microorganisms, they require the inclusion of a preservative. There are several in situ gelation systems currently under investigation. Examples of these systems are ion-activated, pH-activated, and temperature-sensitive gelation systems.[45–47] They combine the advantages of dispensing an aqueous solution with the increased retention time of a high-viscosity formulation.

In the ion-activated gelation system, Gelrite as a polysaccharide, low-acetyl gellan gum forms clear gels in the presence of monovalent or bivalent ions. The concentration of sodium ions in tears is sufficient to cause gelation in the conjunctival sac.[45] The prolonged contact time with the ocular surface increases the bioavailability of the drug.

The pH-activated gelation system is composed of a large amount of an anionic polymer in the form of nanodispersion, which has a very low viscosity at pH <5. On contact with the tear film, which normally has a pH of 7.0–7.4, the particles agglomerate and assume a gel form. The gelation process is due to swelling of the particles from neutralization of the acid groups on the polymer chain and the absorption of water.[46]

Different materials are used to achieve gelation at the temperature of the ocular surface. A 25% poloxamer 407 achieved an increase in viscosity with an increase in temperature from an ambient temperature of 25°C to a temperature at the ocular surface of 32°C to 34°C.[48] Harsh and Gehrke[47] developed a temperature-sensitive hydrogel based on cross-linking cellulose ethers such as hydroxycellulose. Cellulose ethers have been approved by the FDA for food and drug use. They offer an advantage over many synthetic gels based on polymers or monomers, which are carcinogenic or teratogenic.

Another approach to achieve gelation was attempted by a combination of polymers responding simultaneously to two gelating factors, such as pH and temperature. An aqueous solution containing a combination of 0.3% carbopol, a polyacrylic acid polymer that gelates when the pH is raised over its pK_a of 5.5, and a 1.5% methylcellulose that gelates when the temperature is raised above 30°C was reported by Kumar et al.[49] to form a gel under simulated physiologic conditions. This approach may reduce the total polymer content of the delivery system.

1.6 DRUG DELIVERY SYSTEMS

Commonly used ophthalmic drug formulations, such as solutions, gels, suspensions, and ointments, deliver drugs at rates that follow first-order kinetics, in which the concentration of the drug transferred to the eye decreases exponentially with time. To achieve a constant concentration of the drug in the precorneal tear film and create a steady-state concentration in the tissues, an ophthalmic drug delivery system needs to be designed to deliver a specific drug at a zero-order kinetic rate. At a zero-order kinetic rate of delivery, the rate is not proportional to the drug concentration but is related to some functional capacity involved in the transfer of drug.[34] Solid ocular inserts have been designed to achieve this goal.

The release of drug from a solid insert may be controlled by the diffusion rate of the drug through the polymer container.[50] Diffusion-controlled systems are either the reservoir type or the matrix type. In the matrix type of solid insert, the drug is dispersed throughout the polymer matrix and must diffuse through the matrix structure to be released. In contrast, a reservoir type of insert consists of a core of drug encapsulated within polymer layers that are not biodegradable and serve as a rate-controlling barrier to diffusion.[34]

1.6.1 *Ocusert.* Ocusert is a diffusion-controlled, reservoir-type device marketed in the United States that became commercially available in 1974. The device consists of a two-membrane sandwich of ethylene vinyl acetate with a pilocarpine reservoir in the center. A retaining ring of ethylene vinyl acetate impregnated with titanium dioxide for visibility and handling of the insert encloses the drug reservoir circumferentially (figure 1.3).[51] The pilocarpine is bound to alginic acid and is present as a free base, partly in an ionized form and partly in a nonionized form. The device is sterile and contains no preservative.[52,53] The drug release from a reservoir type of diffusion-controlled system is provided by interaction between the polymeric membrane and the drug contained in the reservoir, and the surface area and thickness of the polymer layer.[34,51] The ethylene vinyl acetate membrane is hydrophobic, which allows the nonionized form of pilocarpine to permeate but excludes water from the device.

The major factor in the rate of drug release is the driving force of the concentration gradient between the saturated concentration of drug within the reservoir

A

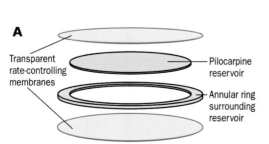

Transparent
rate-controlling
membranes

Pilocarpine
reservoir

Annular ring
surrounding
reservoir

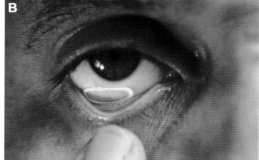

Figure 1.3. Ocusert. (A) Construction of device. Annular ring surrounding reservoir is opaque white for visibility in handling and inserting system. (B) Device in position. Courtesy Akorn, Inc.

and the concentration of drug outside the membrane.[34] Tear flow prevents the buildup of a stagnant layer of drug around the device and therefore maintains the concentration gradient across the membrane. As long as this gradient exists, the drug is released into the tear film at a constant rate over almost the entire lifetime of the device.[54] However, during the initial 6–8 hours following insertion of the device, there is a higher pulsed release of pilocarpine because of the amount of drug previously equilibrated into the barrier membrane. The rate of release in this initial period can be as high as three or four times the desired rate.[55,56]

The device is marketed in two sizes, Ocusert Pilo-20 and Ocusert Pilo-40, representing two different in vitro release rates, 20 and 40 µg/h, respectively. The higher rate for Ocusert Pilo-40 is achieved by making its rate-controlling membranes thinner and by use of the flux enhancer di(2-ethylhexyl)phthalate.[57] The devices are designed to release the drug for approximately 7 days.

Because of individual differences, direct comparisons between the Ocusert systems and various concentrations of pilocarpine drops cannot be made. A majority of patients controlled with pilocarpine 0.5% and 1% drops can usually be controlled with Ocusert Pilo-20. Most patients who required 2% or 4% solution of pilocarpine will require Ocusert Pilo-40.[51,55]

Pilocarpine Ocusert has several advantages over pilocarpine drops. It delivers pilocarpine at a very low constant rate over a 7-day period, except for the higher rate of release in the initial 6–8 hours. During the remainder of the 7-day period, the release rate is within ±20% of the rated value. Satisfactory ocular hypotensive response is maintained around the clock for 7 days. A low baseline amount of miosis and induced myopia persists for the therapeutic life of the Ocusert system. The total amount of drug delivered to the eye is substantially less than with pilocarpine drop instillation.[58] The risk of ocular or systemic pilocarpine toxicity is reduced. Studies have shown that Ocusert Pilo-20 produced less shallowing of the anterior chamber, miosis, accommodation myopia, and reduction in visual acuity than did pilocarpine 2% drops.[59,60] It may provide better compliance because it is inserted only once a week. Because Ocusert offers continuous drug release, diurnal variations of IOP may be stabilized.

Despite these theoretical advantages, Ocusert has not achieved widespread popularity in clinical practice, because it requires detailed instruction and encouragement of patients to use it. Patients are instructed to place the insert in the inferior fornix, but in case of retention difficulty, it may be placed in the superior fornix. The insert may be lost from the eye without the patient noticing it; then the patient does not have the benefit of the drug. In practice, the major complaints with the insert are excessive foreign-body sensation and retention difficulty.[61] Another disadvantage of the insert system is its relatively higher cost compared to pilocarpine drops. Furthermore, cases of sudden leakage of the drug have been reported.[62] Ocusert is no longer commercially available.

1.6.2 *Liposomes.* Liposomes are microscopic vesicular structures consisting of lipid bilayers separated by water or an aqueous buffer compartment used to carry drugs (figure 1.4). They may consist of a single bilayer lipid membrane or a series of concentric multiple bilayer lipid compartments. They are classified as small unilamellar

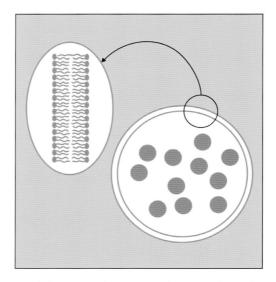

Figure 1.4. Liposome bilayer membranes are formed when phospholipids arrange themselves such that hydrophilic heads are oriented toward aqueous phase and hydrophobic tails are oriented away from aqueous phase. Redrawn with permission from Price CI, Horton J. *Local Liposome Drug Delivery: An Overlooked Application*. Austin, Tex: RG Landes Co; 1992.

vesicles if the size of the unilamellar vesicles is <100nm, or as large unilamellar vesicles if the size is >100nm.[63] Multivesicular liposomes are another type of liposome, consisting of a cluster of numerous monolayered vesicles surrounded by an outer lipid monolayer. An aqueous droplet is entrapped within each vesicle.[64]

Hydrophilic drugs are encapsulated within the internal aqueous compartments, and lipophilic drugs are intercalated with the hydrophobic phospholipid bilayer. The drugs are released by diffusion processes into the surrounding aqueous environment.[65]

Typical phospholipids used to form liposomes are phosphatidylcholine (lecithin), phosphatidylethanolamine (cephalin), phosphatidylserine, phosphatidic acid, sphingomyelins, cardiolipin, plasmalogens, and cerebrosides. Steroid cholesterol and its derivatives are often included as components of liposomal membranes to improve the membrane stability. Liposomes can be prepared by sonication of dispersions of phospholipids, reverse-phase evaporation, solvent injection, detergent removal, or calcium-induced fusion.[34]

Liposomes have been widely investigated as delivery systems for a variety of ocular drugs because of their potential advantages. The major advantage ascribed to liposomal formulation is the ability to circumvent cell membrane permeability barriers by cell membrane–liposome interactions. Liposomes can potentially control the rate of release of the encapsulated drug, protect the drug from metabolic enzymes, reduce drug toxicity, enhance the therapeutic effects, and increase the possibility of ocular drug absorption by the close contact of the liposomes with corneal and conjunctival surfaces. Liposomes are biodegradable and nontoxic.[65] Their drug delivery properties can be manipulated by incorporating and modifying the composition of the lipid bilayer.

The ocular availability to the target tissue of the drug entrapped within the liposomes is associated with the manner in which the drug interacts with the constituents of the vesicles, the interaction of the tissue cells with the liposomes, and the ocular residence time.

The rate of efflux of entrapped drugs from liposomes is governed by the physicochemical characteristics of the drug, in addition to the properties of the liposome membrane. Most phospholipids exhibit a phase change from the gel crystalline state to the liquid crystalline state at a specific temperature, called the *transition temperature*. Varying the phospholipid by adjusting the combination of fatty acid chain length, degree of unsaturation, and polar head group structure can change the transition temperature. The phospholipid bilayer becomes more permeable to the entrapped materials at the liquid crystalline state above the transition temperature. The efflux rate can also be manipulated with incorporation of cholesterol into the bilayer. Decreasing acyl chain length and degree of unsaturation of the phospholipid may increase the permeability of the bilayer. The presence of charged phospholipid in the bilayer may affect the efflux by its interaction with the charged entrapped materials.[65]

Several mechanisms have been proposed for the interactions between the cells and the liposomes and have been reviewed in detail: (1) intermembrane transfer, (2) contact release, (3) adsorption, (4) fusion, and (5) endocytosis.[65–67] The major mechanisms of interaction between liposomes and corneal epithelial cells are probably adsorption and intermembrane transfer.

1. *Intermembrane transfer* is the insertion of the lipophilic materials situated in the liposome membrane into other membranes. It occurs when the distance between the two membranes is small enough.
2. *Contact release* can occur when the membrane of the cell and the liposome experience perturbation as a result of contact. The entrapped aqueous solute molecules leak from the liposome into the cell.
3. *Adsorption* of the liposome to the cell surface takes place as a result of binding by specific receptors or specific cell-surface proteins. Adsorption brings the liposome into close contact with the cell surface.
4. *Fusion* occurs when the cell membrane and the liposome come into close contact. The bilayer can fuse together to release the contents of the liposome into the cytoplasm.
5. *Endocytosis* is considered to be the dominant interaction between liposomes and cells. The cell takes the liposome up into an endosome, which then fuses with a primary lysosome to form a secondary lysosome. Lysosomal enzymes break open the liposome and release the aqueous contents of the liposome. Liposomes may also be taken up by receptor-mediated endocytosis. However, the cornea has been demonstrated to exhibit poor phagocytic activity.

To serve as a topical ocular drug delivery system, liposomes must remain in the conjunctival cul-de-sac long enough to release their contents. Much research has concentrated on methods to increase the precorneal residence of liposomes. At physiologic pH, the corneal epithelium is negatively charged. Therefore, the positive surface charge of a liposome significantly increases the residence time of liposomes in the precorneal region. Retention also increases with smaller mean liposome size.[68] However, there is a lack of specificity of the association of the liposomes for the cornea. The reduced drainage rate of liposomes was also attributed to their affinity for the conjunctival membranes. Specific binding to the cornea surface can be achieved by conjugating ligands on the corneal surface to the liposome. For instance, one approach is the incorporation into the liposomal membranes of a glycoprotein and the subsequent use of lectins to bind the glycoprotein to carbohydrate moieties associated with the target cells.[69] The other possibility is to bind the liposome to the surface of the target tissue with the use of antibodies directed against the target tissue.[65]

Other investigative methods to prolong residence time have been studied. One of the methods is the formulation of a liposome with a positively charged vesicle-forming lipid component, usually an amine-derived phospholipid of a specific structure.[65] These vesicles have been shown to enhance precorneal retention. Viscosity-enhancing polymers such as hydroxypropyl methylcellulose or polyvinyl alcohol have been used to suspend the liposomes. Liposomes suspended in these polymer solutions were retained on the corneal surface for a significantly longer period. Attempts have also been made to coat phospholipid vesicles with a mucoadhesive polymer, poly(acrylic) acid, to enhance the precorneal retention of the vesicles.[65]

Liposomes may be administered subconjunctivally or intravitreally. Liposome-encapsulated antimicrobial agents improve the ocular delivery of antibiotics following subconjunctival administration. Subconjunctival injections of encapsulated gentamicin improved corneal concentration.[70] The liposomal form provided higher drug concentrations in the sclera and cornea up to 24 hours after injection. Studies of liposome-bound cyclosporine injected subconjunctivally found this delivery system to achieve an aqueous concentration about 40% higher than injected free cyclosporine.[71]

Intravitreal injection of liposomes encapsulated with a variety of drugs has demonstrated therapeutic vitreal concentrations of those drugs. The drugs studied so far are gentamicin, amphotericin B, cyclosporine, and antiviral agents.[70,72,73] Liposome-bound cyclosporine administered intravitreally resulted in a prolongation of the half-life of the drug to about 3 days.[74] Several studies also reported a prolongation of vitreal levels of antiviral agents following intravitreous injection of the liposome-encapsulated form.[65] Different methods are available to target liposomes either to promote the interaction between specific cells or tissues and the encapsulated drug or to release the contents of liposomes at specific sites. Liposomes containing acyclovir combined with a monoclonal antibody to herpes simplex virus glycoprotein D were studied to target the antiviral agent specifically to the infected cells.[75,76] Another approach to targeting drug-bound liposomes to a specific site is the use of a heat-sensitive liposome. Triggering mechanisms such as an argon laser or microwaves to elevate the temperature at a specific site to release the contents of liposomes have been studied.[65]

Liposomes present a potential advantage in drug delivery. However, the routine use of liposome formulation as a topical ocular drug delivery is limited by their short

shelf-life, their limited drug-loading capacity, and difficulty in stabilizing the preparation.[65] Liposomes have been shown to achieve a prolonged therapeutic level
when administered subconjunctivally and intravitreally. Much research is needed to
further understand the various parameters that may influence liposomal ocular drug
delivery.

1.6.3 *Slow-Release Contact Lenses.* Ocular bioavailability of conventional ophthalmic
formulations is generally limited because of protective mechanisms, such as tear
drainage and blinking, even with improved formulations such as viscosity enhancers
or in situ gelling system. Medicated contact lenses that can be loaded with drug and
release the drug on the ocular surface may be particularly useful for increasing drug
bioavailability and may also correct impaired vision. The feasibility of this approach depends on whether the drug and contact lens material can be matched so
that the lens absorbs a sufficient quantity of drug and releases it in a controlled
fashion. In general, drug-loading capacity of conventional soft contact lenses is insufficient to be used for ophthalmic drug delivery. To overcome this drawback, the
application of the molecular imprinting technology has been used in the design of
soft contact lenses.[77]

Molecular imprinting refers to the synthesis of a polymer in the presence of the
species to be absorbed in such a way that on removal of these template molecules,
the polymer is left with a high concentration of cavities with special affinity for
the desired absorbate.[77] One of the applications of this technology in ocular drug
delivery is timolol administration from hydrogels in soft contact lenses.[78]

Timolol maleate is a suitable molecule for the imprinting system because of
its multiple sites of interaction with the functional monomer, and it is stable in
solution at the temperatures used for polymerization of hydroxyethyl methacrylate
(HEMA). Poly(hydroxyethyl methacrylate) (poly-HEMA) is the major component
of most soft contact lenses. In a study to evaluate the loading capacity and release
characteristics of timolol-imprinted soft contact lenses, a small proportion of me-
thacrylic (MAA) or methyl methacrylate (MMA) was added as a functional monomer able to interact through ionic and hydrogen bonds with timolol maleate. MMA
is a hydrophobic molecule, polymers of which have been extensively used for non-
foldable intraocular lenses. MAA is the parent acid of MMA and is a hydrophilic
molecule that is ionized above pH 5.5. Hydrogels were prepared by dissolution
of ethylene glycol dimethacrylate, a cross-linker, in HEMA with MMA or MAA
and timolol maleate. The results indicate that the incorporation of MAA as co-
monomer increases the timolol loading capacity to therapeutically useful levels
while sustaining drug release in lacrimal fluid for more than 12 hours, and that
the preparation can be reloaded overnight with timolol and ready to use the next
day.[77,78]

Imprinting systems have an enormous potential in pharmaceutical technology,
although their applications are still incipient. Current research of applying the molecular imprinting technology to manufacture therapeutic contact lenses focuses on
the influence of the backbone monomers on the achievement of the imprinting effect,
finding the ideal proportions of the functional monomer and cross-linker constant,
and keeping the drug binding site stable.[78]

1.6.4 *Implantable Reservoirs.* Implantable reservoirs are devices consisting of a central core of drug encased in layers of permeable and impermeable polymers designed to provide sustained release of the drug when implanted subconjunctivally or intra-vitreally. The device is prepared by compressing a small quantity of an active com-pound, typically 5–6 mg, in a 2.5-mm tablet die. The pellets are then coated entirely in polyvinyl alcohol (permeable polymer) and ethylene vinyl acetate (imperme-able polymer). The device is then heat-treated to change the crystalline structure of the polyvinyl alcohol. The overall release rate is controlled by the layers of ethyl-ene vinyl acetate and polyvinyl alcohol, together with the surface area of the device. The duration and temperature of the heat treatment can also be varied to control the device release rate. Water diffuses into the device to dissolve part of the pellet, forming a saturated drug solution. The device provides a constant rate of release of the active compound.[79]

The potential advantage of an implantable reservoir is the possibility of deliv-ering the active compound directly into the eye and achieving therapeutic drug concentrations. Constant release of a drug over a long period of time eliminates the need and complication of multiple subconjunctival or intravitreal injections for chronic ocular disorders. Clinical applications of implantable reservoirs have been investigated primarily in four areas: (1) AIDS-associated cytomegalovirus ret-initis, (2) chronic uveitis, (3) glaucoma filtering surgery, and (4) proliferative vitreo-retinopathy.

1. Cytomegalovirus retinitis is the most common cause of viral retinitis in pa-tients with AIDS. Intravitreal ganciclovir injection provides a higher intra-ocular drug concentration in the vitreous than does systemic therapy and a reduced systemic exposure to the drug. However, the relatively short intra-vitreal half-life of ganciclovir requires frequent injections to maintain thera-peutic levels in the eye. A ganciclovir intravitreal implant has been developed to provide sustained therapeutic levels in the vitreous for a prolonged period. It is marketed as Vitrasert, a nonerodible drug-delivering implant (figure 1.5). A pellet containing 6 mg of ganciclovir is prepared and coated in polyvinyl alcohol.[80] It is designed to release ganciclovir at two rates: 1 and 2 mg/h. The mean release rate calculated from explanted devices designed to release the drug at 1 mg/h was actually 1.9 mg/h.[81] The device was implanted at the pars plana in a 30-minute procedure. It was reported to control cytomegalovirus retinitis in 90% to 95% of cases. Complications include retinal detachment, endophthalmitis, vitreous hemorrhage, and postoperative inflammation.[79] When the device becomes depleted, it can be replaced. It can be exchanged after 32 weeks, or earlier if progression of retinitis occurs.[81]
2. Devices containing cyclosporin A, dexamethasone, or a combination of cy-closporin A and dexamethasone have been prepared and implanted into the vitreous cavity of a rabbit model of uveitis. The devices were reported to be effective in suppressing inflammation.[79,82,83]
3. Failure of glaucoma filtering procedure is usually due to the proliferation of fibroblasts, which leads to scarring and subsequent blockage of the filter. Subconjunctival injections of 5-fluorouracil (5-FU) have been shown to in-crease the success rate of glaucoma filtering procedures in patients with poor prognoses. However, multiple injections are required, and there is a high

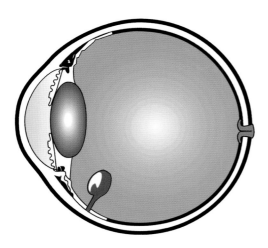

Figure 1.5. Illustration of position of Vitrasert implant in the vitreous after suturing the device into sclera at the pars plana. The Retisert device can also be implanted in this position. Image provided courtesy Bausch & Lomb Surgical, Inc.

incidence of toxicity to the corneal epithelium and the conjunctival wound. A 5-FU sustained-release device was designed to maintain low therapeutic levels when implanted subconjunctivally. Pellets containing 12 mg of 5-FU were coated in a mixture of permeable and impermeable polymers. When implanted subconjunctivally in the rabbit, the pellet released 5-FU at a rate of approximately 1 mg/day for 10 days. In the phase I clinical study to evaluate the safety and efficacy of the device in high-risk glaucoma surgical patients, the implants were placed subconjunctivally in four patients undergoing trabeculectomy. Three of the four patients maintained functioning filters, while the fourth failed within 2 months of surgery. No untoward events were linked to the implant.[84] The device is not bioerodible and would remain implanted in the eye indefinitely.

4. An intravitreal implant containing corticosteroid and 5-FU conjugate was studied in a rabbit model of experimental proliferative vitreoretinopathy. The corticosteroids studied included triamcinolone and dexamethasone. Both the intravitreal sustained-release implant containing triamcinolone/5-FU codrug and that containing dexamethasone/5-FU codrug were found to be effective in inhibiting the progression of proliferative vitreoretinopathy in the rabbit model.[85,86] Retisert (fluocinolone acetonide intravitreal implant) 0.59 mg is a sterile intravitreal implant designed to release fluocinolone acetonide locally to the posterior segment of the eye at a nominal initial rate of 0.6 µg/day, decreasing over the first month to a steady state between 0.3 and 0.4 µg/day over approximately 30 months. The implant consists of a fluocinolone acetonide tablet in a silicone elastomer cup containing a release orifice and a polyvinyl alcohol membrane positioned between the tablet and the orifice. The silicone cup is attached to a suture tab for surgical implantation into the posterior segment through a pars plana incision. Each implant is approximately 3 mm × 2 mm × 5 mm. It is indicated for the treatment of chronic noninfectious uveitis affecting the posterior segment of the eye. Following depletion of fluocinolone acetonide from Retisert as evidenced by recurrence of uveitis, it can be replaced. Phase III randomized, double-masked, multicenter-controlled clinical trials showed that the rate of recurrence of uveitis affecting the posterior segment of the study eye ranged from approximately 7% to 14% for

a 34-week period postimplantation as compared to approximately 40% to 54% for the 34-week period preimplantation. Based on the clinical trials, within 34 weeks postimplantation, approximately 60% of patients required medications to control IOP. Within an average postimplantation period of 2 years, approximately 32% of patients are expected to require filtering procedures to control IOP, and nearly all phakic eyes are expected to develop cataracts and require cataract surgery.[87,88]

Implantable reservoirs have been shown to achieve a sustained release of a variety of drugs, particularly in the delivery of drugs into the vitreous cavity. However, risks of endophthalmitis, retinal detachment, vitreous hemorrhage, inflammation, device dislocation or extrusion, cataract formation, and astigmatism have to be extensively studied. At present, the clinical application of these devices is likely to be restricted to sight-threatening diseases requiring long-term drug therapy.

1.7 OCULAR USE OF STEROIDS

1.7.1 *Pharmacology of Steroids.* Most of the known effects of the glucocorticoids are mediated by widely distributed glucocorticoid receptors. Glucocorticoid enters a target cell as a free molecule. In the absence of the hormonal ligand, intracellular glucocorticoid receptors bound to stabilizing proteins are incapable of activating transcription. When a molecule of glucocorticoid binds to the receptor, the complex undergoes conformational changes that allow it to dissociate from the stabilizing protein. The ligand-bound receptor complex, as a homodimer, then is actively transported into the nucleus, where it binds to the glucocorticoid response element (GRE) in the promoter and other non-GRE-containing promoters of the responsive gene and regulates transcription by RNA polymerase II and associated transcription factors. The resulting mRNA is exported to the cytoplasm for the production of protein that brings about the final hormone response.[89]

The anti-inflammatory and immunosuppressive effect of glucocorticoids has been used widely in medical management. The dramatic reduction of the manifestation of inflammation by glucocorticoids is due to their profound effects in the concentration, distribution, and function of peripheral leukocytes and to their suppressive effects on the inflammatory cytokines and chemokines and on other lipid and glucolipid mediators of inflammation. Inflammation is characterized by the extravasation and infiltration of leukocytes into the affected tissue mediated by a complex series of interactions of white cell adhesion molecules with those on endothelial cells. Glucocorticoids inhibit these interactions. Glucocorticoids also inhibit the functions of tissue macrophages and other antigen-presenting cells. The ability of macrophages to phagocytose and kill microorganisms and to produce tumor necrosis factor-α, interleukin-1, metalloproteinases, and plasminogen activator is limited by glucocorticoids. Glucocorticoids can influence the inflammatory response by reducing the prostaglandin, leukotriene, and platelet-activating factor synthesis that results from activation of phospholipase A$_2$. Glucocorticoids also reduce expression of cyclooxygenase II in inflammatory cells, reducing the amount of enzyme to produce prostaglandins.[89]

Glucocorticoids have important dose-related effects on carbohydrate, protein, and fat metabolism. Glucocorticoids increase serum glucose levels and thus stimulate insulin release and inhibit the uptake of glucose by muscle cells, while they stimulate hormone-sensitive lipase and thus lipolysis. The increased insulin secretion stimulates lipogenesis and, to a lesser degree, inhibits lipolysis, leading to a net increase in fat deposition combined with increased release of fatty acids and glycerol into the circulation. Glucocorticoids promote fat redistribution in the body.

Glucocorticoids have catabolic and antianabolic effects in lymphoid and connective tissue, muscle, fat, and skin. Supraphysiologic amounts of glucocorticoids lead to decreased muscle mass and weakness, thinning of the skin, osteoporosis, and reduce growth in children. They appear to antagonize the effect of vitamin D on calcium absorption.

Glucocorticoids have important effects on the nervous system, including behavior and intracranial pressure. Large doses of glucocorticoids have been associated with the development of peptic ulcer, possibly by suppressing the local immune response against *Helicobactor pylori*. Glucocorticoids given chronically suppress the pituitary release of adrenocorticotropic hormone, growth hormone, thyroid-stimulating hormone, and leutinizing hormone.

1.7.2 *Steroids in Ocular Use*. The actions of the synthetic steroids used therapeutically are similar to those of cortisol. They bind to the specific intracellular receptor proteins and produce the same effects but have different ratios of glucocorticoid to mineralocorticoid potency. The anti-inflammatory and immunosuppressive effects of glucocorticoids are used for a variety of ocular conditions, such as postoperative inflammation, uveitis, macular edema, hyphema, and ocular trauma. The most common route of administration is topical as solution, suspension, or ointment. Other routes of administration include subconjunctival, subtenon, intraocular, or intravitreal injection. Occasionally, glucocorticoids are administered systemically in ocular-related diseases such as optic neuritis and giant cell arteritis.

1.7.3 IOP *Response With Steroid Use*. A rise of IOP may occur as an adverse effect of corticosteroid therapy, including all routes of administration, such as topical, inhaled, and systemic administration. The type and potency of the agent, the means and frequency of its administration, and the susceptibility of the patient all affect the duration of time before the IOP rises and the extent of this rise. The higher steroid potency is associated with greater and earlier ocular hypertensive effect.[90,91] Approximately one-third of all patients demonstrate some responsiveness to corticosteroid. Although only a small percentage will have a clinically significant elevation in IOP, patients with primary open-angle glaucoma are more likely to demonstrate this response. Topical steroids have been shown to produce a steroid response over a period of weeks in both normal and glaucomatous eyes.[91–93] However, a more acute onset of IOP rise can occur with intensive topical dexamethasone or systemic steroid therapy.[90,94] Corticosteroid-induced IOP elevation may develop at any time during long-term corticosteroid administration, and regular IOP monitoring is warranted. Although some corticosteroid preparations such as fluorometholone, rimexolone (Vexol), medrysone (HMS), or loteprednol (Lotemax), which are less potent than prednisolone or dexamethasone, may be less likely to raise IOP, it cannot be overemphasized that even weaker corticosteroids or lower concentrations of stronger drugs can raise IOP in susceptible individuals.

Recently, intraocular injection of depot steroid is shown to be effective in management of a number of retina pathologies with associated improvement of visual outcome. It should be remembered that since the depot steroid cannot be removed, it may result in a prolonged exposure of the ocular tissue to the effect of steroid, and an extended IOP monitoring for several months is required. Studies have reported a high rate of up to 40% of steroid response associated with intraocular injection of triamcinolone.[95] Special attention should be paid to patients who are known steroid responders or who already have a glaucomatous optic neuropathy. Furthermore, topical corticosteroid treatment may not be useful as a screening method to exclude any subsequent pressure response with depot steroid injections.[96]

Although most corticosteroid response of increase in IOP resolved after stopping corticosteroid, the ocular hypertensive response has been shown to be irreversible in about 3% of cases, and particularly when there is a family history of glaucoma or chronic use of steroid.[90,94,97]

A number of risk factors for developing corticosteroid-induced increase of IOP have been identified. Greater risk of corticosteroid response is noted in patients who have glaucoma or have been diagnosed as glaucoma suspects, patients who are older, and patients with certain types of connective tissue diseases, type I diabetes mellitus, high myopia, and a first-degree relative with primary open-angle glaucoma.[98]

REFERENCES

1. Shell JW. Pharmacokinetics of topically applied ophthalmic drugs. *Surv Ophthalmol.* 1982;26:207–218.

2. Plazonnet B, Grove J, Durr M, et al. Pharmacokinetics and biopharmaceutical aspects of some anti-glaucoma drugs. In: Saettone MF, Bucci M, Speiser P, eds. *Ophthalmic Drug Delivery: Biopharmaceutical, Technological, and Clinical Aspects.* New York: Springer-Verlag; 1987:117–119.

3. Wagner JG. Kinetics of pharmacologic response, I: proposed relationships between response and drug concentration in the intact animal and man. *J Theor Biol.* 1968; 20:173–201.

4. Maurice DM, Mishima S. Ocular pharmacokinetics. In: Sears ML, ed. *Pharmacology of the Eye.* New York: Springer-Verlag; 1984:19–102. *Handbook of Experimental Pharmacology*; Vol 69.

5. Schoenwald RD. Ocular drug delivery pharmacokinetic considerations. *Clin Pharmacokinet.* 1990;18:255–269.

6. Schaeffer BE, Zadunaisky JA. Stimulation of chloride transport by fatty acids in corneal epithelium and relation to changes in membrane fluidity. *Biochim Biophys Acta.* 1979;556:131–143.

7. Schoenwald R. The control of drug bioavailability from ophthalmic dosage forms. In: Smolen VF, Ball LA, eds. *Controlled Drug Bioavailability.* New York: John Wiley & Sons; 1985;3:257–306.

8. Schoenwald RD. Ocular pharmacokinetics/pharmacodynamics. In: Mitra AK, ed. *Ophthalmic Drug Delivery Systems*. New York: Dekker; 1993:83–110. *Drugs and the Pharmaceutical Sciences*; Vol 58.

9. Wagner JG. Half-life and volume of distribution. In: *Biopharmaceutics and Relevant Pharmacokinetics*. Hamilton, IL: Drug Intelligence Publishing; 1979:52–53.

10. Holly FJ. Tear film physiology. *Int Ophthalmol Clin.* 1987;27:2–6.

11. Farris RL, Stuchell RN, Mandel ID. Basal and reflex human tear analysis, I: Physical measurements: osmolarity, basal volumes, and reflex flow rate. *Ophthalmology.* 1981;88:852–857.

12. Stuchell RN, Farris RL, Mandel ID. Basal and reflex human tear analysis, II: Chemical analysis: lactoferrin and lysozyme. *Ophthalmology.* 1981;88:858–861.

13. Mishima S, Gasset A, Klyce SD Jr, et al. Determination of tear volume and tear flow. *Invest Ophthalmol.* 1966;5:264–276.

14. Lee VH, Robinson JR. Topical ocular drug delivery: recent developments and future challenges. *J Ocul Pharmacol.* 1986;2:67–108.

15. Raviola G. The structural basis of the blood–ocular barriers. *Exp Eye Res.* 1977;25(suppl):27–63.

16. Zaki I, Fitzgerald P, Hardy JG, et al. A comparison of the effect of viscosity on the precorneal residence of solutions in rabbit and man. *J Pharm Pharmacol.* 1986;38:463–466.

17. Mishima S. Clinical pharmacokinetics of the eye [Proctor lecture]. *Invest Ophthalmol Vis Sci.* 1981;21:504–541.

18. Chen KK, Poth EJ. Racial difference of the mydriatic action of ephedrines, cocaine and euphthalmine. *J Pharmacol Exp Ther.* 1929;36:429–445.

19. Lee VH, Smith RE. Effect of substrate concentration, product concentration, and peptides on the in vitro hydrolysis of model ester prodrugs by corneal esterases. *J Ocul Pharmacol.* 1985;1:269–278.

20. Lee VH, Chang SC, Oshiro CM, et al. Ocular esterase composition in albino and pigmented rabbits: possible implications in ocular prodrug design and evaluation. *Curr Eye Res.* 1985;4:1117–1125.

21. Ariens EJ. Stereoselectivity, a natural aspect of molecular biology: a blind spot in clinical pharmacology and pharmacokinetics. *Eur J Drug Metab Pharmacokinet.* 1988;13:307–308.

22. Patil PN, Miller DD, Trendelenburg U. Molecular geometry and adrenergic drug activity. *Pharmacol Rev.* 1974;26:323–392.

23. Gabelt BT, Kaufman PL. Aqueous humor hydrodynamics. In: Kaufman PL, Alm A, eds. *Adler's Physiology of the Eye Clinical Application.* 10th ed. St Louis, MO: Mosby; 2003:237–289.

24. Brubaker RF. Measurement of uveoscleral outflow in humans. *J Glaucoma.* 2001;10(suppl 1):S45–S48.

25. Chrai SS, Makoid MC, Eriksen SP, et al. Drop size and initial dosing frequency problems of topically applied ophthalmic drugs. *J Pharm Sci.* 1974;63:333–338.

26. Patton TF, Francoeur M. Ocular bioavailability and systemic loss of topically applied ophthalmic drugs. *Am J Ophthalmol.* 1978;85:225–229.

27. Huang TC, Lee DA. Punctal occlusion and topical medications for glaucoma. *Am J Ophthalmol.* 1989;107:151–155.

28. Zimmerman TJ, Sharir M, Nardin GF, et al. Therapeutic index of pilocarpine, carbachol, and timolol with nasolacrimal occlusion. *Am J Ophthalmol.* 1992;114:1–7.

29. Fraunfelder FT. Extraocular fluid dynamics: how best to apply topical ocular medication. *Trans Am Ophthalmol Soc.* 1977;74:457–487.

30. Olejnik O. Conventional systems in ophthalmic drug delivery. In: Mitra AK, ed. *Ophthalmic Drug Delivery Systems.* New York: Dekker; 1993:177–198. *Drugs and the Pharmaceutical Sciences*; Vol 58.

31. Sieg JW, Robinson JR. Vehicle effects on ocular drug bioavailability, I: Evaluation of fluorometholone. *J Pharm Sci.* 1975;64:931–936.

32. Schoenwald RD, Stewart P. Effect of particle size on ophthalmic bioavailability of dexamethasone suspensions in rabbits. *J Pharm Sci.* 1980;69:391–394.

33. Sieg JW, Robinson JR. Vehicle effects on ocular drug bioavailability, II: Evaluation of pilocarpine. *J Pharm Sci.* 1977;66:1222–1228.

34. DeSantis LM, Patil PN. Pharmacokinetics. In: Mauger TF, Craig EL, eds. *Havener's Ocular Pharmacology.* 6th ed. St Louis, MO: CV Mosby Co; 1994:22–52.

35. Mitra AK, Mickelson TJ. Mechanism of transcorneal permeation of pilocarpine. *J Pharm Sci.* 1988;77:771–775.

36. Norn MS. Tear fluid pH in normals, contact lens wearers, and pathological cases. *Acta Ophthalmol.* 1988;66:485–489.

37. Coles WH, Jaros PA. Dynamics of ocular surface pH. *Br J Ophthalmol.* 1984;68:549–552.

38. Van Ooteghem MM. Factors influencing the retention of ophthalmic solutions on the eye surface. In: Saettone MF, Bucci M, Speiser P, eds. *Ophthalmic Drug Delivery: Biopharmaceutical, Technological, and Clinical Aspects.* New York: Springer-Verlag; 1987:7.

39. Bar-Ilan A, Neumann R. Basic considerations of ocular drug-delivery systems. In: Zimmerman TJ, ed. *Textbook of Ocular Pharmacology.* Philadelphia, PA: Lippincott-Raven; 1997:139–150.

40. Patton TF, Robinson TR. Ocular evaluation of polyvinyl alcohol vehicle in rabbits. *J Pharm Sci.* 1975;64:1312–1316.

41. Burstein NL. Preservative alteration of corneal permeability in humans and rabbits. *Invest Ophthalmol Vis Sci.* 1984;25:1453–1457.

42. Hughes PM, Mitra AK. Overview of ocular drug delivery and iatrogenic ocular cytopathologies. In: Mitra AK, ed. *Ophthalmic Drug Delivery Systems.* New York: Dekker; 1993:1–27. *Drugs and the Pharmaceutical Sciences*; Vol 58.

43. Fraunfelder FT. *Drug-Induced Ocular Side Effects and Drug Interactions.* Philadelphia, PA: Lea & Febiger; 1976.

44. Bar-Ilan A, Aviv H, Friedman D, et al. Improved performance of ocular drugs formulated in submicron emulsions. *Invest Ophthalmol Vis Sci.* 1993(suppl);34:1488.

45. Roziere A, Mazuel C, Grove J, Plazonnet B. Gelrite: a novel, ion-activated, in-situ gelling polymer for ophthalmic vehicles: effect on bioavailability of timolol. *Int J Pharm.* 1989;57:163–168.

46. Ibrahim H, Gurny R, Buri P, et al. Ocular bioavailability of pilocarpine from phase transition latex system triggered by pH. *Eur J Drug Metab Pharmacokinet.* 1990; 15(suppl):206.

47. Harsh DC, Gehrke SH. Controlling the swelling characteristics of temperature-sensitive cellulose ether hydrogels. *J Controlled Release.* 1991;17:175–185.

48. Miller SC, Donovan MD. Effect of poloxamer 407 gel on the miotic activity of pilocarpine nitrate in rabbits. *Int J Pharmacol.* 1982;12:147–152.

49. Kumar S, Haglund BO, Himmelstein KJ. In situ–forming gels of ophthalmic drug delivery. *J Ocul Pharmacol.* 1994;10:47–56.

50. Heller J. Controlled drug release from monolithic systems. In: Saettone MF, Bucci M, Speiser P, eds. *Ophthalmic Drug Delivery: Biopharmaceutical, Technological, and Clinical Aspects*. New York: Springer-Verlag; 1987:179.

51. Bartlett JD, Cullen AP. Clinical administration of ocular drugs. In: Bartlett JD, Jaanus SD, eds. *Clinical Ocular Pharmacology*. 2nd ed. Boston, MA: Butterworths; 1989:46–48.

52. Lamberts DW. Solid delivery devices. *Int Ophthalmol Clin*. 1980;20:63–77.

53. Bawa R. Ocular inserts. In: Mitra AK, ed. *Ophthalmic Drug Delivery Systems*. New York: Dekker; 1993:232–234. *Drugs and the Pharmaceutical Sciences*; Vol 58.

54. Zimmerman TJ, Leader B, Kaufman HE. Advances in ocular pharmacology. *Annu Rev Pharmacol Toxicol*. 1980;20:415–428.

55. Quigley HA, Pollack IP, Harbin TS. Pilocarpine Ocuserts: long-term clinical trials and selected pharmacodynamics. *Arch Ophthalmol*. 1975;93:771–775.

56. Shell JW, Baker RW. Diffusional systems for controlled release of drugs to the eye. *Ann Ophthalmol*. 1974;6:1037–1043,1045.

57. Urquhart J. Development of the Ocusert pilocarpine ocular therapeutic systems: a case history in ophthalmic product development. In: Robinson JR, ed. *Ophthalmic Drug Delivery Systems*. Washington, DC: American Pharmaceutical Association; 1980:105.

58. Hitchings RA, Smith RJ. Experience with pilocarpine Ocuserts. *Trans Ophthalmol Soc UK*. 1977;97:202–205.

59. Drance SM, Mitchell DW, Schulzer M. The effects of Ocusert pilocarpine on anterior chamber depth, visual acuity and intraocular pressure in man. *Can J Ophthalmol*. 1977;12:24–28.

60. Francois J, Goes F, Zagorski Z. Comparative ultrasonographic study of the effect of pilocarpine 2% and Ocusert P 20 on the eye components. *Am J Ophthalmol*. 1978; 86:233–238.

61. Novak S, Stewart RH. The Ocusert system in the management of glaucoma. *Tex Med*. 1975;71:63–65.

62. Armaly MF, Rao KR. The effect of pilocarpine Ocusert with different release rates on ocular pressure. *Invest Ophthalmol*. 1973;12:491–496.

63. Weiner N, Martin F, Riaz M. Liposomes as a drug delivery system. *Drug Dev Indust Pharm*. 1989;15:1523–1554.

64. Schulman JA, Peyman GA. Intracameral, intravitreal and retinal drug delivery. In: Mitra AK, ed. *Ophthalmic Drug Delivery Systems*. New York: Dekker; 1993:395–397. *Drugs and the Pharmaceutical Sciences*; Vol 58.

65. Davis NM, Kellaway IW, Greaves JL, Wilson CG. Advanced corneal delivery systems: liposomes. In: Mitra AK, ed. *Ophthalmic Drug Delivery Systems*. New York: Dekker; 1993:289–303. *Drugs and the Pharmaceutical Sciences*; Vol 58.

66. New RRC, Black CDV, Parker RJ, et al. Liposomes in biological systems. In: New RRC, ed. *Liposome*. Oxford: IRL Press at Oxford University; 1990:221.

67. Lee VH, Urrea PT, Smith RE, Schanzlin DJ. Ocular drug bioavailability from topically applied liposomes. *Surv Ophthalmol*. 1985;29:335–348.

68. Schaeffer HE, Krohn DL. Liposomes in topical drug delivery. *Invest Ophthalmol Vis Sci*. 1982;22:220–227.

69. Juliano RL, Stamp D. Lectin-mediated attachment of glycoprotein-bearing liposomes to cells. *Nature*. 1976;261:235–238.

70. Barza M, Baum J, Szoka F Jr. Pharmacokinetics of subconjunctival liposome-encapsulated gentamicin in normal rabbit eyes. *Invest Ophthalmol Vis Sci*. 1984;25: 486–490.

71. Alghadyan AA, Peyman GA, Khoobehi B, et al. Liposome-bound cyclosporine: aqueous and vitreous level after subconjunctival injection. *Int Ophthalmol.* 1988;12:101–104.

72. Fishman PH, Peyman GA, Lesar T. Intravitreal liposome-encapsulated gentamicin in a rabbit model: prolonged therapeutic levels. *Invest Ophthalmol Vis Sci.* 1986;27:1103–1106.

73. Tremblay C, Barza M, Szoka F, et al. Reduced toxicity of liposome-associated amphotericin B injected intravitreally in rabbits. *Invest Ophthalmol Vis Sci.* 1985;26:711–718.

74. Alghadyan AA, Peyman GA, Khoobehi B, et al. Liposome-bound cyclosporine: clearance after intravitreal injection. *Int Ophthalmol.* 1988;12:109–112.

75. Norley SG, Huang L, Rouse BT. Targeting of drug loaded immunoliposomes to herpes simplex virus infected corneal cells: an effective means of inhibiting virus replication in vitro. *J Immunol.* 1986;136:681–685.

76. Norley SG, Sendele D, Huang L, Rouse BT. Inhibition of herpes simplex virus replication in the mouse cornea by drug containing immunoliposomes. *Invest Ophthalmol Vis Sci.* 1987;28:591–595.

77. Alvarez-Lorenzo C, Hiratani H, Gomez-Amoza JL, et al. Soft contact lenses capable of sustained delivery of timolol. *J Pharm Sci.* 2002;91:2182–2192.

78. Alvarez-Lorenzo C, Concheiro A. Molecularly imprinted polymers for drug delivery. *J Chromatogr B.* 2004;804:231–245.

79. Ashton P, Blandford DL, Pearson PA, et al. Review: implants. *J Ocul Pharmacol.* 1994;10:691–701.

80. Smith TJ, Pearson PA, Blandford DL, et al. Intravitreal sustained-release ganciclovir. *Arch Ophthalmol.* 1992;110:255–258.

81. Martin DF, Ferris FL, Parks DJ, et al. Ganciclovir implant exchange: timing, surgical procedure, and complications. *Arch Ophthalmol.* 1997;115:1389–1394.

82. Jaffe GJ, Yang CS, Wang XC, et al. Intravitreal sustained-release cyclosporine in the treatment of experimental uveitis. *Ophthalmology.* 1998;105:46–56.

83. Enyedi LB, Pearson PA, Ashton P, Jaffe GJ. An intravitreal device providing sustained release of cyclosporine and dexamethasone. *Curr Eye Res.* 1996;15:549–557.

84. Smith TJ, Ashton P. Sustained-release subconjunctival 5-fluorouracil. *Ophthalmic Surg Lasers.* 1996;27:763–767.

85. Yang CS, Khawly JA, Hainsworth DP, et al. An intravitreal sustained-release triamcinolone and 5-fluorouracil codrug in the treatment of experimental proliferative vitreoretinopathy. *Arch Ophthalmol.* 1998;116:69–77.

86. Berger AS, Cheng CK, Pearson PA, et al. Intravitreal sustained release corticosteroid–5-fluorouracil conjugate in the treatment of experimental proliferative vitreoretinopathy. *Invest Ophthalmol Vis Sci.* 1996;37:2318–2325.

87. Lim LL, Smith JR, Rosenbaum JT. Retisert (Bausch & Lomb/control delivery system). *Cur Opin Invest Drugs.* 2005;6:1159–1167.

88. Fluocinolone acetonide ophthalmic-Bausch & Lomb: fluocinolone acetonide Envision TD implant. *Drugs R D.* 2005;6:116–119.

89. Chrousos GP. Adrenocorticosteroids and adrenocortical antagonists. In: Katzung B ed. *Basic and Clinical Pharmacology.* 9th ed. New York: Large Medical Books/McGraw-Hill; 2004:641–660.

90. Francois J. Corticosteroid glaucoma. *Ann Ophthalmol.* 1977;9:1075–1080.

91. Cantrill HL, Palmberg, Zink HA, et al. Comparison of in vitro potency of corticosteroids with ability to raise intraocular pressure. *Am J Ophthalmol.* 1975;79:1012–1017.

92. Armaly MF. Effect of corticosteroids on intraocular pressure and fluid dynamics: I. The effect of desamethasone in the normal eye. *Arch Ophthalmol*. 1963;70:482–491.

93. Armaly MF. Effect of corticosteroids on intraocular pressure and fluid dynamics: II. The effect of desamethasone on the glaucomatous eye. *Arch Ophthalmol*. 1963;70:492–499.

94. Weinreb RN, Polansky JR, Kramer SG, et al. Acute effects of dexamethasone on introcular pressure in glaucoma. *Invest Ophthalmol Vis Sci*. 1985;26:170–175.

95. Smithen LM, Ober MD, Maranan L, et al. Intravitreal triamcinolone acetonide and intraocular pressure. *Am J Ophthalmol*. 2004;138:740–743.

96. Herschler J. Increased intraocular pressure induced by repository corticosteroids. *Am J Ophthalmol*. 1976;82:90–93.

97. Espildora J, Vicuna P, Diaz E. Cortisone-induced glaucoma: a report on 44 affected eyes. *J Fr Ophthalmol*. 1981;4:503–508.

98. Kersey JP, Broadway DC. Corticosteroid-induced glaucoma: a review of the literature. *Eye*. 2006;20:407–416.

2

Prostaglandin Analogs

THOMAS W. HEJKAL AND CARL B. CAMRAS

*P*rostaglandin (PG) analogs, originally introduced for glaucoma therapy in the United States with latanoprost in 1996, have rapidly become the most commonly used ocular hypotensive agents. As a class, PG analogs are the most effective topical agents currently available for lowering intraocular pressure (IOP).[1-4] Four PG analogs are available for clinical use: latanoprost (Xalatan 0.005%, Pfizer, New York, NY), travoprost (Travatan 0.004%, Alcon, Fort Worth, Tex.), bimatoprost (Lumigan 0.03%, Allergan, Irvine, Calif.), and unoprostone (Rescula 0.15%, Novartis Ophthalmics, Basel, Switzerland). All have similar structures and are prodrugs of prostaglandin $F_{2\alpha}$ ($PGF_{2\alpha}$) analogs. The structures of these drugs are compared in figure 2.1. Latanoprost, travoprost, and unoprostone are ester prodrugs that are hydrolyzed by corneal esterases to become biologically active. Latanoprost and travoprost are selective agonists for the $F_{2\alpha}$ prostaglandin (FP) prostanoid receptor. Bimatoprost has been described as a prostamide, although the structure is similar to that of the other two PG analogs. It has been shown to be an amide prodrug.[5] The free acid of bimatoprost has a structure almost identical to the free acid of latanoprost, is a potent FP receptor agonist, and appears to be the active form of this drug.[5-7] Unoprostone is an analog of a pulmonary metabolite of $PGF_{2\alpha}$, and the affinity of unoprostone for the FP receptor is 100-fold less than that of latanoprost. It has been demonstrated to be less effective than the other three analogs in clinical trials.[8,9] Unoprostone was withdrawn from the U.S. market in 2004; however, it continues to be commercially available in Japan and in some other countries.

The first study to demonstrate a reduction in IOP after topical application of PGs was published in 1977.[10] This study demonstrated that the dose is an important factor influencing the effect in rabbits, since other early studies on the ocular effects

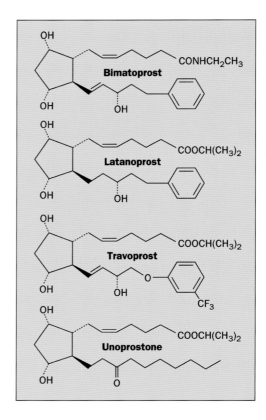

Figure 2.1. Chemical structures of the prostaglandin analogs.

of PGs consistently showed that very high doses of topical or intracameral PGs raised IOP. Studies over the next two decades led to the development of a PG analog that was effective and well tolerated, and the development of other PG analogs followed.

Because their mechanism of action is different from most other glaucoma medications, PGs can produce a substantial additional reduction in IOP when added to treatment regimens consisting of other topical and/or systemic ocular hypotensive agents.

2.1 MECHANISM OF ACTION

The primary mechanism by which most PGs reduce IOP is by increasing outflow, especially through the uveoscleral outflow pathway (figure 2.2). Numerous animal and human studies have confirmed this mechanism of action.[11,12] In several studies, PGs have been demonstrated to increase outflow facility.[12–17] PGs do not reduce aqueous production.

The mechanism by which PGs increase uveoscleral outflow is continuing to be elucidated. One mechanism may be the relaxation of the ciliary muscle. This is supported by studies in monkeys that have shown pilocarpine pretreatment blocks the effect of PGs on uveoscleral outflow or IOP.[11,12,15] An increase in ciliary body

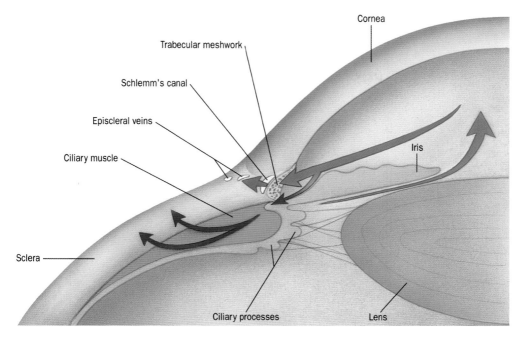

Figure 2.2. Two major routes aqueous outflow. Prostaglandin analogs act by increasing outflow, primarily through the uveoscleral pathway (blue arrows), with some contribution through the conventional trabecular outflow pathway (green arrows).

thickness has been measured by ultrasound biomicroscopy in human eyes treated with latanoprost.[18] Additionally, PGs may cause dilated spaces between ciliary muscle bundles. This is thought to result from PG-induced stimulation of collagenases and other matrix metalloproteinases.[11,19] However, other studies, using both light and electron microscopy, have found no evidence of dilated spaces between ciliary muscle bundles or other alterations in the ciliary muscle or other ocular tissues in monkeys treated with $PGF_{2\alpha}$.[20]

2.2 INDICATIONS

Originally approved for second-line therapy when introduced in 1996, latanoprost has been FDA approved as a first-line treatment of open-angle glaucoma or ocular hypertension since 2002. Travoprost and bimatoprost were initially approved by the FDA for second-line therapy, and subsequently both drugs have been approved for first-line treatment.

Clinical studies have also demonstrated that PGs lower IOP in patients with normal tension glaucoma,[21–24] exfoliation syndrome,[25–31] pigment dispersion syndrome,[17,27,31] and chronic angle-closure glaucoma.[32–35] There are limited reports of clinical experience with the use of latanoprost in other types of glaucoma.[28] Caution is recommended in uveitic glaucoma, although some studies demonstrate safety and efficacy of PGs in uveitic glaucoma.[36] PGs, like other glaucoma medications, may be less effective in pediatric patients.[37]

PG analogs have several advantages over other ocular hypotensive medications. Their main advantage over the beta blockers is the apparent lack of systemic side effects. Compared with beta blockers, PG analogs are more potent and effective ocular hypotensive agents with once-a-day dosing, and they are equally well tolerated by patients. Whereas beta blockers do not reduce aqueous flow during sleep, PGs are as effective at night as during the day.[38,39] Reducing IOP at night may have the added advantage of reducing glaucomatous damage during sleep when ocular perfusion pressure may be reduced secondary to decreased systemic blood pressure.[40] Because of their mechanism of action, PG analogs potentially can reduce IOP below episcleral venous pressure, unlike medications that increase outflow facility. This, along with their more favorable effect on ocular perfusion pressure, presents a potential advantage in normal tension glaucoma, which may require very low IOPs for adequate control.[22–24]

2.3 CONTRAINDICATIONS

PG analogs are contraindicated in any patient who is allergic or sensitive to these drugs. Patients who are pregnant or nursing should use caution. There are limited studies in pediatric patients, and although side effects are infrequent and mild, some children have had an inadequate response to PGs.[37] Although limited studies are available, it remains unclear what effect PGs have on ocular inflammation in postoperative patients and what role PGs may have in treating patients with elevated IOP following cataract surgery or other intraocular surgery.[41] There have been some reports of an association of latanoprost with cystoid macular edema (CME), which is discussed in section 2.5.5.[36] Although the controlled clinical trials have not shown a causal relationship between PGs and these problems, PGs should be used with caution in patients with multiple risk factors for CME, with iritis or herpes simplex keratitis, or in the immediate postoperative period following intraocular surgery.[36] Until further clinical studies have clarified the relationship between the PGs and CME, it should not be the drug of first choice in complicated aphakic or pseudophakic eyes with torn posterior capsules and other known risk factors for CME.[36,42,43]

2.4 TREATMENT REGIMEN

The recommended treatment regimen for latanoprost, travoprost, and bimatoprost is one drop applied topically once daily in the evening. Evening, rather than morning, administration appears to be more efficacious and may block the early morning diurnal spike in IOP that may be observed in many patients.[29] With the exception of unoprostone, which has a recommended dosage of twice daily, none of the other PGs should be used more than once daily since more frequent dosage decreases the IOP-lowering effect.[2,4,44]

2.5 SIDE EFFECTS

The side effect profiles of the various PG analogs are compared in table 2.1. Eye irritation, conjunctival hyperemia, and eyelash changes are the most frequently reported side effects. Eye irritation, burning, and pain are reported with variable frequency in the various studies, and the rates of these symptoms with the various PG analogs are not substantially different from each other or from timolol. A wide range of other signs or symptoms such as superficial punctate keratitis, blurred vision, cataract, and headache have been reported at low rates in various clinical studies. The side effects of iris color changes, eyelash changes, and periocular skin color changes are specifically associated with the PG analogs.

Bimatoprost and travoprost have been reported to give a higher incidence of hyperemia and eyelash changes compared to latanoprost,[2,3,45,46] and package insert labeling reflects this difference. There is no clear evidence that the incidence or severity of other side effects vary substantially among these medications. At the time this chapter was prepared, peer-reviewed reports were not available regarding benzalkonium chloride-free travoprost ophthalmic solution 0.004% (Travatan Z). More experience is required with the newer PG analogs to determine whether the incidence of rare side effects is different among the PGs.

2.5.1 *Conjunctival Hyperemia.* Conjunctival hyperemia is reported significantly more frequently with bimatoprost and travoprost than with latanoprost (table 2.1).[2,3,45,46] In general, the level of hyperemia is very mild for most patients and usually is not noticed by the patient and not severe enough to require discontinuation of the medication.[2,3,29,45–49] Based on the phase III clinical trials and as stated in the package inserts, 3% of patients required discontinuation of therapy with travoprost or bimatoprost because of intolerance to conjunctival hyperemia, whereas

Table 2.1 Percentage of Patients in Comparative Trials Exhibiting Specific Ocular Signs and Symptoms

Signs or Symptoms	Latanoprost[3,45,46,117] (0.005%)	Bimatoprost[45,46,117] (0.03%)	Travoprost[3,45] (0.004%)
Conjunctival hyperemia	12–47	31–69[a]	32–58[a]
Eye Symptoms			
Irritation	3–7	11	4–8
Burning	6	5	NR
Itching	0–6	0–10[a]	2–8
Pain	2–4	1	3–8
Iris Color Change	5	NR	3
Eyelash Change	0–26	3–11[a]	1–57[a]
Skin Pigmentation	2	3	3

NR, Not reported
[a]Significant differences compared to latanoprost in at least one study.

less than 1% of those treated with latanoprost required discontinuation because of these symptoms.

2.5.2 *Iris Color Changes.* Iris pigment changes are a well-documented side effect of chronic topical PG use in certain patients.[28,50] Patients exhibiting darkening of the iris are most commonly those with a concentric brown ring of pigmentation around the pupil and a light gray, green, or blue color of the peripheral iris (figure 2.3).[28,50,51] In open-label clinical trials, the overall incidence of increased iris pigmentation detectable by serial photographs over 3 years of treatment with latanoprost was 30%, with higher rates in patients with blue/gray-brown (45%), green-brown (69%), or yellow-brown (70%) eyes than in those with blue/gray (8%) or brown (17%) eyes.[28,50] Similarly, in a 5-year, open-label multicenter study, 38% of patients had increases in iris pigmentation with onset occurring within 8 months in 70% of patients who developed darkening.[28] While the overall incidence may be up to 30% to 40%, most cases are mild, and only about half the patients with documented changes reported this as a noticeable effect.[28,50] Increases in iris pigmentation have also been reported with travoprost,[3,49] bimatoprost,[4,48] and unoprostone.[52] Thus, increased iris pigmentation in patients with hazel or heterochromic irides appears to be a side effect of this entire class of medications.

It is thought that PGs may increase iris pigmentation by substituting for sympathetic innervation to the iris, which is required to maintain the level of pigmentation in iris melanocytes.[53] PGs increase the melanin content of melanocytes in the iris, but not the total number of melanocytes.[50,54] Specimens of irides from latanoprost-treated eyes with and without hyperpigmentation have revealed no pathologic changes.[54–57]

There is no evidence that PGs increase intraocular melanin other than in the stromal melanocytes in the iris. Changes in pigmentation in the iris pigment epithelium or in the trabecular meshwork have not been observed.[50,55,58,59] Therefore, PGs would not be expected to worsen pigmentary dispersion glaucoma or induce uveitis through pigment release.

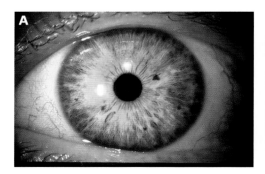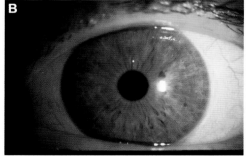

Figure 2.3. (A) Eye before treatment. Note the brown ring of pigmentation around the pupil and light pigmentation in the periphery. This baseline iris color is most likely to exhibit darkening during treatment. (B) Same eye following latanoprost treatment. Reprinted with permission from Camras CB, Neely DG, Weiss EL. Latanoprost-induced iris color darkening: a case report with long-term follow-up. *J Glaucoma.* 2000;9:95–98.

2.5.3 *Eyelash Changes*. Topical PG analogs have been reported to increase length, number, thickness, and pigmentation of eyelashes and adjacent hair (figure 2.4).[2,3,44,48,49,60,61] Although phase III clinical trials for latanoprost did not find eyelash changes, one study reported that each of the 43 subjects treated with latanoprost in one eye for 11 to 40 weeks showed hypertrichosis and increased eyelash pigmentation.[60] The incidence in a larger scale clinical trial with latanoprost was 14%.[28] Eyelash changes have also been documented with travoprost and bimatoprost both in phase III clinical trials and in subsequent reports.[3,44,48,49] Subsequent comparative studies have documented a higher incidence of these changes with bimatoprost and travoprost than with latanoprost.[2,3,45,46]

2.5.4 *Uveitis*. There have been anecdotal and retrospective reports of the possible association of PG analogs with anterior uveitis.[36,62–65] Earlier reports of anterior uveitis associated with latanoprost use have been summarized by Schumer et al.[36] Although these reports have raised the possibility of an association between PG analogs and iritis, no clear causal relationship has been established. Several multicenter, randomized, masked clinical trials have failed to demonstrate a difference in ocular inflammation with PG analogs compared to timolol.[3,4,12,21,26,29,30,44,47–49] In a multicenter trial with 198 patients, there were 10 patients in whom a few cells

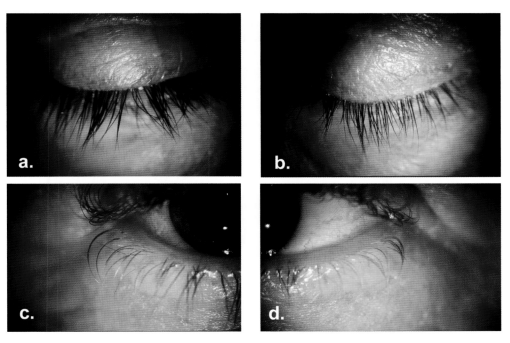

Figure 2.4. (a) Eyelashes of upper eyelid after latanoprost treatment, and (b) untreated fellow eye of same patient. (c) Lashes of lower eyelid after latanoprost treatment, and (d) untreated fellow eye. Treated lashes are longer, thicker, darker, and more numerous. Reprinted with permission from Johnstone MA, Albert DM. Prostaglandin-induced hair growth. *Surv Ophthalmol.* 2002;47(suppl 1):S185–S202.

were observed in the anterior chamber at least once during 12 months of treatment with latanoprost. Two of the 10 patients also had cells observed at baseline prior to treatment.[27] There was no difference between patients treated with latanoprost or timolol in the incidence of aqueous flare or an anterior chamber cellular response during the randomized, masked, 6-month phase of the trial.[29,47] Multiple studies using sensitive techniques such as fluorophotometry or laser-flare meters to determine the status of the blood–aqueous barrier or protein concentration in aqueous humor showed no significant effect following PG treatment for as long as 12 months.[12,36,66] Comparative studies evaluating the effects of different PG analogs on flare and cellularity have failed to demonstrate a clear difference among them.[42,67]

Thus, it appears that the risk of developing significant uveitis with PG analogs is low and might be no higher than the risk of uveitis with other topical glaucoma medications such as pilocarpine, dorzolamide, or brimonidine.[36] However, one should be aware of the possibility of a uveitic reaction and use caution in treating patients with risk factors for uveitis. PG analogs should be discontinued in patients who develop a significant uveitis when there is no other evident cause.

2.5.5 *Cystoid Macular Edema.*

There have been anecdotal reports of CME associated with PG analog use.[36,42,43,68–70] Cases of CME reported with topical latanoprost were compiled and analyzed, and almost all of the reported cases had other known risk factors for CME.[36] These risk factors included open posterior capsules, recent intraocular surgery, complicated surgery with vitreous loss, a prior history of CME, concomitant dipivefrin therapy, or recent iritis.[36,43] In a review of anecdotal, retrospective reports from which total numbers of eyes treated could be estimated, a total of two cases of CME occurred in at least 894 eyes of patients treated with latanoprost.[71] A causal relationship between PG treatment and CME has still not been clearly established. As with uveitis, no controlled clinical studies support the speculation that latanoprost causes CME. There were no cases of CME attributable to PG use in more than 1,000 patients treated in phase III latanoprost clinical trials,[30,36] nor were any cases of CME observed in the clinical trials for bimatoprost[44,48] or travoprost.[3,49]

Topical PGs do not appear to affect the retinal vasculature. Monkeys treated with high doses of latanoprost and $PGF_{2\alpha}$ analogs showed no evidence of CME or leakage on fluorescein angiography in either phakic or aphakic eyes treated 2 weeks to 6 months.[20,72,73] In pseudophakic eyes with elevated IOP, treated with latanoprost twice daily for 4 weeks, there was no angiographic evidence of leakage or changes in the retinal vasculature.[73]

Other prospective studies have found some evidence for angiographic CME in patients treated with PG analogs. In a prospective study of pseudophakic and aphakic patients, 4 of 16 latanoprost-treated eyes, 1 of 16 bimatoprost-treated eyes, and 1 of 17 travoprost-treated eyes developed angiographic CME.[42] Other studies have found an increased incidence of angiographic CME with latanoprost, timolol, and preserved vehicle, but not with preservative-free vehicle.[74] They concluded that the benzalkonium chloride preservative was the probable cause of the increased incidence of CME.

Overall, the literature indicates that the risk of developing CME from PG use is low. However, in eyes with risk factors for CME, PGs should be used with caution until controlled trials have further defined the risk of this potential side effect.[36,43]

2.5.6 *Other Local Side Effects*. Increased pigmentation of periorbital skin has been associated with topical PG use in some studies.[36,48,75] There was a 5% rate of eyelid skin darkening with bimatoprost compared to 0.4% with timolol in the phase III trials.[48] A histopathologic study on patients with increased skin pigmentation following bimatoprost use demonstrated that the increased pigmentation was associated with increased melanogenesis but found no evidence of melanocyte proliferation or inflammation.[76]

Deepening of the lid sulcus has been anecdotally reported in patients being treated with bimatoprost.[77] This side effect has not been clearly substantiated.

Rare anecdotal reports have described reactivation of herpes simplex virus keratitis or dermatitis in patients treated with topical PG.[36] Although a couple of studies in rabbits provided equivocal evidence that latanoprost increased the severity and recurrence rate of herpes simplex keratitis, later studies have refuted this contention.[36,78] There is no evidence from any of the numerous controlled clinical trials or from a retrospective, population-based cohort study of claims records that PG analogs increase the risk of herpes simplex virus reactivation.[36,79]

2.5.7 *No Systemic Side Effects*. One would not expect significant systemic effects based on the pharmacokinetics of topically applied latanoprost. The biologically active acid of latanoprost that reaches the systemic circulation is metabolized primarily in the liver by fatty acid beta-oxidation and is rapidly eliminated primarily by the kidneys; its half-life is 17 minutes in human plasma. Latanoprost is measurable in human plasma only during the first hour after administration. There have been no systemic side effects attributed to topical PGs in any of the clinical trials. In contrast to timolol, PG analogs have no effect on blood pressure, heart rate, or pulmonary function.[29,30,47,80] Topical beta blockers are well known to lower blood pressure, decrease heart rate, and worsen pulmonary function, and to exacerbate depression, cause impotence, and produce other serious side effects in some patients. The apparent lack of systemic side effects might be the most significant advantage that topical PGs have over beta blockers in glaucoma therapy. However, since rare side effects might not be discovered until a drug is in widespread use for many years, the possibility of a systemic side effect in the rare individual exists, especially for the newer PG analogs, as has been anecdotally reported.

2.6 DRUG INTERACTIONS

Eye drops containing thimerosal form a precipitate when mixed with latanoprost. Therefore, it is recommended that patients using both latanoprost and drops containing thimerosal should administer these drugs at least 5 minutes apart. There are no known adverse interactions with other drugs. The additivity of the effect of PGs when used in combination with other ocular hypotensive medications is discussed in section 2.8.

2.7 IOP REDUCTION IN CLINICAL TRIALS

Numerous clinical trials have demonstrated the efficacy of PG analogs in lowering IOP. Clinical trials with latanoprost,[1,2,29,31,47,81] bimatoprost,[1,2,44,48] and travoprost[1-3,49] have all shown that these drugs given once daily are more effective than timolol 0.5% given twice a day in reducing mean diurnal IOP in patients with ocular hypertension or glaucoma (figure 2.5). PGs have also been shown to be as effective or more effective and often better tolerated than other topical glaucoma

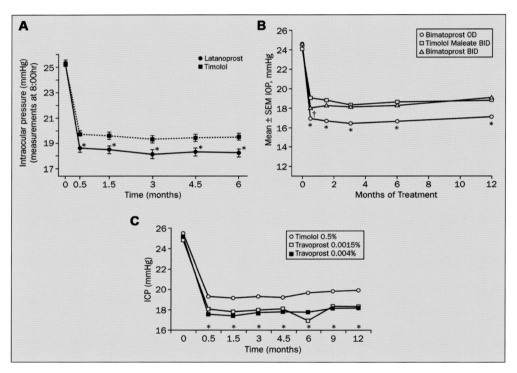

Figure 2.5. Efficacy of PG analogs compared to timolol 0.5% twice daily in reducing IOP. (A) Latanoprost 0.005% once daily. Reprinted with permission from Camras CB. Comparison of latanoprost and timolol in patients with ocular hypertension and glaucoma: a six-month, masked, multicenter trial in the United States. United States Latanoprost Study Group. *Ophthalmology.* 1996;103:138–147. (B) Bimatoprost 0.03% once daily. Reprinted with permission from Higginbotham EJ, Schuman EK, Goldberg I, et al. One-year, randomized study comparing bimatoprost and timolol in glaucoma and ocular hypertension. *Arch Ophthalmol.* 2002;120:1286–1293. (C) Travoprost 0.004% or 0.0015% once daily. Reprinted with permission from Netland PA, Landry T, Sullivan EK, et al. Travoprost compared with latanoprost and timolol in patients with open-angle glaucoma or ocular hypertension. *Am J Ophthalmol.* 2001;132:472–484.

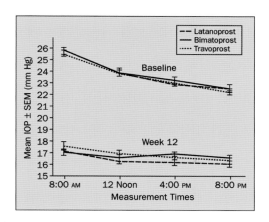

Figure 2.6. Comparison of latanoprost 0.005%, bimatoprost 0.03%, and travoprost 0.004% in lowering IOP. Reprinted with permission from Parrish RK, Palmberg P, Sheu WP, et al. A comparison of latanoprost, bimatoprost, and travoprost in patients with elevated intraocular pressure: a 12-week, randomized, masked-evaluator multicenter study. XLT Study Group. *Am J Ophthalmol.* 2003;135:688–703.

medications,[1] including pilocarpine, dorzolamide,[82,83] timolol–dorzolamide combinations,[84–87] and brimonidine.[88]

Based on pooled data from eight clinical trials ($n = 1,389$), latanoprost reduces mean diurnal IOP an average of 7.9 mm Hg, or 32% (from a baseline of 24.6 mm Hg).[81] This is 1.6 mm Hg more than the effect achieved by timolol. Unlike timolol, which shows a mild contralateral effect, PG analogs do not affect the IOP in untreated fellow eyes.[30,47] Clinical trials with bimatoprost[4,48] and travoprost[49] show similar efficacy for these drugs (figure 2.5). The higher the baseline IOP, the greater the IOP reduction, as is the case for other ocular hypotensive drugs.

Several prospective, randomized clinical trials have demonstrated that the IOP reductions achieved by latanoprost, bimatoprost, and travoprost are similar (figure 2.6).[1–3,38,45] In spite of isolated studies showing some modest differences,[41,46] the bulk of the clinical evidence shows no substantial differences in IOP-lowering effect among these three drugs.[1–3,38,45] Unoprostone, however, has significantly lower efficacy compared to the other PG analogs.[8,9]

PG analogs appear to be effective in a variety of ethnic groups. There is little difference in efficacy between African Americans and U.S. Caucasians.[3,47,89,90] Prostaglandin analogs are more effective compared with timolol in African Americans.[3,90] Clinical studies in the United States (in either African Americans or Caucasians), United Kingdom, Scandinavia, Japan, Philippines, Mexico, Korea, and China consistently show latanoprost to be more effective than timolol in each of these patient populations,[81] and the other PG analogs have shown similar efficacies when tested in various populations.

Prolonged treatment with PG analogs shows no loss of effect over a 1- to 2-year period,[3,27,31,44] and 5-year data for latanoprost show continued efficacy.[28]

2.8 CLINICAL STUDIES ON ADDITIVITY

Because PG analogs have a different mechanism of action than other ocular hypotensive drugs, the IOP reduction from PGs can be expected to be additive to that of other glaucoma medications. Multiple clinical studies have demonstrated that the effect of PGs is additive to the effect of other ocular hypotensive agents, including timolol, pilocarpine, topical and oral carbonic anhydrase inhibitors (CAIs), alpha-2 agonists, and dipivefrin[91–98] and when used in patients on otherwise maximally tolerated medical therapy.[8,99] Also, patients on a nonselective beta blocker with pilocarpine or dorzolamide achieved significantly lower IOP when latanoprost was added to the regimen.[99]

2.8.1 *Beta Blockers.* Beta-adrenergic antagonists reduce IOP by inhibiting the production of aqueous humor, whereas PGs work by increasing uveoscleral outflow. Thus, it is expected that the effects of beta blockers and PGs on IOP reduction would be additive, and this has been confirmed in clinical studies. In several trials in which latanoprost once daily was added to timolol twice daily, additional IOP reductions of 24% to 37% were achieved.[91] The additive effect is less with twice-daily dosing of latanoprost or when timolol is added to latanoprost. Interestingly, when patients are switched from timolol to latanoprost monotherapy, they experience almost as much IOP reduction (21% to 25%) as when latanoprost is added to timolol therapy. The additive effect of pilocarpine and timolol is not as great as with latanoprost and timolol.[91] Studies with the other PG analogs also demonstrate an additive effect when used in combination with beta blockers.[94–96] Fixed combinations of PGs and timolol are discussed in section 2.8.5.

PG analogs and beta blockers are often used together, typically with morning dosing of a beta blocker and evening dosing of a PG analog.

2.8.2 *Carbonic Anhydrase Inhibitors.* The additivity of PG analogs to oral and topical CAIs has been demonstrated in clinical studies.[83,91,99,100] Oral CAIs combined with PG analogs can give a dramatic decrease in IOP. For example, latanoprost 0.005% once daily gives an additional 15% decrease in IOP when added to an acetazolamide regimen of 250 mg twice daily.[100] Latanoprost gives an additional 24% reduction in IOP when added to dorzolamide three times a day,[83] and dorzolamide gives an additional 15% to 20% reduction in IOP when added to latanoprost.[82,101] It has also been demonstrated that latanoprost further reduces IOP when added to a fixed combination of timolol and dorzolamide.[102] The other PG analogs also have an additive effect when used with CAIs.[103,104]

2.8.3 *Cholinergic Agonists.* Cholinergic agonists, such as pilocarpine, act by increasing trabecular outflow facility. This increase is accomplished through contraction of the ciliary muscle, which pulls on the scleral spur and opens channels in the trabecular meshwork. The contraction of the ciliary muscle also contracts the spaces between the muscle bundles and causes a reduction in uveoscleral outflow. Therefore, theoretically, pilocarpine could reduce the increase in uveoscleral outflow caused by PGs. Although this effect has been observed with pilocarpine and $PGF_{2\alpha}$ in monkeys, human studies show no blockage of the PG effect with concurrent pilocarpine treatment.[15,105] Clinical studies have demonstrated that latanoprost produces an additional reduction in IOP when added to pilocarpine or physostigmine.[15,91] When added to a regimen of pilocarpine 2%, latanoprost reduces IOP an additional 14% to 18% compared to pilocarpine alone; conversely, pilocarpine reduces IOP an additional 7% when added to latanoprost alone.[15,105] A study with 13 patients in which pilocarpine up to 6% four times daily was added to bimatoprost once daily showed no significant additive or antagonistic effect from the added pilocarpine.[92] In general, the PG analogs produce a substantial additional IOP reduction when added to regimens with pilocarpine; however, less additional effect can be expected when adding pilocarpine to a PG regimen.[15,92,105]

2.8.4 Adrenergic Agonists.

Epinephrine increases trabecular outflow facility and uveoscleral outflow. There is evidence that PGs are involved in the ocular hypotensive effects of epinephrine, which may stimulate the production of endogenous PGs.[106] In any case, clinical studies have demonstrated that latanoprost is indeed additive to dipivefrin, an epinephrine prodrug.[91,99] Studies in which latanoprost has been added to dipivefrin show an additional reduction in IOP of 19% to 28%. When dipivefrin is added to latanoprost the additional IOP reduction is less (15% to 16%) but still significant.[91] Dipivefrin and latanoprost are both analogs of mediators that are naturally present in the eye (epinephrine and $PGF_{2\alpha}$). They may work by modulating normal physiologic mechanisms. The combination of these two medications is very effective in lowering IOP, producing total IOP reduction of up to 47% from initial baseline.[91]

Brimonidine has a significant additional effect when added to PG analogs.[101,104,107,108] In one study, brimonidine added to latanoprost seems to have an effect similar to that of adding topical dorzolamide to latanoprost.[108] Also, concomitant therapy with brimonidine and latanoprost has been reported to have a similar effect on IOP compared with latanoprost–timolol fixed combination.[109] However, another study reported a lesser effect from brimonidine than either timolol or brinzolamide when added to a regimen of once-daily travoprost.[104] Studies with bimatoprost have also shown an additive effect with brimonidine.[93]

2.8.4 Fixed Combinations With PG Analogs.

Because of the potent additive effect that PG analogs have when combined with other ocular hypotensive agents and the common clinical usage of PG analogs with beta blockers, much attention has been given to the development of fixed combinations of PGs with other medications, especially timolol (table 2.2).

A fixed-combination of latanoprost 0.005% and timolol 0.5% (Xalacom) is available in some countries but is not yet approved in the United States. There is substantial evidence that the fixed-combination product is more effective than either timolol or

Table 2.2 Prostaglandin Fixed-Combination Products Either Commercially Available or Under Investigation

PG analog	Combination Drug	Brand Name	Manufacturer
Latanoprost 0.005%	Timolol 0.5%	Xalacom	Pfizer
Bimatoprost 0.03%	Timolol 0.5%	Ganfort	Allergan
Travoprost 0.004%	Timolol 0.5%	DuoTrav, Extravan	Alcon

latanoprost alone.[91,97,98,110–113] Fixed combinations of latanoprost and timolol reduce IOP an additional 15% to 25% below a timolol-treatment baseline or a latanoprost-treatment baseline.[91,97,98,110–113] The reduction in IOP achieved with the fixed-combination product dosed once daily either in the morning or in the evening is not substantially less than that achieved with concomitant treatment of once-daily latanoprost with twice-daily timolol.[97,113,114] Other studies have shown that the latanoprost–timolol combination is at least as effective as twice-daily dorzolamide–timolol (Cosopt).[115,116]

Fixed-combination travoprost–timolol and bimatoprost–timolol products are under investigation. Fixed combinations of travoprost 0.004% and timolol 0.5% used once daily in the morning have been reported to be as effective as concomitant therapy with the individual drugs and significantly more effective than timolol alone.[94–96]

Fixed-combination products have the advantage of being more convenient and potentially less expensive for patients, and therefore have the potential advantage of improving patient compliance. They also reduce preservative exposure by decreasing the number of daily drops. Beta blockers and PG analogs are especially well suited for a fixed-combination product. Since nonselective beta blockers or PG analogs both are effective when given once daily, a fixed combination of these products given once daily does not compromise circadian efficacy based on the duration of action of each component. Other fixed combinations may be less effective since other glaucoma medications require more frequent administration to maintain efficacy, and a combination product with a PG analog given once daily would sacrifice circadian efficacy.

REFERENCES

1. van der Valk R, Webers CA, Schouten JS, et al. Intraocular pressure-lowering effects of all commonly used glaucoma drugs: a meta-analysis of randomized clinical trials. *Ophthalmology*. 2005;112:1177–1185.

2. Eisenberg DL, Toris CB, Camras CB. Bimatoprost and travoprost. a review of recent studies of two new glaucoma drugs. *Surv Ophthalmol*. 2002;47(suppl 1):S105–S115.

3. Netland PA, Landry T, Sullivan EK, et al. Travoprost compared with latanoprost and timolol in patients with open-angle glaucoma or ocular hypertension. *Am J Ophthalmol*. 2001;132:472–484.

4. Sherwood M, Brandt J. Six-month comparison of bimatoprost once-daily and twice-daily with timolol twice-daily in patients with elevated intraocular pressure. *Surv Ophthalmol*. 2001;45(suppl 2):S361–S368.

5. Camras CB, Toris CB, Sjoquist B, et al. Detection of the free acid of bimatoprost in aqueous humor samples from human eyes treated with bimatoprost before cataract surgery. *Ophthalmology*. 2004;111:2193–2198.

6. Crowston JG, Lindsey JD, Morris CA, et al. Effect of bimatoprost on intraocular pressure in prostaglandin FP receptor knockout mice. *Invest Ophthalmol Vis Sci*. 2005;46:4571–4577.

7. Ota T, Aihara M, Narumiya S, Araie M. The effects of prostaglandin analogues on IOP in prostanoid FP-receptor-deficient mice. *Invest Ophthalmol Vis Sci*. 2005;46: 4159–4163.

8. Susanna R, Jr., Chew P, Kitazawa Y. Current status of prostaglandin therapy: lata-noprost and unoprostone. *Surv Ophthalmol.* 2002;47(suppl 1):S97–S104.

9. Jampel HD, Bacharach J, Sheu WP, et al. Randomized clinical trial of latanoprost and unoprostone in patients with elevated intraocular pressure. *Am J Ophthalmol.* 2002; 134:863–871.

10. Camras CB, Bito LZ, Eakins KE. Reduction of intraocular pressure by prostaglandins applied topically to the eyes of conscious rabbits. *Invest Ophthalmol Vis Sci.* 1977;16: 1125–1134.

11. Weinreb R, Toris C, Gabelt B, et al. Effects of prostaglandins on the aqueous humor outflow pathways. *Surv Ophthalmol.* 2002;47(suppl 1):S53–S64.

12. Toris CB, Camras CB, Yablonski ME, Brubaker RF. Effects of exogenous pros-taglandins on aqueous humor dynamics and blood-aqueous barrier function. *Surv Ophthalmol.* 1997;41(suppl 2):S69–S75.

13. Toris CB, Zhan G, Camras CB. Increase in outflow facility with unoprostone treat-ment in ocular hypertensive patients. *Arch Ophthalmol.* 2004;122:1782–1787.

14. Christiansen GA, Nau CB, McLaren JW, Johnson DH. Mechanism of ocular hypo-tensive action of bimatoprost (Lumigan) in patients with ocular hypertension or glaucoma. *Ophthalmology.* 2004;111:1658–1662.

15. Toris CB, Alm A, Camras CB. Latanoprost and cholinergic agonists in combination. *Surv Ophthalmol.* 2002;47(suppl 1):S141–S147.

16. Dinslage S, Hueber A, Diestelhorst M, Krieglstein G. The influence of latanoprost 0.005% on aqueous humor flow and outflow facility in glaucoma patients: a double-masked placebo-controlled clinical study. *Graefes Arch Clin Exp Ophthalmol.* 2004; 242:654–660.

17. Mastropasqua L, Carpineto P, Ciancaglini M, Gallenga PE. A 12-month, random-ized, double-masked study comparing latanoprost with timolol in pigmentary glau-coma. *Ophthalmology.* 1999;106:550–555.

18. Marchini G, Ghilotti G, Bonadimani M, Babighian S. Effects of 0.005% latanoprost on ocular anterior structures and ciliary body thickness. *J Glaucoma.* 2003;12:295–300.

19. Weinreb RN, Lindsey JD. Metalloproteinase gene transcription in human ciliary muscle cells with latanoprost. *Invest Ophthalmol Vis Sci.* 2002;43:716–722.

20. Camras CB, Friedman AH, Rodrigues MM, et al. Multiple dosing of prostaglandin $F_{2\alpha}$ or epinephrine on cynomolgus monkey eyes. III. Histopathology. *Invest Oph-thalmol Vis Sci.* 1988;29:1428–1436.

21. Tomita G, Araie M, Kitazawa Y, Tsukahara S. A three-year prospective, randomized and open comparison between latanoprost and timolol in Japanese normal-tension glaucoma patients. *Eye.* 2004;18:984–989.

22. Hoyng PF, Kitazawa Y. Medical treatment of normal tension glaucoma. *Surv Ophthalmol.* 2002;47(suppl 1):S116–S124.

23. Ang A, Reddy MA, Shepstone L, Broadway DC. Long term effect of latanoprost on intraocular pressure in normal tension glaucoma. *Br J Ophthalmol.* 2004;88:630–634.

24. Liu CJ, Ko YC, Cheng CY, et al. Changes in intraocular pressure and ocular perfusion pressure after latanoprost 0.005% or brimonidine tartrate 0.2% in normal-tension glaucoma patients. *Ophthalmology.* 2002;109:2241–2247.

25. Konstas AG, Mylopoulos N, Karabatsas CH, et al. Diurnal intraocular pressure reduction with latanoprost 0.005% compared to timolol maleate 0.5% as mono-therapy in subjects with exfoliation glaucoma. *Eye.* 2004;18:893–899.

26. Nordmann JP, Mertz B, Yannoulis NC, et al. A double-masked randomized com-parison of the efficacy and safety of unoprostone with timolol and betaxolol in

patients with primary open-angle glaucoma including pseudoexfoliation glaucoma or ocular hypertension. 6 month data. *Am J Ophthalmol.* 2002;133:1–10.

27. Camras CB, Alm A, Watson PG, et al. Latanoprost, a prostaglandin analog, for glaucoma therapy: efficacy and safety after one year of treatment in 198 patients. *Ophthalmology.* 1996;103:1916–1924.

28. Alm A, Schoenfelder J, McDermott J. A 5-year, multicenter, open-label, safety study of adjunctive latanoprost therapy for glaucoma. *Arch Ophthalmol.* 2004;122:957–965.

29. Alm A, Stjernschantz J, the Scandinavian Latanoprost Study Group. Effects on intraocular pressure and side-effects of 0.005% latanoprost applied once daily, evening or morning. A comparison with timolol. *Ophthalmology.* 1995;102:1743–1752.

30. Alm A, Camras CB, Watson PG. Phase III latanoprost studies in Scandinavia, the United Kingdom and the United States. *Surv Ophthalmol.* 1997;41(suppl 2):S105–S110.

31. Hedman K, Watson PG, Alm A. The effect of latanoprost on intraocular pressure during 2 years of treatment. *Surv Ophthalmol.* 2002;47(suppl 1):S65–S76.

32. Sakai H, Shinjyo S, Nakamura Y, et al. Comparison of latanoprost monotherapy and combined therapy of 0.5% timolol and 1% dorzolamide in chronic primary angle-closure glaucoma (CACG) in Japanese patients. *J Ocul Pharmacol Ther.* 2005;21:483–489.

33. Chew PT, Aung T, Aquino MV, Rojanapongpun P. Intraocular pressure-reducing effects and safety of latanoprost versus timolol in patients with chronic angle-closure glaucoma. *Ophthalmology.* 2004;111:427–434.

34. Sihota R, Saxena R, Agarwal HC, Gulati V. Crossover comparison of timolol and latanoprost in chronic primary angle-closure glaucoma. *Arch Ophthalmol.* 2004;122:185–189.

35. Chew PT, Hung PT, Aung T. Efficacy of latanoprost in reducing intraocular pressure in patients with primary angle-closure glaucoma. *Surv Ophthalmol.* 2002;47(suppl 1):S125–S128.

36. Schumer RA, Camras CB, Mandahl AK. Putative side effects of prostaglandin analogs. *Surv Ophthalmol.* 2002;47(suppl 1):S219–S230.

37. Enyedi LB, Freedman SF. Latanoprost for the treatment of pediatric glaucoma. *Surv Ophthalmol.* 2002;47(suppl 1):S129–S132.

38. Orzalesi N, Rossetti L, Bottoli A, Fogagnolo P. Comparison of the effects of latanoprost, travoprost, and bimatoprost on circadian intraocular pressure in patients with glaucoma or ocular hypertension. *Ophthalmology.* 2006;113:239–246.

39. Larsson L-I, Mishima HK, Takamatsu M, et al. The effect of latanoprost on circadian intraocular pressure. *Surv Ophthalmol.* 2002;47(suppl 1):S90–S96.

40. Choi J, Jeong J, Cho HS, Kook MS. Effect of nocturnal blood pressure reduction on circadian fluctuation of mean ocular perfusion pressure: a risk factor for normal tension glaucoma. *Invest Ophthalmol Vis Sci.* 2006;47:831–836.

41. Arici MK, Erdogan H, Toker I, et al. The effect of latanoprost, bimatoprost, and travoprost on intraocular pressure after cataract surgery. *J Ocul Pharmacol Ther.* 2006;22:34–40.

42. Arcieri ES, Santana A, Rocha FN, et al. Blood-aqueous barrier changes after the use of prostaglandin analogues in patients with pseudophakia and aphakia: a 6-month randomized trial. *Arch Ophthalmol.* 2005;123:186–192.

43. Wand M, Shields BM. Cystoid macular edema in the era of ocular hypotensive lipids. *Am J Ophthalmol.* 2002;133:393–397.

44. Cohen JS, Gross RL, Cheetham JK, et al. Two-year double-masked comparison of bimatoprost with timolol in patients with glaucoma or ocular hypertension. *Surv Ophthalmol.* 2004;49(suppl 1):S45–S52.

45. Parrish RK, Palmberg P, Sheu WP, XLT Study Group. A comparison of latanoprost, bimatoprost, and travoprost in patients with elevated intraocular pressure: a 12-week, randomized, masked-evaluator multicenter study. *Am J Ophthalmol.* 2003; 135:688–703.

46. Noecker RS, Dirks MS, Choplin NT, et al. A six-month randomized clinical trial comparing the intraocular pressure-lowering efficacy of bimatoprost and latanoprost in patients with ocular hypertension or glaucoma. *Am J Ophthalmol.* 2003;135:55–63.

47. Camras CB; the United States Latanoprost Study Group. Comparison of latanoprost and timolol in patients with ocular hypertension and glaucoma. A six-month, masked, multicenter trial in the United States. *Ophthalmology.* 1996;103:138–147.

48. Higginbotham EJ, Schuman JS, Goldberg I, et al. One-year, randomized study comparing bimatoprost and timolol in glaucoma and ocular hypertension. *Arch Ophthalmol.* 2002;120:1286–1293.

49. Fellman RL, Sullivan EK, Ratliff M, et al. Comparison of travoprost 0.0015% and 0.004% with timolol 0.5% in patients with elevated intraocular pressure: a 6-month, masked, multicenter trial. *Ophthalmology.* 2002;109:998–1008.

50. Stjernschantz J, Albert D, Hu D, et al. Mechanism and clinical significance of prostaglandin-induced iris pigmentation. *Surv Ophthalmol.* 2002;47(suppl 1):S162–S175.

51. Camras CB, Neely DG, Weiss EL. Latanoprost-induced iris color darkening: a case report with long-term follow-up. *J Glaucoma.* 2000;9:95–98.

52. Yamamoto T, Kitazawa Y. Iris-color change developed after topical isopropyl unoprostone treatment. *J Glaucoma.* 1997;6:430–432.

53. Zhan GL, Toris CB, Meza JL, Camras CB. Unoprostone isopropyl ester darkens iris color in pigmented rabbits with sympathetic denervation. *J Glaucoma.* 2003;12:383–389.

54. Albert DM, Gangnon RE, Zimbric ML, et al. A study of iridectomy histopathologic features of latanoprost- and non-latanoprost-treated patients. *Arch Ophthalmol.* 2004; 122:1680–1685.

55. Grierson I, Pfeiffer N, Cracknell KPB, Appleton P. Histology and fine structure of the iris and outflow system following latanoprost therapy. *Surv Ophthalmol.* 2002; 47(suppl 1):S176–S184.

56. Cracknell KP, Grierson I, Hogg P, et al. Latanoprost-induced iris darkening: a morphometric study of human peripheral iridectomies. *Exp Eye Res.* 2003;77:721–730.

57. Pfeiffer N, Grierson I, Goldsmith H, et al. Fine structural evaluation of the iris after unilateral treatment with latanoprost in patients undergoing bilateral trabeculectomy (the Mainz II study). *Arch Ophthalmol.* 2003;121:23–31.

58. Nakamura Y, Nakamura Y, Morine-Shinjo S, et al. Assessment of chamber angle pigmentation during longterm latanoprost treatment for open-angle glaucoma. *Acta Ophthalmol.* 2004;82:158–160.

59. Cracknell KP, Grierson I, Hogg P, et al. Melanin in the trabecular meshwork is associated with age, POAG but not latanoprost treatment. A masked morphometric study. *Exp Eye Res.* 2006;82:986–993.

60. Johnstone MA. Hypertrichosis and increased pigmentation of eyelashes and adjacent hair in the region of the ipsilateral eyelids of patients treated with unilateral topical latanoprost. *Am J Ophthalmol.* 1997;124:544–547.

61. Johnstone MA, Albert DM. Prostaglandin-induced hair growth. *Surv Ophthalmol.* 2002;47(suppl 1):S185–S202.

62. Packer M, Fine IH, Hoffman RS. Bilateral nongranulomatous anterior uveitis associated with bimatoprost. *J Cataract Refract Surg.* 2003;29:2242–2243.

63. Parentin F. Granulomatous anterior uveitis associated with bimatoprost: a case report. *Ocul Immunol Inflamm.* 2003;11:67–71.

64. Suominen S, Valimaki J. Bilateral anterior uveitis associated with travoprost. *Acta Ophthalmol.* 2006;84:275–276.

65. Kumarasamy M, Desai SP. Anterior uveitis is associated with travoprost. *BMJ.* 2004;329:205.

66. Martin E, Martinez-de-la-Casa JM, Garcia-Feijoo J, et al. A 6-month assessment of bimatoprost 0.03% vs timolol maleate 0.5%: hypotensive efficacy, macular thickness and flare in ocular-hypertensive and glaucoma patients. *Eye* 2007;21:164–168.

67. Cellini M, Caramazza R, Bonsanto D, et al. Prostaglandin analogs and blood-aqueous barrier integrity: a flare cell meter study. *Ophthalmologica.* 2004;218:312–317.

68. Carrillo MM, Nicolela MT. Cystoid macular edema in a low-risk patient after switching from latanoprost to bimatoprost. *Am J Ophthalmol.* 2004;137:966–968.

69. Wand M, Gaudio AR. Cystoid macular edema associated with ocular hypotensive lipids. *Am J Ophthalmol.* 2002;133:403–405.

70. Yeh PC, Ramanathan S. Latanoprost and clinically significant cystoid macular edema after uneventful phacoemulsification with intraocular lens implantation. *J Cataract Refract Surg.* 2002;28:1814–1818.

71. Camras CB. CME and anterior uveitis with latanoprost use. *Ophthalmology.* 1998;105:1978–1981.

72. Camras CB, Bhuyan KC, Podos SM, et al. Multiple dosing of prostaglandin $F_{2\alpha}$ or epinephrine on cynomolgus monkey eyes. II. Slit-lamp biomicroscopy, aqueous humor analysis, and fluorescein angiography. *Invest Ophthalmol Vis Sci.* 1987;28: 921–926.

73. Hoyng PFJ, Rulo AH, Greve EL, et al. Fluorescein angiographic evaluation of the effect of latanoprost treatment on blood-retinal barrier integrity: a review of studies conducted on pseudophakic glaucoma patients and on phakic and aphakic monkeys. *Surv Ophthalmol.* 1997;41(suppl 2):S83–S88.

74. Miyake K, Ibaraki N, Goto Y, et al. ESCRS Binkhorst lecture 2002: Pseudophakic preservative maculopathy. *J Cataract Refract Surg.* 2003;29:1800–1810.

75. Herndon LW, Robert DW, Wand M, Asrani S. Increased periocular pigmentation with ocular hypotensive lipid use in African Americans. *Am J Ophthalmol.* 2003;135:713–715.

76. Kapur R, Osmanovic S, Toyran S, Edward DP. Bimatoprost-induced periocular skin hyperpigmentation: histopathological study. *Arch Ophthalmol.* 2005;123:1541–1546.

77. Peplinski LS, Albiani SK. Deepening of lid sulcus from topical bimatoprost therapy. *Optom Vis Sci.* 2004;81:574–577.

78. Gordon YJ, Yates KA, Mah FS, Romanowski EG. The effects of Xalatan on the recovery of ocular herpes simplex virus type 1 (HSV-1) in the induced reactivation and spontaneous shedding rabbit models. *J Ocul Pharmacol Ther.* 2003;19:233–245.

79. Bean G, Reardon G, Zimmerman TJ. Association between ocular herpes simplex virus and topical ocular hypotensive therapy. *J Glaucoma.* 2004;13:361–364.

80. Inan UU, Ermis SS, Orman A, et al. The comparative cardiovascular, pulmonary, ocular blood flow, and ocular hypotensive effects of topical travoprost, bimatoprost, brimonidine, and betaxolol. *J Ocul Pharmacol Ther.* 2004;20:293–310.

81. Hedman K, Larsson LI. The effect of latanoprost compared with timolol in African-American, Asian, Caucasian, and Mexican open-angle glaucoma or ocular hypertensive patients. *Surv Ophthalmol.* 2002;47(suppl 1):S77–S89.

82. O'Donoghue EP. A comparison of latanoprost and dorzolamide in patients with glaucoma and ocular hypertension: a 3 month, randomised study. *Br J Ophthalmol.* 2000;84:579–582.

83. Kimal Arici M, Topalkara A, Güler C. Additive effect of latanoprost and dorzolamide in patients with elevated intraocular pressure. *Int Ophthalmol.* 1998;22:37–42.

84. Day DG, Sharpe ED, Beischel CJ, et al. Safety and efficacy of bimatoprost 0.03% versus timolol maleate 0.5%/dorzolamide 2% fixed combination. *Eur J Ophthalmol.* 2005;15:336–342.

85. Coleman AL, Lerner F, Bernstein P, Whitcup SM. A 3-month randomized controlled trial of bimatoprost (LUMIGAN) versus combined timolol and dorzolamide (Cosopt) in patients with glaucoma or ocular hypertension. *Ophthalmology.* 2003;110:2362–2368.

86. Chiselita D, Antohi I, Medvichi R, Danielescu C. Comparative analysis of the efficacy and safety of latanoprost, travoprost and the fixed combination timolol-dorzolamide; a prospective, randomized, masked, cross-over design study. *Oftalmologia.* 2005;49:39–45.

87. Fechtner RD, McCarroll KA, Lines CR, Adamsons IA. Efficacy of the dorzolamide/timolol fixed combination versus latanoprost in the treatment of ocular hypertension or glaucoma: combined analysis of pooled data from two large randomized observer and patient-masked studies. *J Ocul Pharmacol Ther.* 2005;21:242–249.

88. Camras CB, Sheu WP. Latanoprost or brimonidine as treatment for elevated intraocular pressure: multicenter trial in the United States. *J Glaucoma.* 2005;14:161–167.

89. Camras CB. Travoprost compared with latanoprost and timolol in patients with open-angle glaucoma or ocular hypertension. *Am J Ophthalmol.* 2002;133:732.

90. Netland PA, Robertson SM, Sullivan EK, et al. Response to travoprost in black and nonblack patients with open-angle glaucoma or ocular hypertension. *Adv Ther.* 2003;20:149–163.

91. Higginbotham EJ, Diestelhorst M, Pfeiffer N, et al. The efficacy and safety of unfixed and fixed combinations of latanoprost and other antiglaucoma medications. *Surv Ophthalmol.* 2002;47(suppl 1):S133–S140.

92. Toor A, Chanis RA, Polikoff LA, et al. Additivity of pilocarpine to bimatoprost in ocular hypertension and early glaucoma. *J Glaucoma.* 2005;14:243–248.

93. Netland PA, Michael M, Rosner SA, et al. Brimonidine purite and bimatoprost compared with timolol and latanoprost in patients with glaucoma and ocular hypertension. *Adv Ther.* 2003;20:20–30.

94. Hughes BA, Bacharach J, Craven ER, et al. A three-month, multicenter, double-masked study of the safety and efficacy of travoprost 0.004%/timolol 0.5% ophthalmic solution compared to travoprost 0.004% ophthalmic solution and timolol 0.5% dosed concomitantly in subjects with open angle glaucoma or ocular hypertension. *J Glaucoma.* 2005;14:392–399.

95. Schuman JS, Katz GJ, Lewis RA, et al. Efficacy and safety of a fixed combination of travoprost 0.004%/timolol 0.5% ophthalmic solution once daily for open-angle glaucoma or ocular hypertension. *Am J Ophthalmol.* 2005;140:242–250.

96. Barnebey HS, Orengo-Nania S, Flowers BE, et al. The safety and efficacy of travoprost 0.004%/timolol 0.5% fixed combination ophthalmic solution. *Am J Ophthalmol.* 2005;140:1–7.

97.   Diestelhorst M, Larsson LI. A 12-week, randomized, double-masked, multicenter study of the fixed combination of latanoprost and timolol in the evening versus the individual components. *Ophthalmology*. 2006;113:70–76.

98.   Hamacher T, Schinzel M, Scholzel-Klatt A, et al. Short term efficacy and safety in glaucoma patients changed to the latanoprost 0.005%/timolol maleate 0.5% fixed combination from monotherapies and adjunctive therapies. *Br J Ophthalmol*. 2004; 88:1295–1298.

99.   Gandolfi SA, Rossetti L, Cimino L, et al. Replacing maximum-tolerated medications with latanoprost versus adding latanoprost to maximum-tolerated medications: a two-center randomized prospective trial. *J Glaucoma*. 2003;12:347–353.

100. Rulo AH, Greve EL, Hoyng PFJ. Additive ocular hypotensive effect of latanoprost and acetazolamide. A short-term study in patients with elevated intraocular pressure. *Ophthalmology*. 1997;104:1503–1507.

101. O'Connor DJ, Martone JF, Mead A. Additive intraocular pressure lowering effect of various medications with latanoprost. *Am J Ophthalmol*. 2002;133:836–837.

102. Akman A, Cetinkaya A, Akova YA, Ertan A. Comparison of additional intraocular pressure-lowering effects of latanoprost vs brimonidine in primary open-angle glaucoma patients with intraocular pressure uncontrolled by timolol-dorzolamide combination. *Eye*. 2005;19:145–151.

103. Martinez-de-la-Casa JM, Castillo A, Garcia-Feijoo J, et al. Concomitant administration of travoprost and brinzolamide versus fixed latanoprost/timolol combined therapy: three-month comparison of efficacy and safety. *Curr Med Res Opin*. 2004; 20:1333–1339.

104. Reis R, Queiroz CF, Santos LC, et al. A randomized, investigator-masked, 4-week study comparing timolol maleate 0.5%, brinzolamide 1%, and brimonidine tartrate 0.2% as adjunctive therapies to travoprost 0.004% in adults with primary open-angle glaucoma or ocular hypertension. *Clin Ther*. 2006;28:552–559.

105. Toris CB, Zhan GL, Zhao J, et al. Potential mechanism for the additivity of pilocarpine and latanoprost. *Am J Ophthalmol*. 2001;131:722–728.

106. Camras CB, Feldman SG, Podos SM, et al. Inhibition of the epinephrine-induced reduction of intraocular pressure by systemic indomethacin in humans. *Am J Ophthalmol*. 1985;100:169–175.

107. Erdogan H, Toker I, Arici MK, et al. A short-term study of the additive effect of latanoprost 0.005% and brimonidine 0.2%. *Jpn J Ophthalmol*. 2003;47:473–478.

108. Konstas AG, Karabatsas CH, Lallos N, et al. 24-hour intraocular pressures with brimonidine purite versus dorzolamide added to latanoprost in primary open-angle glaucoma subjects. *Ophthalmology*. 2005;112:603–608.

109. Stewart WC, Stewart JA, Day DG, et al. Efficacy and safety of the latanoprost/timolol maleate fixed combination vs concomitant brimonidine and latanoprost therapy. *Eye*. 2004;18:990–995.

110. Higginbotham EJ, Feldman R, Stiles M, et al. Latanoprost and timolol combination therapy vs monotherapy: one-year randomized trial. *Arch Ophthalmol*. 2002;120: 915–922.

111. Pfeiffer N. A comparison of the fixed combination of latanoprost and timolol with its individual components. *Graefes Arch Clin Exp Ophthalmol*. 2002;240:893–899.

112. Konstas AG, Boboridis K, Tzetzi D, et al. Twenty-four-hour control with latanoprost-timolol-fixed combination therapy vs latanoprost therapy. *Arch Ophthalmol*. 2005;123:898–902.

113. Konstas AG, Banyai L, Blask KD, et al. Intraocular pressure and safety in glaucoma patients switching to latanoprost/timolol maleate fixed combination from mono- and adjunctive therapies. *J Ocul Pharmacol Ther.* 2004;20:375–382.

114. Diestelhorst M, Larsson LI. A 12 week study comparing the fixed combination of latanoprost and timolol with the concomitant use of the individual components in patients with open angle glaucoma and ocular hypertension. *Br J Ophthalmol.* 2004; 88:199–203.

115. Konstas AG, Kozobolis VP, Lallos N, et al. Daytime diurnal curve comparison between the fixed combinations of latanoprost 0.005%/timolol maleate 0.5% and dorzolamide 2%/timolol maleate 0.5%. *Eye.* 2004;18:1264–1269.

116. Shin DH, Feldman RM, Sheu WP. Efficacy and safety of the fixed combinations latanoprost/timolol versus dorzolamide/timolol in patients with elevated intraocular pressure. *Ophthalmology.* 2004;111:276–282.

117. Gandolfi S, Simmons ST, Sturm R, et al. Three-month comparison of bimatoprost and latanoprost in patients with glaucoma and ocular hypertension. *Adv Ther.* 2001;18:110–121.

3

Beta Blockers

ALBERT S. KHOURI, PAUL J. LAMA, AND ROBERT D. FECHTNER

*I*n 1948, Raymond P. Ahlquist proposed that two distinct classes of adrenergic receptors exist in the autonomic nervous system, which he classified as alpha and beta.[1] In 1958, adrenergic receptor antagonists were developed, initiating the pursuit of pharmaceutical agents designed to take advantage of manipulation of these receptors. Propranolol, introduced in 1964, was the first beta-adrenergic antagonist with widespread clinical application. This medication was used for the treatment of systemic hypertension, angina, and cardiac arrhythmias. Phillips et al.[2] observed that intraocular pressure (IOP) was lowered in patients with glaucoma following systemic administration of propranolol. Others observed similar IOP-lowering effect when the medication was administered intravenously, orally, and topically. However, local adverse effects, such as ocular stinging, irritation, and corneal anesthesia, limited the development of this drug as an IOP-lowering medication. Practolol, a beta-1–selective antagonist, exerted IOP-lowering effects similar to those of propranolol but without the corneal anesthetic activity. Other adverse effects were related to an immunologically mediated oculomucocutaneous syndrome limiting the utility of this drug.

Investigations of timolol as an IOP-lowering drug were initiated in the 1970s. The current era of topical glaucoma therapy began when timolol maleate was granted approval by the FDA in the United States in 1978. The ocular beta blockers (OBBs) are topical beta-adrenergic antagonists. These drugs have been approved for use in the US since 1978. With more than three decades of accumulated experience, the OBBs remained the favored choice for initial monotherapy for lowering IOP, even well after the introduction of topical prostaglandin analogues. The OBBs are well accepted due to their efficacy at lowering IOP, generally well-tolerated local and systemic adverse effects, and familiarity. Prior to the introduction of the OBB, available IOP-lowering medications included the nonselective adrenergic agonists, the parasympathomimetic agonists, and the oral carbonic anhydrase inhibitors (CAIs). Each of these classes of drugs had significant limitations. In recent years, the prostaglandin analogues have largely replaced OBBs as initial monotherapy, but the OBBs remain an alternative and a popular choice for adjunctive therapy.

3.1 GENERAL PHARMACOLOGY

Beta-adrenoreceptors have been categorized into subclasses beta-1, beta-2, and beta-3. Beta-1 receptors are principally found in the heart. Stimulation of beta-1 receptors increases heart rate, cardiac contractility, and atrioventricular conduction rate. Beta-2 receptors are located in bronchial muscle, blood vessels, and the uterus. Stimulating beta-2 receptors causes dilation of bronchi and blood vessels. Beta-3 receptors, recently identified in mammals, are involved in the mediation of lipolysis. Available beta blockers have a low affinity for $beta_3$ receptors.

Beta-adrenergic antagonists are competitive inhibitors at the beta-receptor site. They are classified as selective or nonselective based on relative affinity to the beta-1 and beta-2 receptors. The nonselective antagonists inhibit both beta-1 and beta-2 receptors, while the selective antagonists inhibit preferentially only one subtype of receptor. This selectivity is relative; at high concentrations, selective beta-adrenergic antagonists inhibit other beta receptors.

3.2 MECHANISM OF ACTION

The OBBs lower IOP through a reduction in aqueous formation. There appears to be no change in aqueous outflow. Aqueous formation can decrease by as much as 50%.[3-8]

Despite the fact that OBBs have been in clinical use for more than 30 years, the exact mechanism of action has not been entirely elucidated. In normal physiology, when a beta-adrenergic agonist binds to its receptor, activation of a regulatory protein (G-protein) results. This stimulates membrane-bound adenyl cyclase, catalyzing conversion of adenosine triphosphate (ATP) to cyclic adenosine monophosphate (cAMP). In the classic model for the mechanisms of action of OBBs, the intracellular cAMP acts as a second messenger that, through additional steps, ultimately stimulates production of aqueous from the ciliary processes.

It has been demonstrated that timolol and other beta blockers inhibit cAMP production in the ciliary body. However, the direct relationship between beta blocker effect on cAMP and IOP effect is not supported in all studies. In one study, there was no relationship between reduction of cAMP and IOP lowering.[9] Further, IOP can decrease in response to drugs that increase cAMP.[10] The dextro-isomer of timolol has a low affinity for beta receptors, yet this compound decreases aqueous flow as well as the higher affinity levo-isomer in the clinically available preparations.[11] These observations suggest that the IOP-lowering effect of OBBs may not be mediated directly through competitive inhibition of beta receptors in the ciliary body. While it is accepted that OBBs lower IOP through a decrease in aqueous production, some evidence suggests we must not assume this is simply beta-adrenergic blockade mediated through the classic second-messenger system.

Alternative mechanisms have been suggested. One postulates that there is endogenous adrenergic tone controlling aqueous production mediated by epinephrine. In this model, ciliary processes are under continuous tonic stimulation to produce aqueous. Beta blockers are hypothesized to exert an effect by interfering with this tonic stimulation of normal aqueous production.[12] The basis for such tonic stimulation remains speculative since there is no identified anatomic basis, but a model such as this could explain some of the inconsistencies discussed above.

3.3 INDICATIONS

The indications for use for all OBBs as approved by the FDA are quite similar, although the language in the approved labeling differs. In general, OBBs are indicated for the treatment of elevated IOP in patients with ocular hypertension or open-angle glaucoma. The drugs may be used alone or in combination with other IOP-lowering medications. Specific information about each drug can be found in the package insert or in a reference such as the *Physicians' Desk Reference for Ophthalmic Medications*.

While the product labeling lists only ocular hypertension and open-angle glaucoma as indications for use, the OBBs have been accepted and can be effective for treatment of other causes of elevated IOP such as secondary glaucomas and angle closure.

3.4 CONTRAINDICATIONS

Several contraindications to use are listed in the FDA-approved labeling for these drugs. They can be grouped in a few categories. Specific differences are noted below in the sections on adverse effects and in the sections on each compound. There is a relative or absolute contraindication in patients with pulmonary disease such as bronchial asthma and severe chronic obstructive pulmonary disease (COPD; this contraindication is not listed for betaxolol). Beta blockers affect the heart and may be contraindicated in patients with conditions such as sinus bradycardia, overt uncompensated cardiac failure, cardiogenic shock, or second- or third-degree atrioventricular block who do not have a pacemaker. As with all drugs, each OBB is contraindicated in patients with a hypersensitivity to any component of the product.

In addition to being aware of the contraindications listed on the product labeling, the physician must regularly reassess the health status of the patient. While it is clear that OBBs are contraindicated in patients with reactive airway disease, heart block (greater than first degree), overt congestive heart failure, and symptomatic sinus bradycardia, any patient who develops one of these conditions while using an OBB should have the OBB discontinued to see if the condition improves.

3.5 TREATMENT REGIMENS

OBBs are used once or twice daily. There exists a difference between the approved labeling and current clinical practice where once-daily use is often recommended. For the branded OBBs, all but Istalol (timolol), Timoptic-XE (timolol in gel-forming solution), and Betagan (levobunolol) are recommended initially as twice daily. Istalol and Timoptic-XE are recommended once daily. Betagan is recommended once or twice daily. For timolol maleate solution, the labeling indicates that if the IOP is controlled at a satisfactory level, dosing can be changed to once daily.

Although the large controlled clinical trial examining once-daily dosing for nonselective OBBs studied only levobunolol and timolol, it has become common to initiate therapy with nonselective beta blockers once daily rather than twice daily. If IOP control is not satisfactory, dosing frequency can be increased to twice daily. This offers the opportunity to titrate the dose while minimizing the potential for adverse effects.[13]

3.6 SIDE EFFECTS

Most of the significant side effects of the OBBs are thought to be explained by beta blockade. While not every adverse effect has been reported with every drug, this discussion does not associate specific events with specific drugs unless there is a unique relationship reported between one drug and the effect.

3.6.1 *Local Adverse Effects.* Corneal anesthesia was a significant adverse effect associated with topical propranolol. No significant corneal anesthesia effect has been observed with current OBBs in the majority of patients.[14] However, individual patients can have a significant corneal anesthesia effect that may exacerbate existing ocular surface disease.[15,16]

Discomfort upon instillation (burning and stinging) is an adverse effect associated with every drug used to lower IOP. This effect is a function of several factors: active molecule, pH, preservative, and vehicle. There has been a higher incidence of transient discomfort associated with betaxolol solution and with metipranolol than with timolol.[17–19] The betaxolol suspension appears to be better tolerated than the solution.[20]

Almost all OBBs have benzalkonium chloride (BAK) as their preservative (table 3.1). Sensitivity to BAK is not uncommon. Patients may become symptomatic, particularly if they are taking multiple medications with BAK. The branded preparations of carteolol, levobunolol, and metipranolol have lower concentrations of BAK than do branded betaxolol and timolol maleate solution. Timolol maleate is available without preservatives. Timoptic-XE has benzododecinium bromide as a preservative. An awareness of the preservatives may help the clinician choose a tolerable OBB for the BAK-sensitive patient.

Timolol use has been associated with decreased tear production and decreased goblet cell density.[21,22] These alterations may result in dry eye symptoms. Use of

Table 3.1 Available Ophthalmic Beta-Blockers

Drug	Comment	Concentration (%)	Supplied (mL)	Preservative
Timolol	Maleate generic	0.25, 0.5	5, 10, 15	BAK 0.01%
Timoptic	Maleate	0.25, 0.5	5, 10	BAK 0.01%
Timoptic	Ocudose unit dose	0.25, 0.5	0.2	Preservative-free
Betimol	Hemihydrate	0.25, 0.5	5, 10, 15	BAK 0.01%
Istalolol		0.5	5	BAK 0.005%
Timoptic-XE	Gellan gum gel-forming solution	0.25, 0.5	5	Benzododecinium bromide 0.012%
Timolol GFS	Xantham gum	0.25, 0.5	2.5, 5	Benzododecinium bromide 0.012%
Carteolol	Generic	1.0	5, 10, 15	BAK 0.005%
Ocupress	Not available			
Levobunolol	Generic	0.25, 0.5	5, 10, 15	BAK 0.004%
Betagan		0.25, 0.5	2, 5, 10, 15	BAK 0.004%
Metipranolol	Generic	0.3	5, 10	BAK 0.004%
OptiPranolol		0.3	5, 10	BAK 0.004%
Betaxolol				
Betaxolol solution	Not available	0.5		
Betoptic S	Suspension	0.25	2.5, 5, 10, 15	BAK 0.01%

Data from *Physicians' Desk Reference for Ophthalmic Medicines*, 34th edition, 2006.

topical timolol has occasionally been associated with more serious ocular surface disease such as cicatricial pemphigoid.[23] Allergic blepharoconjunctivitis develops in about 3% of patients using OBBs.[24]

Transient blurred vision following administration is a common adverse side effect associated with OBBs. With timolol gel-forming solutions, blurring is likely due to the gel, which can also cause crusting of the lashes.

Metipranolol as manufactured in the United Kingdom was associated with granulomatous uveitis that was confirmed upon rechallenge in some eyes.[25-27] The exact cause was not determined, although the manufacturing process was implicated. There have been only isolated case reports of this association in the United States.[28,29]

3.6.2 *Systemic Adverse Effects.* Many of the systemic adverse effects of OBBs can be predicted by an understanding of the sympathetic nervous system. Topically applied OBBs are absorbed systemically, largely via drainage into the nasolacrimal system and absorption through the nasal mucosa.[30] This is analogous to an intravenous dose of medication.

Topically applied timolol can be detected in the systemic circulation, but levels do not approach those achieved with common oral doses. A typical dose of oral timolol for the treatment of systemic hypertension is 20 to 60 mg daily. Although the oral dose undergoes first-pass hepatic metabolism, the bioavailability is still approximately

50% (10 to 30 mg). Each 1 µL of timolol 0.5% ophthalmic solution contains 5 µg timolol. Assuming a drop volume of approximately 30 µL, if the entire drop were absorbed, the total daily systemic exposure of timolol 0.5% administered in both eyes twice daily would be approximately 600 µg. Thus, the systemic burden of timolol 0.5% used in both eyes twice daily is less than 6% of a 20-mg oral dose of timolol.

Peak plasma concentrations following chronic systemic administration of timolol (7 days) in seven normal volunteers was 64 ± 4 ng/mL.[31] When 20 mg was administered as a single dose in seven normal volunteers (mean body weight = 67.5 kg), the range of peak values was between 50 and 103 ng/mL, and trough levels were between 0.8 and 7.2 ng/mL.[32] In contrast, following ocular administration of two drops of 0.5% timolol solution in adults, plasma levels achieved a range from 5.0 to 9.6 ng/mL.[33,34] Thus, plasma levels of topically applied timolol can approach trough levels of systemic administration but are typically much less than peak plasma levels following systemic administration of therapeutic doses of timolol. This strongly suggests that while systemic adverse effects are possible with ophthalmic beta blockers, thoughtful patient selection should make this relatively uncommon compared with oral use of this very popular class of medications.

Systemic absorption of timolol (and other topical ophthalmic drugs) and the likelihood of systemic effects can be decreased through passive eyelid closure or active nasolacrimal occlusion. This has been shown to decrease plasma levels of timolol by 60%.[35] Patients should be instructed in these techniques.

3.6.3 *Central Nervous System Adverse Effects.* Central nervous system (CNS) adverse effects are often overlooked because of their subjective and sometimes subtle nature. Only a detailed history is likely to elicit these complaints. The list of CNS effects associated with OBBs is long: anxiety, depression, fatigue, lethargy, confusion, sleep disturbance, memory loss, and dizziness.[36–39] The beta-1–selective OBB betaxolol may be associated with fewer CNS effects, particularly in susceptible individuals.[40,41] This may be due to the higher volume of distribution of betaxolol.

Sexual dysfunction associated with OBB use has been reported. Symptoms include decreased libido in men and women and impotence in men.[40] With physicians' improved awareness of drug effects on quality of life, it is the responsibility of the physician to elicit this complaint. Patients are often reluctant to discuss sexual dysfunction, or they may attribute it to different causes. With the popularity of oral medications for the treatment of erectile dysfunction, it may be easier to broach this topic, especially with symptomatic male patients. Certainly, any patient using a medication for erective dysfunction should be considered for a beta blocker holiday or a switch to another therapeutic class.

3.6.4 *Cardiovascular System Adverse Effects.* The effects of systemic beta blockade are used therapeutically in the treatment of conditions such as systemic hypertension, angina, and supraventricular as well as ventricular arrhythmias, as prophylaxis after myocardial infarction, and as a disease-modifying agent as well as for mortality reduction in congestive heart failure (CHF).[42] The mortality reduction following myocardial infarction and in CHF appears to be largely due to a reduction in sudden arrhythmic death. In addition, beta blockers also reduce pathologic ventricular re-modeling and improve cardiac function in such patients.[43–46]

Blocking the beta-1 receptors interferes with normal sympathetic stimulation of the heart. The results are lower heart rate and blood pressure, decreased myocardial contractility, and slowed conduction time. However, these same effects may become adverse effects in susceptible patients or in those with other underlying illnesses.

Topical OBB use may be associated with decrease in heart rate.[47,48] In some individuals, particularly those with conduction system abnormalities, this decrease may lead to a significant bradycardia. In early experience with timolol, 41% of 32 deaths attributed to ocular timolol use were classified as cardiovascular. Half of these occurred within 2 days of initiation of therapy.[49] These associations were circumstantial, not causative, and were reported during an era of increased vigilance for possible adverse effects of OBBs. Better understanding of relative contraindications for this class of drugs and the availability of other classes has decreased the likelihood of such events.

Resting heart rate and blood pressure are statistically significantly reduced following short- or long-term dosing with timolol maleate solution in healthy individuals.[47,48] Timolol also decreases exercise-induced tachycardia in healthy individuals.[50] Betaxolol, however, was no different from placebo in cardiovascular effects in one study.[51] However, these studies were conducted in healthy individuals. Patients requiring IOP-lowering therapy are often of advanced age and have coexisting systemic medical conditions, making them more susceptible to beta blockade.

While betaxolol is classified as a relatively cardioselective (beta-1) beta blocker, it is less potent in its beta-blocking activity than either timolol or levobunolol. That does not make it free of cardiovascular adverse effects. There are isolated case reports of betaxolol use associated with effects such as sinus arrest and symptomatic bradycardia.[38,52] Causality could not be ascertained.

In a small crossover study of timolol maleate solution and Timoptic-XE, plasma levels and heart-rate effects from the gel-forming preparation were less than those from the solution following 1 week of therapy.[53] One interpretation of this finding is that the gel-forming solution may decrease systemic absorption and adverse effects.

Carteolol (Ocupress) is a beta blocker with intrinsic sympathomimetic activity (ISA). It has partial agonist activity, which has not uniformly translated into a more favorable cardiovascular adverse effect profile. Rather, carteolol has been demonstrated to reduce heart rate and blood pressure similar to other OBBs without ISA. It is interesting to note that carteolol reduced heart rate for subjects with a resting rate above 70 beats per minute but did not affect heart rate for those with rates below 70 beats per minute.[54,55] It has not been demonstrated that this translates into an advantage for glaucoma patients.

3.6.5 *Pulmonary Adverse Effects.* Subjects with pulmonary disease were excluded in the preapproval trials of timolol. The original package labeling approved by the FDA warned against use in patients with pulmonary disease, but these precautions were not widely disseminated. It was only after the widespread use of ophthalmic timolol that the potential for pulmonary complications became better appreciated.[56,57] In the first 8 years of timolol use in the United States, 12 deaths were attributed to respiratory adverse events from the drug. More than 50% of these patients had a history of pulmonary disease.[51] In one early case report, respiratory arrest was reported within 30 minutes after the initial dose of timolol 0.5% solution in a 67-year-old man with stable COPD.[58]

The published data regarding topical and systemic beta blockers and pulmonary disease are not entirely consistent. Topical nonselective OBBs are reported to have the potential to exacerbate reactive airway disease in patients who are previously controlled. In a study of a large group of patients receiving bronchodilator therapy, those who were using timolol were 47% more likely to need additional broncho-dilator drugs.[59] Of greater concern is the administration of OBBs to patients with undetected or asymptomatic reactive airway disease. Severe asthmatic attacks have been reported in association with OBB use in such patients.[60]

Betaxolol is a beta-1–selective adrenergic antagonist. Because the pulmonary adverse effects of OBBs are mediated through beta-2 receptor blockade, it is expected that betaxolol should have a more favorable pulmonary adverse effect profile. This has been supported in clinical trials. In a masked crossover study of patients with reactive airway disease challenged with timolol or betaxolol, timolol produced a significant decrease in forced expiratory volume in 1 second (FEV_1), while betaxolol produced no such decrease in the same subjects.[61] In a group of asymptomatic elderly patients, pulmonary function improved when they were switched from a nonselective OBB to betaxolol.[62]

Betaxolol has been used successfully in patients with pulmonary disease,[63–65] but it is not entirely free of potential pulmonary adverse effects: There have been several reports of pulmonary symptoms associated with betaxolol use.[38,66,67]

There are interesting data more recently published in the medical literature from a meta-analysis evaluating the use of systemic beta-1–selective beta blockers in asthmatics and patients with COPD. Acute administration in asthmatics reduced FEV_1 by 7.46%, indicating increased airway resistance, but chronically FEV_1 did not change. Symptoms and inhaler use were no different between those on beta blockers and placebo. In patients with COPD, there was no difference between those that received beta blockers versus those that received placebo acutely and chronically with respect to FEV_1, symptoms, and inhaler use. Responsiveness to inhalers was in fact better in the beta blocker group, presumably as a result of beta receptor up-regulation mediated by chronic beta blockade.[68,69] Despite these reports, the potential for pulmonary adverse effects exists, and we do not advocate the use of OBBs in asthmatics and patients with COPD. With the introduction of new classes of drugs such as the topical CAIs and prostaglandin analogues, there are attractive alternatives to OBB therapy as initial treatment to lower IOP in patients with pulmonary disease.

3.6.6 *Metabolic Adverse Effects.* The OBBs have been reported to affect lipid metabolism. In normal volunteers taking topical timolol, triglyceride levels increased 12%, and high-density lipoproteins decreased 9%. Theoretically, this negative alteration in the blood-lipid profile could increase the risk of coronary heart disease.[70] Similar information has not been collected in older patients with glaucoma. A different study did not reproduce these results.[71] These studies had marked limitations:

They lacked placebo control, and only two lipid measurements were made, one at baseline and a second 6 weeks later. In another study, carteolol was shown to have less effect on blood-lipid parameters, possibly due to its ISA.[72] In summary, the evidence regarding the effects of OBBs on the lipid profile is inconclusive.

3.7 DRUG–DRUG INTERACTIONS

While not generally considered an interaction, additivity of IOP-lowering medications is a topic of considerable interest. More than 50% of glaucoma patients in the United States are taking multiple IOP-lowering medications. The OBBs are now commonly used as an adjunct to prostaglandins and are a component of all modern fixed-combination products (see chapter 7).

As the first available OBB, timolol maleate solution became a de facto gold standard against which new drugs are compared for regulatory approval. Usually, phase III drug development trials include a study demonstrating drug efficacy compared to timolol and often another demonstrating drug additivity to timolol. These tend to be well-designed, large, prospective studies. In general, after the drug is approved, there remains little incentive for its sponsor to initiate similar studies exploring its additivity to other compounds. Therefore, most additivity data for OBBs examine the efficacy of a second drug to timolol. This no longer reflects common practice, where prostaglandins are a more popular initial monotherapy. It is worth emphasizing that the mean IOP response of a study population does not predict how a drug will act in an individual. While we have previously advocated using a one-eye trial to determine efficacy and additivity within an individual, new data about spontaneous and unilateral IOP fluctuations open valid debate about the value of the one-eye trial. At present, the best strategy to determine efficacy is to measure IOP a few times before and a few times after a change in therapy rather than base efficacy judgment on single IOP measurements.[73–75]

Reports have provided mixed results concerning the additivity of nonselective OBBs and nonselective adrenergic agonists. In a short-term study, the additivity of timolol to epinephrine was transient.[76] Although the majority of patients taking either drug did not have a clinically significant reduction of IOP with the addition of the other, about one-fifth to one-third had an additional reduction of 3 mm Hg in IOP when epinephrine was added to timolol.[77,78] Epinephrine compounds had greater additivity with betaxolol than with timolol, but the former combination had about the same IOP-lowering effect as timolol alone.[79,80] These studies were performed when topical glaucoma therapy consisted of OBBs, epinephrine compounds, and parasympathomimetic drugs. The nonselective adrenergic agonists have been largely replaced by newer classes of drugs.

The OBBs have been demonstrated to be additive in combination with all other classes of IOP-lowering drugs, including parasympathomimetics, topical and oral CAIs, alpha-2–adrenergic agonists, and prostaglandin analogues.[81–89] It is interesting to note that while the prostaglandin analogues latanoprost and travoprost have been shown to be additive in subjects receiving OBBs, similar studies demonstrating additivity of OBBs in patients already on prostaglandins are lacking.

It was the observation that oral beta blockers lower IOP that stimulated development of OBBs. With the common use of oral beta blockers, there is a possibility for some patients to be prescribed both oral and topical beta blockers. Ophthalmic timolol lowered IOP to an equal extent in subjects taking oral placebo and 80 mg propranolol but had no additive effect on subjects taking 160 mg propranolol.[90] Similarly, while 20 mg oral timolol administered twice daily lowered IOP, the addition of topical timolol did not further reduce IOP.[91] Clinically, this finding can be important. A patient taking oral beta blockers may have little or no additional IOP effect from OBBs. With the advent of new drugs for systemic hypertension, a patient in whom an oral beta blocker is discontinued may appear to have loss of IOP control. In such patients, OBBs may restore IOP to previous levels. It is important to maintain an accurate and current history of systemic medications.

OBBs can have significant interactions with drugs used to treat cardiac disease. Severe bradycardia has been reported in patients taking OBBs in combination with verapamil or quinidine.[92] In one case, a patient who was stable when taking quinidine developed symptomatic bradycardia when timolol was added. Normal sinus rhythm returned when both drugs were discontinued. Timolol alone did not induce a recurrence of the bradycardia, but it returned when quinidine was added.[93] Quinidine inhibits the CYP2D6 enzyme of the cytochrome P-450 system involved in the metabolism of timolol.[94]

3.8 DRUG–DISEASE INTERACTIONS

The potential CNS adverse effects of OBBs are discussed in section 3.6.3. In patients with subtle changes in mental status, OBBs may contribute to symptoms. This effect is reversible with discontinuation of OBBs. Depression, a common condition, is also commonly listed as a CNS adverse effect of beta blockers. Most of the data propagating the notion that beta blockers cause depression emanate from individual case reports or short case series in the late 1960s and 1970s. In contrast, there are at least 10 published studies that used standardized rating assessments for depression, such as the Hamilton Rating Scale for Depression, Profile of Mood States, and Zung Self-Rating Depression Scale, rather than less rigorous methods of assessment, such as using the isolated symptom "depression" or providing simple checklist responses. Eight of these 10 studies were prospective studies. Four were double-masked, randomized, placebo-controlled trials, and another had a placebo arm but used a crossover design. Nine of these 10 studies did not demonstrate an association between beta-adrenergic blockers and depression. Three of these were relatively large and had between 312 and 487 subjects. The only one that reported a positive association had only 20 patients randomized, and the agents were administered for only 4 days. This detailed illustration shows how case reports may not be supported by appropriately designed studies. This is summarized in reviews.[95,96]

Use of OBBs is contraindicated in the presence of several cardiovascular diseases as mentioned in section 3.6.4. In a patient with uncompensated heart failure, sick sinus syndrome, or undetected bradycardia, OBBs may cause adverse symptoms or even be life-threatening. They can also lower blood pressure, potentially worsening symptoms in patients with orthostatic hypotension, cerebrovascular insufficiency, or peripheral vascular disease.

The OBBs should be avoided in patients with known reactive airway disease. As discussed in section 3.6.5, pulmonary function can be affected even in healthy asymptomatic individuals. While betaxolol formerly was considered relatively safe for use in those individuals, now newer classes of drugs offer safer alternatives.

Oral beta blockers can mask symptoms of thyrotoxicosis. Similarly, abrupt withdrawal of OBBs can exacerbate symptoms of hyperthyroidism. In a labile diabetic patient with known history of hypoglycemic unawareness, OBBs could theoretically mask the symptoms of hypoglycemia, which are mediated by catecholamines. Patients with non-insulin-dependent diabetes mellitus receiving systemic beta blockers do not appear to be at increased risk of hypoglycemic unawareness, nor have beta blockers been shown to be associated with prolonged hypoglycemia due to blockade of catecholamine-mediated recovery. However, patients with insulin-dependent diabetes or labile diabetes may be potentially at greater risk for prolonged hypoglycemia when receiving systemic doses of beta blockers.[97–99]

3.9 SPECIFIC OCULAR BETA BLOCKERS

In the United States, five topical OBBs have been approved for lowering IOP. These compounds are similar, although there are some differences among the individual compounds and their activity and pharmaceutics. Figure 3.1 depicts the chemical structures of these OBBs, and table 3.1 summarizes them.

3.9.1 *Nonselective Beta Blockers.*

3.9.1.1 *Timolol solution* is available as timolol maleate 0.25% and 0.5% (Timoptic, Istalol) and as timolol hemihydrate 0.5% (Betimol). A timolol maleate gel-forming solution 0.25% and 0.5% is also available (Timoptic-XE). The timolol maleate preparations are also available as generics. Timolol maleate solution, the prototype OBB in the United States, was the first OBB approved by the FDA in 1978. As the prototype, it is discussed in greater detail than other OBBs. Many of the observations relating to timolol are relevant to the other OBBs.

The introduction of OBB drugs provided an attractive alternative to the other agents previously available. The adrenergic agonists, parasympathomimetics, and oral CAIs had adverse effect profiles that limited their tolerability. Timolol rapidly advanced to become the most commonly used first-line therapy for the treatment of elevated IOP, replaced in recent years by prostaglandin analogues.

Timolol is a nonselective beta-adrenergic antagonist. It and the other OBBs lack the membrane-stabilizing property (local anesthesia) that limited the usefulness of propranolol as an IOP-lowering medication. Timolol was demonstrated to have greater efficacy at lowering IOP than either pilocarpine or epinephrine.[100,101] Timolol maleate has been demonstrated to lower IOP in normal, ocular hypertensive, and glaucomatous eyes.[102–104]

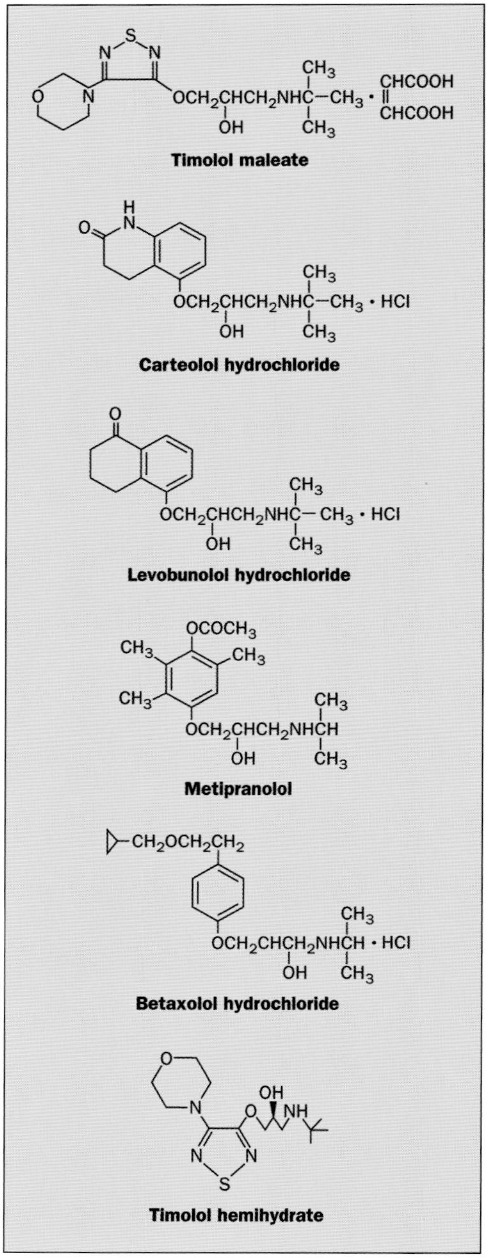

Figure 3.1. Chemical structures of beta blockers.

Timolol is available commercially at 0.25% and 0.5% concentrations in the United States. The 0.5% concentration is most commonly used; however, lower concentrations may be equally effective. (Timolol is available as 0.1% solution and gel outside the U.S.) When interpreted in the context of the knowledge we have gained about timolol, it becomes clear that early studies to establish the dose response of timolol had what we can now recognize as design flaws.

There is no clearly defined dose–response effect for reduction of IOP by timolol with concentrations ranging from 0.1% to 1.5%. A single-dose, incomplete block design study of 20 patients showed almost equivalent peak IOP reduction (no significant difference) with timolol 0.1% to 1.5% compared with fellow eyes receiving placebo or no drug. All subject received timolol at varying doses, or placebo in the study eye. The study had a somewhat complex design but is the best reported among the dose-ranging studies. There were significant IOP reductions for 24 hours with timolol at concentration of 0.25% and higher, but IOP began to increase after 8 hours with timolol 0.1% single dose. Interestingly, all concentrations maintained 25% IOP reduction or greater at 24 hours.[103] Another double-blind study compared epinephrine to timolol 0.1%, 0.25%, and 0.5% twice daily in 119 glaucoma patients. Intraocular pressure measurements were performed on weeks 2, 4, 10, and 14. Timolol was superior to epinephrine, and interestingly, 68% of subjects on timolol 0.1% had an IOP below 22 mm Hg.[105] One of the key limitations of early studies was the lack of appreciation of the need for a run-in period; the full IOP effect is not achieved with a single dose or even with a week of therapy.

In none of the dose-ranging studies or single-dose studies is there comment on eye color. Clearly, the studies and comments are silent on the issue of the time to reach steady state with pigment binding. This may represent another fundamental error in early decisions about dosing; the 0.25% concentration may have maximal efficacy, particularly in less pigmented eyes, and lower incidence of systemic side effects.[106] Despite these limitations in the early studies, clinicians in the United States most commonly prescribe timolol 0.5%.

With topical timolol maleate use, there is a contralateral effect when the drug is used in one eye. This IOP lowering in the untreated eye is believed to be due to systemic absorption of the drug.[107,108]

The onset of action of timolol maleate is about 30 minutes following instillation, with maximum effect after 2 hours.[103] This maximal effect can persist for 12 hours following application, with measurable IOP lowering persisting for 24 hours.

Studies of aqueous flow have demonstrated that timolol reduces aqueous production below baseline levels when taken in the morning but does not reduce it below baseline levels following an evening dose.[109] There is a normal physiologic decrease in aqueous flow at night, and timolol did not reduce flow below this level. Recent sleep laboratory data have further suggested a lack of nocturnal efficacy of timolol. When IOP is measured in habitual position (upright during daytime and supine at night), timolol dosed once daily in the morning lowered daytime IOP below baseline values but did not lower nocturnal IOP below the baseline.[110]

The prolonged duration of action and the lack of effect on aqueous flow with dosing at night and the sleep laboratory data have raised questions about the dosing frequency of OBBs. Although the labeled indication for the drug specifies twice-daily dosing, clinical studies and practical experience have demonstrated that once-daily administration may be effective and, in fact, preferable.[111–113]

In some patients, the efficacy of timolol maleate may decrease over time. It has been hypothesized that the decrease may be due to the response of beta receptors to constant exposure to an antagonist. Initially, most patients have a substantial reduction in IOP in response to timolol maleate, but after several weeks IOP response may lessen. This phenomenon is called short-term escape. It has been suggested that, in response to the beta-receptor antagonism, there is drug-induced up-regulation of beta receptors in the target tissue.

Over a longer time period of months to years, some patients who were initially well controlled by timolol maleate evidenced reduced IOP control. This effect, termed long-term drift, does not occur in all patients. Following a several-week drug holiday, earlier levels of IOP lowering can be restored. One might also wonder if this is an acquired lack of efficacy or poor adherence and a lack of using the eye drops.

The effects of timolol may persist for weeks after discontinuation of the drug. Some IOP lowering may persist for up to 2 weeks, and aqueous flow may be affected for up to 6 weeks. For clinical studies, 4 weeks is accepted as a "washout" for timolol maleate.

Timolol has been demonstrated to be additive to most other IOP medications. As mentioned above, newer IOP-lowering agents have been studied in comparison to timolol and were often studied as an adjunct to timolol. This is not because of any particular advantage of timolol over other nonselective beta blockers. Because of its widespread acceptance, timolol became a benchmark to which new IOP-lowering therapies are compared. It would be reasonable to expect that additivity of other nonselective beta blockers would be similar (see section 3.7).

Timolol maleate is available in gel-forming solutions. The first of these (Timoptic-XE) is formulated in gellan gum. This vehicle forms a gel when it comes in contact with cations in tear film. It has been proposed that this would increase bioavailability and decrease systemic absorption.

In clinical trials, the IOP-lowering effect of once-daily Timoptic-XE was compared to that of twice-daily timolol maleate solution and found to be similar.[53] No large trials are available comparing Timoptic-XE once daily with timolol maleate solution once daily. Timoptic-XE has as its preservative benzododecinium bromide rather than BAK, which is found in other beta blocker preparations. This may be useful for a patient with sensitivity to BAK. A generic equivalent to the gel-forming solution is available. Timolol in xantham gum gel-forming solution (Timolol GFS) was approved by the FDA as an A-B equivalent.

As mentioned above, the once-daily administration of timolol in gel-forming solution should decrease the amount available for systemic absorption through nasolacrimal drainage and thus decrease adverse effects. In a small crossover study comparing Timoptic-XE 0.5% once daily to timolol maleate 0.5% solution twice daily, plasma levels of timolol were lower in patients receiving once-daily gel-forming solution.[114] It is not clear if this result is due to the gel or the less frequent dosing.

Timolol hemihydrate (Betimol) is a timolol solution available as 0.25% and 0.5% in which hemihydrate has been substituted for the maleate anion. Timolol hemihydrate is similar to timolol maleate in IOP-lowering effect and is expected to have a similar adverse effect profile.[115]

Timolol maleate 0.5% has been formulated with potassium sorbate (Istalol), with a claim to enhance bioavailability and with a lower concentration of BAK. This formulation administered once daily in the morning was compared with timolol maleate 0.5% solution administered twice daily, with 290 patients completing the

12-month study. At none of the visits did the 95% confidence intervals for between-treatment comparisons exceed 1.5 mm Hg, and at most of the visits, these intervals did not exceed 1.0 mm Hg.[116] Istalol is the only timolol maleate solution compared with twice-daily dosing of the original formulation and received an indication for once-daily dosing. No studies are available that compare once-daily with twice-daily dosing of the original formulation of timolol maleate.

3.9.1.2 *Carteolol hydrochloride* 1% (*Ocupress*) is a nonselective beta blocker approved in 1992 for use in the United States. The branded product is no longer marketed in the United States. Generic carteolol is available.

Carteolol differs from the other nonselective OBBs by having ISA. This means that, while acting as a competitive antagonist, carteolol binds to the adrenergic receptor and results in partial agonist activity. This effect appears to be due to a metabolite that is also a potent IOP-lowering agent. An OBB with ISA offers the theoretical advantage of causing less frequent or less severe adverse effects of beta blockade. Such benefits have not been clearly established in clinical practice.

Carteolol lowers IOP within 1 hour of administration, with peak effect at 4 hours. Significant IOP lowering persists for 12 hours.[117,118] Carteolol appears to be as effective as other nonselective OBBs.[119,120]

The side effects associated with carteolol can be expected to be similar to those of other OBBs, although the intrinsic sympathomimetic activity (ISA) of carteolol may confer some advantages. As noted above, in some studies, the effect on heart rate and lipid profile with carteolol was more favorable than that with timolol. However, in stark contrast with other beta blockers, those with ISA in fact are not favored systemically because the ISA component results in a significant reduction in the survival advantage that beta blockers as a class have in patients with a history of myocardial infarction.[121]

3.9.1.3 *Levobunolol hydrochloride* (*Betagan*) is a nonselective OBB derived from propranolol. It was approved for use in the United States in 1985. The commercial preparation is formulated in 0.25% and 0.5% concentrations and contains only the levo-isomer. Generic preparations are available.

As with other OBBs, levobunolol decreases IOP in normal subjects and in those with elevated IOP. The IOP-lowering effect begins within 1 hour of administration and reaches peak in 2 to 6 hours.[122] A significant effect can be maintained for 24 hours.[112,123,124] A metabolite of levobunolol, dihydrobunolol, possesses beta-blocking activity and may account for the sustained effect. As noted above, levobunolol is indicated for once-daily or twice-daily dosing.

In short-term studies, levobunolol twice daily was equivalent to other OBBs in IOP-lowering ability.[125–127] However, in a 3-month, double-masked trial comparing once-daily levobunolol 0.5% and 1% with once-daily timolol 0.5%, the levobunolol groups had a significantly greater mean reduction in IOP than did the timolol group (7 and 6.5 mm Hg vs 4.5 mm Hg). It is interesting to note that 72% (18 of 25) of the levobunolol 0.5% group and 64% (16 of 25) of the timolol 0.5% group were considered to have satisfactory IOP control on the once-daily regimen.[112] Additivity and adverse effects with levobunolol are similar to those of other nonselective OBBs.

3.9.1.4 *Metipranolol 0.3%* (*Optipranolol*) is a nonselective beta blocker approved in 1991 for use in the United States. It is available only as a generic preparation.

The IOP-lowering effect of metipranolol is similar to that of other nonselective OBBs.[19,128] Onset of action is within 30 minutes of administration, with peak effect at 2 hours. A detectable IOP effect can last for 24 hours.[129] Like levobunolol, metipranolol has an active metabolite that may contribute to prolonged action.

Additivity and adverse effects of metipranolol are similar to those of other nonselective OBBs. As mentioned in section 3.6.1, there may be an association between metipranolol and granulomatous uveitis.

3.9.2 *Selective Beta Blockers*

3.9.2.1 *Betaxolol hydrochloride* is a relatively selective beta-1–adrenergic antagonist. It was initially introduced as a 0.5% solution (Betoptic) and approved for use in the United States in 1985. A new vehicle was introduced in 1991, consisting of betaxolol 0.25% in a suspension of resin-coated beads designed to allow a gradual release of drug. It is marketed under the trade name Betoptic S (suspension). The commercial product is a racemic mixture of the dextro- and levo-isomers. It is available as a 0.25% suspension. (The 0.5% solution is no longer marketed in the U.S.) In clinical trials, betaxolol was effective at lowering IOP.[130–133] In most studies, it lowers IOP slightly less than timolol or other nonselective beta blockers.[17,134,135,136] The betaxolol 0.25% suspension has the same IOP-lowering effect as the 0.5% solution, and it seems to cause less ocular irritation.[20]

In an intriguing study, the long-term effects on visual fields in patients taking betaxolol were compared with those in patients taking timolol. Even though the IOP was higher in the betaxolol group, the visual fields were judged slightly better.[137,138] Similar results were found in another study.[139] These small studies have not been verified with larger, prospective studies.

Betaxolol may possess other interesting properties. There is some evidence that it possesses calcium channel blocker properties.[140,141] Preliminary limited evidence raised the possibility that the drug may also have neuroprotective effects under certain conditions.[142–145] The significance of these observations to human glaucoma, if any, remains to be established.

Betaxolol is highly lipid soluble and has a large volume of distribution. It binds well to plasma proteins. This may explain in part the lower incidence of CNS side effects with betaxolol than with timolol.[40,41]

3.9.3 *Combination Drugs.* Timolol has been tested as a component of several fixed-combination products, which are discussed in chapter 7.

3.10 CONCLUSION

Since the introduction of timolol in 1978, OBBs have been a popular choice for monotherapy for elevated IOP. They are now viewed as an alternative to prostaglandin analogues for initial monotherapy, an adjunctive therapy, or as a component of fixed-combination therapy. As such, they remain a useful class of medication. After only a few years, it was widely appreciated that OBBs had the potential to cause the same constellation of adverse effects as did systemic beta blockers. The population with glaucoma tends to be older and may be more susceptible to subtle effects, or may have other medical conditions that could interact with drugs in this class. However, at least one review of the available literature has suggested that the evidence for adverse effects from OBBs has not been rigorously analyzed or accurately represented.[95] The routine use of timolol 0.5% twice daily should be reconsidered by clinicians. This once-popular regimen may be excessive for at least some patients, both in concentration and in frequency. It is essential to obtain a thorough medical history before prescribing OBBs for a patient. It is also appropriate to measure and record heart rate and blood pressure. Communication with the primary medical care provider is essential to help avoid possible drug–drug and drug–disease interactions. Once-daily dosing, starting treatment with lower concentrations, teaching nasolacrimal occlusion techniques, and prescribing gel-forming solutions may help decrease systemic exposure to the drugs.

REFERENCES

1. Alquist RP. A study of the adrenotropic receptors. *Am J Physiol.* 1948;153:586–600.
2. Phillips CI, Howitt G, Rowlands DJ. Propranolol as ocular hypotensive agent. *Br J Ophthalmol.* 1967;51:222–226.
3. Yablonski ME, Zimmerman TJ, Waltman SR, Becker B. A fluorophotometric study of the effect of topical timolol on aqueous humor dynamics. *Exp Eye Res.* 1978;27:135–142.
4. Neufeld AH, Bartels SP, Liu JH. Laboratory and clinical studies on the mechanism of action of timolol. *Surv Ophthalmol.* 1983;28(suppl):286–292.
5. Coakes RL, Brubaker RF. The mechanism of timolol in lowering intraocular pressure: in the normal eye. *Arch Ophthalmol.* 1978;96:2045–2048.
6. Gaul GR, Will NJ, Brubaker RF. Comparison of a noncardioselective beta-adrenoceptor blocker and a cardioselective blocker in reducing aqueous flow in humans. *Arch Ophthalmol.* 1989;107:1308–1311.
7. Reiss GR, Brubaker RF. The mechanism of betaxolol, a new ocular hypotensive agent. *Ophthalmology.* 1983;90:1369–1372.
8. Yablonski ME, Novack GD, Burke PJ, et al. The effect of levobunolol on aqueous humor dynamics. *Exp Eye Res.* 1987;44:49–54.
9. Schmitt C, Lotti VJ, DeDouarec JC. Beta-adrenergic blockers: lack of relationship between antagonism of isoproterenol and lowering of intraocular pressure in rabbits. In: Sears ML, ed. *New Directions in Ophthalmic Research.* New Haven, CT: Yale University Press; 1981:147–162.
10. Caprioli J, Sears M, Bausher L, et al. Forskolin lowers intraocular pressure by reducing aqueous inflow. *Invest Ophthalmol Vis Sci.* 1984;25:268–277.
11. Keates EU, Stone R. The effect of d-timolol on intraocular pressure in patients with ocular hypertension. *Am J Ophthalmol.* 1984;98:73–78.
12. Polansky JR, Cherksey BD, Alvarado JA. Update on -adrenergic drug therapy. In: Drance SM, Van Buskirk EM, Neufeld AH, eds. *Pharmacology of Glaucoma.* Baltimore, MD: Williams & Wilkins; 1992:301–321.

13. Zimmerman TJ, Fechtner RD. Maximal medical therapy for glaucoma [editorial]. *Arch Ophthalmol.* 1997;115:1579–1580.

14. Kitazawa Y, Tsuchisaka H. Effects of timolol on corneal sensitivity and tear production. *Int Ophthalmol.* 1980;3:25–29.

15. Van Buskirk EM. Corneal anesthesia after timolol maleate therapy. *Am J Ophthalmol.* 1979;88:739–743.

16. Wilson RP, Spaeth GL, Poryzees E. The place of timolol in the practice of ophthalmology. *Ophthalmology.* 1980;87:451–454.

17. Berry DP Jr, Van Buskirk EM, Shields MB. Betaxolol and timolol: a comparison of efficacy and side effects. *Arch Ophthalmol.* 1984;102:42–45.

18. Allen RC, Hertzmark E, Walker AM, Epstein DL. A double-masked comparison of betaxolol vs timolol in the treatment of open-angle glaucoma. *Am J Ophthalmol.* 1986;101:535–541.

19. Mills KB, Wright G. A blind randomised cross-over trial comparing metipranolol 0.3% with timolol 0.25% in open-angle glaucoma: a pilot study. *Br J Ophthalmol.* 1986;70:39–42.

20. Weinreb RN, Caldwell DR, Goode SM, et al. A double-masked three-month comparison between 0.25% betaxolol suspension and 0.5% betaxolol ophthalmic solution. *Am J Ophthalmol.* 1990;110:189–192.

21. Bonomi L, Zavarise G, Noya E, Michieletto S. Effects of timolol maleate on tear flow in human eyes. *Graefes Arch Klin Exp Ophthalmol.* 1980;213:19–22.

22. Herreras JM, Pastor JC, Calonge M, Asensio VM. Ocular surface alteration after long-term treatment with an antiglaucomatous drug. *Ophthalmology.* 1992;99:1082–1088.

23. Fiore PM, Jacobs IH, Goldberg DB. Drug-induced pemphigoid: a spectrum of diseases. *Arch Ophthalmol.* 1987;105:1660–1663.

24. Novack GD. Ophthalmic beta-blockers since timolol. *Surv Ophthalmol.* 1987;31:307–327.

25. Kinshuck D. Glauline (metipranolol) induced uveitis and increase in intraocular pressure. *Br J Ophthalmol.* 1991;75:575.

26. Akingbehin T, Villada JR. Metipranolol-associated granulomatous anterior uveitis. *Br J Ophthalmol.* 1991;75:519–523.

27. Akingbehin T, Villada JR, Walley T. Metipranolol-induced adverse reactions, I: the rechallenge study. *Eye.* 1992;6:277–279.

28. Schultz JS, Hoenig JA, Charles H. Possible bilateral anterior uveitis secondary to metipranolol (OptiPranolol) therapy. *Arch Ophthalmol.* 1993;111:1606–1607.

29. Melles RB, Wong IG. Metipranolol-associated granulomatous iritis. *Am J Ophthalmol.* 1994;118(6):712–715.

30. Shell JW. Pharmacokinetics of topically applied ophthalmic drugs. *Surv Ophthalmol.* 1982;26:207–218.

31. Bobik A, Jennings GL, Asley P, et al. Timolol pharmacokinetics and effects on heart rate and blood pressure after acute and chronic administration. *Eur J Clin Pharmacol.* 1979;16:243–249.

32. Vuori ML, Kaila T. Plasma kinetics and antagonist activity of topical ocular timolol in elderly patients. *Arch Clin Exp Ophthalmol.* 1995;233:131–134.

33. Affrime MB, Lowenthal DT, Tobert JA, et al. Dynamics and kinetics of ophthalmic timolol. *Clin Pharmacol Ther.* 1980;27:471–477.

34. Alvan G, Calissendorff B, Seideman P, et al. Absorption of ocular timolol. *Clin Pharmacokinet.* 1980;5:95–100.

35. Zimmerman TJ, Kooner KS, Kandarakis AS, Ziegler LP. Improving the therapeutic index of topically applied ocular drugs. *Arch Ophthalmol.* 1984;102:551–553.

36. Van Buskirk EM. Adverse reactions from timolol administration. *Ophthalmology.* 1980;87:447–450.

37. McMahon CD, Shaffer RN, Hoskins HD Jr, Hetherington J Jr. Adverse effects experienced by patients taking timolol. *Am J Ophthalmol.* 1979;88:736–738.

38. Nelson WL, Kuritsky JN. Early postmarketing surveillance of betaxolol hydrochloride, September 1985–September 1986. *Am J Ophthalmol.* 1987;103:592.

39. Shore JH, Fraunfelder FT, Meyer SM. Psychiatric side effects from topical ocular timolol, a beta-adrenergic blocker. *J Clin Psychopharmacol.* 1987;7:264–267.

40. Lynch MG, Whitson JT, Brown RH, et al. Topical beta-blocker therapy and central nervous system side effects: a preliminary study comparing betaxolol and timolol. *Arch Ophthalmol.* 1988;106:908–911.

41. Cohen JB. A comparative study of the central nervous system effects of betaxolol versus timolol [letter]. *Arch Ophthalmol.* 1989;107:633–634.

42. Hoffman BB, Lefkowitz RJ. Catecholamines, sympathomimetic drugs, and adrenergic receptor antagonists. In: Hardman JG, Limbird LE, Molinoff PB, et al, eds. *The Pharmacologic Basis of Therapeutics.* New York: McGraw-Hill; 1996:199–248.

43. Hjalmarson A. Prevention of sudden cardiac death with beta blockers. *Clin Cardiol.* 1999;22(suppl 5):V11–V15.

44. Yan AT, Yan RT, Liu PP. Narrative review. pharmacotherapy for chronic heart failure: evidence from recent clinical trials. *Ann Intern Med.* 2005;142(2):132–145.

45. Teerlink JR, Massie BM. Beta-adrenergic blocker mortality trials in congestive heart failure. *Am J Cardiol.* 1999;84:94R–102R.

46. Domanski MJ, Krause-Steinrauf H, Massie BM, et al; BEST Investigators. A comparative analysis of the results from 4 trials of beta-blocker therapy for heart failure. BEST, CIBIS-II, MERIT-HF, and COPERNICUS. *J Card Fail.* 2003;9(5):354–363.

47. Burggraf GW, Munt PW. Topical timolol therapy and cardiopulmonary function. *Can J Ophthalmol.* 1980;15:159–160.

48. Leier CV, Baker ND, Weber PA. Cardiovascular effects of ophthalmic timolol. *Ann Intern Med.* 1986;104:197–199.

49. Nelson WL, Fraunfelder FT, Sills JM, et al. Adverse respiratory and cardiovascular events attributed to timolol ophthalmic solution, 1978–1985. *Am J Ophthalmol.* 1986; 102:606–611.

50. Doyle WJ, Weber PJ, Meeks RH. Effects of topical timolol maleate on exercise performance. *Arch Ophthalmol.* 1984;102:1517–1518.

51. Atkins JM, Pugh BR Jr, Timewill RM. Cardiovascular effects of topical beta-blockers during exercise. *Am J Ophthalmol.* 1985;99:173–175.

52. Zabel RW, MacDonald IM. Sinus arrest associated with betaxolol ophthalmic drops. *Am J Ophthalmol.* 1987;104:431.

53. Rosenlund EF. The intraocular pressure lowering effect of timolol in gel-forming solution [published correction appears in *Acta Ophthalmol Scand.* 1996;74(4):416]. *Acta Ophthalmol Scand.* 1996r;74(2):160–162.

54. Kitazawa Y. Multicenter double-blind comparison of carteolol and timolol in primary open-angle glaucoma and ocular hypertension. *Adv Ther.* 1993;10:95–131.

55. Netland PA, Weiss HS, Stewart WC, et al. Cardiovascular effects of topical carteolol hydrochloride and timolol maleate in patients with ocular hypertension and primary open-angle glaucoma. *Am J Ophthalmol.* 1997;123:465–477.

56. Jones FL Jr, Ekberg NL. Exacerbation of asthma by timolol [letter]. *N Engl J Med.* 1979;301:270.

57. Schoene RB, Martin TR, Charan NB, French CL. Timolol-induced bronchospasm in asthmatic bronchitis. *JAMA.* 1981;245:1460–1461.

58. Prince DS, Carliner NH. Respiratory arrest following first dose of timolol ophthalmic solution. *Chest.* 1983;84:640–641.

59. Avorn J, Glynn RJ, Gurwitz JH, et al. Adverse pulmonary effects of topical beta blockers used in the treatment of glaucoma. *J Glaucoma.* 1993;2:158–165.

60. Charan NB, Lakshminarayan S. Pulmonary effects of topical timolol. *Arch Intern Med.* 1980;140:843–844.

61. Schoene RB, Abuan T, Ward RL, Beasley CH. Effects of topical betaxolol, timolol, and placebo on pulmonary function in asthmatic bronchitis. *Am J Ophthalmol.* 1984;97:86–92.

62. Diggory P, Heyworth P, Chau G, et al. Improved lung function tests on changing from topical timolol: non-selective beta-blockade impairs lung function tests in elderly patients. *Eye.* 1993;7:661–663.

63. Van Buskirk EM, Weinreb RN, Berry DP, et al. Betaxolol in patients with glaucoma and asthma. *Am J Ophthalmol.* 1986;101:531–534.

64. Ofner S, Smith TJ. Betaxolol in chronic obstructive pulmonary disease. *J Ocul Pharmacol.* 1987;3:171–176.

65. Weinreb RN, Van Buskirk EM, Cherniack R, Drake MM. Long-term betaxolol therapy in glaucoma patients with pulmonary disease. *Am J Ophthalmol.* 1988;106:162–167.

66. Harris LS, Greinstein SH, Bloom AF. Respiratory difficulties with betaxolol. *Am J Ophthalmol.* 1986;102:274–275.

67. Berger WE. Betaxolol in patients with glaucoma and asthma [letter]. *Am J Ophthalmol.* 1987;103:600–601.

68. Salpeter SR, Ormiston TM, Salpeter EE. Cardioselective beta-blockers in patients with reactive airway disease. a meta-analysis. *Ann Intern Med.* 2002;137(9):715–725.

69. Salpeter SR, Ormiston TM, Salpeter EE, Poole PJ, Cates CJ. Cardioselective beta-blockers for chronic obstructive pulmonary disease. a meta-analysis. *Respir Med.* 2003;97(10):1094–1101.

70. Coleman AL, Diehl DL, Jampel HD, et al. Topical timolol decreases plasma high-density lipoprotein cholesterol level. *Arch Ophthalmol.* 1990;108:1260–1263.

71. West J, Longstaff S. Topical timolol and serum lipoproteins. *Br J Ophthalmol.* 1990;74:663–664.

72. Freedman SF, Freedman NJ, Shields MB, et al. Effects of ocular carteolol and timolol on plasma high-density lipoprotein cholesterol level. *Am J Ophthalmol.* 1993;116:600–611.

73. Realini T, Barber L, Burton D. Frequency of asymmetric intraocular pressure fluctuations among patients with and without glaucoma. *Ophthalmology.* 2002;109:1367–1371.

74. Realini T, Fechtner RD, Atreides, SP, Gollance S. The uniocular drug trial and second-eye response to glaucoma medications. *Ophthalmology.* 2004;111:421–426.

75. Liu JHK, Sit AJ, Weinreb RN. Variation of 24-hour intraocular pressure in healthy individuals. *Ophthalmology.* 2005;112:1670–1675.

76. Goldberg I, Ashburn FS Jr, Palmberg PF, et al. Timolol and epinephrine: a clinical study of ocular interactions. *Arch Ophthalmol.* 1980;98:484–486.

77. Korey MS, Hodapp E, Kass M, et al. Timolol and epinephrine: long-term evaluation of concurrent administration. *Arch Ophthalmol.* 1982;100:742–745.

78. Cyrlin MN, Thomas JV, Epstein DL. Additive effect of epinephrine to timolol therapy in primary open angle glaucoma. *Arch Ophthalmol.* 1982;100:414–418.

79. Weinreb RN, Ritch R, Kushner FH. Effect of adding betaxolol to dipivefrin therapy. *Am J Ophthalmol.* 1986;101:196–198.

80. Allen RC, Epstein DL. Additive effect of betaxolol and epinephrine in primary open angle glaucoma. *Arch Ophthalmol.* 1986;104:1178–1184.

81. Airaksinen PJ, Valkonen R, Stenborg T, et al. A double-masked study of timolol and pilocarpine combined. *Am J Ophthalmol.* 1987;104:587–590.

82. Kass MA, Korey M, Gordon M, Becker B. Timolol and acetazolamide: a study of concurrent administration. *Arch Ophthalmol.* 1982;100:941–942.

83. Smith JP, Weeks RH, Newland EF, Ward RL. Betaxolol and acetazolamide: combined ocular hypotensive effect. *Arch Ophthalmol.* 1984;102:1794–1795.

84. Adamsons I, Clineschmidt D, Polis A, et al. The efficacy and safety of dorzolamide as adjunctive therapy to timolol maleate gellan solution in patients with elevated intraocular pressure. Additivity Study Group. *J Glaucoma.* 1998;7:253–260.

85. Clineschmidt CM, Williams RD, Snyder E, Adamsons IA. A randomized trial in patients inadequately controlled with timolol alone comparing the dorzolamide–timolol combination to monotherapy with timolol or dorzolamide. Dorzolamide–Timolol Combination Study Group. *Ophthalmology.* 1998;105:1952–1959.

86. Racz P, Ruzsonyi MR, Nagy ZT, et al. Around-the-clock intraocular pressure reduction with once-daily application of latanoprost by itself or in combination with timolol. *Arch Ophthalmol.* 1996;114:268–273.

87. Alm A,Widengard I, Kjellgren D, et al. Latanoprost administered once daily caused a maintained reduction of intraocular pressure in glaucoma patients treated concomitantly with timolol. *Br J Ophthalmol.* 1995;79:12–16.

88. Rulo AH, Greve EL, Hoyng PF. Additive effect of latanoprost, a prostaglandin F2 alpha analogue, and timolol in patients with elevated intraocular pressure. *Br J Ophthalmol.* 1994;78:899–902.

89. Orengo-Nania S,Landry T, Von Tress M, et al. Evaluation of travoprost as adjunctive therapy in patients with uncontrolled intraocular pressure while using timolol 0.5%. *Am J Ophthalmol.* 2001;132:860–868.

90. Blondeau P, Côté M, Tetrault L. Effect of timolol eye drops in subjects receiving systemic propranolol therapy. *Can J Ophthalmol.* 1983;18:18–21.

91. Batchelor ED, O'Day DM, Shand DG, Wood AJ. Interaction of topical and oral timolol in glaucoma. *Ophthalmology.* 1979;86:60–65.

92. Pringle SD, MacEwen CJ. Severe bradycardia due to interaction of timolol eye drops and verapamil. *BMJ.* 1987;294:155–156.

93. Dinai Y, Sharir M, Naveh N, Halkin H. Bradycardia induced by interaction between quinidine and ophthalmic timolol. *Ann Intern Med.* 1985;103:890–891.

94. Edeki TI, He H, Wood AJ. Pharmacogenetic explanation for excessive beta-blockade following timolol eye drops: potential for oral–ophthalmic drug interaction. *JAMA.* 1995;274:1611–1613.

95. Lama PJ. Systemic adverse effects of beta-adrenergic blockers. an evidence-based assessment. *Am J Ophthalmol.* 2002;134(5):749–760.

96. Kohn RJ. Beta-blockers an important cause of depression. a medical myth without evidence. *Med Health R I.* 2001;84:92–95.

97. Paauw DS. Did we learn evidenced-based medicine in medical school? Some common medical mythology. *J Am Board Fam Prac.* 1999;12:143–149.

98. United Kingdom Prospective Diabetes Study Group. Efficacy of atenolol and captopril in reducing risk of macrovascular and microvascular complications in type 2 diabetes. *BMJ.* 1998;317:713–720.

99. Shorr RS, Ray WA, Daugherty JR, Griffin MR. Antihypertensives and the risk of serious hypoglycemia in older persons using insulin or sulfonylureas. *JAMA.* 1997; 278:40–43.

100. Boger WP III, Steinert RF, Puliafito CA, Pavan-Langston D. Clinical trial comparing timolol ophthalmic solution to pilocarpine in open-angle glaucoma. *Am J Ophthalmol.* 1978;86:8–18.

101. Sonntag JR, Brindley GO, Shields MB, et al. Timolol and epinephrine: comparison of efficacy and side effects. *Arch Ophthalmol.* 1979;97:273–277.

102. Katz IM, Hubbard WA, Getson AJ, Gould AL. Intraocular pressure decrease in normal volunteers following timolol ophthalmic solution. *Invest Ophthalmol.* 1976;15: 489–492.

103. Zimmerman TJ, Kaufman HE. Timolol: dose response and duration of action. *Arch Ophthalmol.* 1977;95:605–607.

104. Zimmerman TJ, Kass MA, Yablonski ME, Becker B. Timolol maleate: efficacy and safety. *Arch Ophthalmol.* 1979;97:656–658.

105. Demailly P, Lehner MA, Etienne R, et al. Results of a double-blind medium-term study comparing effects of timolol maleate and epinephrine in 120 patients with chronic open-angle glaucoma. *J Fr Ophthalmol.* 1978;1:727–732.

106. Katz IM, Berger ET. Effects of iris pigmentation on response of ocular pressure to timolol. *Surv Ophthalmol.* 1979;23:395–398.

107. Zimmerman TJ, Kaufman HE. Timolol: a beta-adrenergic blocking agent for the treatment of glaucoma. *Arch Ophthalmol.* 1977;95:601–604.

108. Shin DH. Bilateral effects of monocular timolol treatment. *Am J Ophthalmol.* 1986;102:275–276.

109. Topper JE, Brubaker RF. Effects of timolol, epinephrine, and acetazolamide on aqueous flow during sleep. *Invest Ophthalmol Vis Sci.* 1985;26:1315–1319.

110. Liu JH, Kripke DF, Weinreb RN. Comparison of the nocturnal effects of once-daily timolol and latanoprost on intraocular pressure. *Am J Ophthalmol.* 2004;138:389–395.

111. Letchinger SL, Frohlichstein D, Glieser DK, et al. *Can the concentration of timolol or the frequency of its administration be reduced?* Ophthalmology. 1993;100: 1259–1262.

112. Wandel T, Charap AD, Lewis RA, et al. Glaucoma treatment with once-daily levobunolol. *Am J Ophthalmol.* 1986;101:298–304.

113. Soll DB. Evaluation of timolol in chronic open-angle glaucoma: once a day vs twice a day. *Arch Ophthalmol.* 1980;98:2178–2181.

114. Shedden AH, Laurence J, Barrish A, Olah TV. Plasma timolol concentrations of timolol maleate. timolol gel-forming solution (TIMOPTIC-XE) once daily versus timolol maleate ophthalmic solution twice daily. *Doc Ophthalmol.* 2001;103(1):73–79.

115. Mundorf TK, Cate EA, Sine CS, et al. The safety and efficacy of switching timolol maleate 0.5% solution to timolol hemihydrate 0.5% solution given twice daily. *J Ocul Pharmacol Ther.* 1998;14:129–135.

116. Mundorf TK, Ogawa T, Naka H, Novack GD, Crockett RS; US Istalol Study Group. A 12-month, multicenter, randomized, double-masked, parallel-group comparison of

timolol-LA once daily and timolol maleate ophthalmic solution twice daily in the treatment of adults with glaucoma or ocular hypertension. *Clin Ther.* 2004;26(4): 541–551.

117. Araie M, Takase M. Effects of S-596 and carteolol, new beta-adrenergic blockers, and flurbiprofen on the human eye: a fluorophotometric study. *Graefes Arch Klin Exp Ophthalmol.* 1985;222:259–262.

118. Negishi C, Ueda S, Kanai A, et al. Effects of beta-blocking agent carteolol on healthy volunteers and glaucoma patients. *Acta Soc Ophthalmol Jpn.* 1981;25:464–476.

119. Stewart WC, Cohen JS, Netland PA, et al. Efficacy of carteolol hydrochloride 1% vs timolol maleate 0.5% in patients with increased intraocular pressure. *Am J Ophthalmol.* 1997;124:498–505.

120. Scoville B, Mueller B, White BG, Krieglstein GK. A double-masked comparison of carteolol and timolol in ocular hypertension. *Am J Ophthalmol.* 1988;105:150–154.

121. Soriano JB, Hoes AW, Meems L, Grobbee DE. Increased survival with beta-blockers. importance of ancillary properties. *Prog Cardiovasc Dis.* 1997;39(5):445–456.

122. Duzman E, Ober M, Scharrer A, Leopold IH. A clinical evaluation of the effects of topically applied levobunolol and timolol on increased intraocular pressure. *Am J Ophthalmol.* 1982;94:318–327.

123. Rakofsky SI, Melamed S, Cohen JS, et al. A comparison of the ocular hypotensive efficacy of once-daily and twice-daily levobunolol treatment. *Ophthalmology.* 1989;96:8–11.

124. Derick RJ, Robin AL, Tielsch J, et al. Once-daily versus twice-daily levobunolol (0.5%) therapy: a crossover study. *Ophthalmology.* 1992;99:424–429.

125. Berson FG, Cohen HB, Foerster RJ, et al. Levobunolol compared with timolol for the long-term control of elevated intraocular pressure. *Arch Ophthalmol.* 1985;103: 379–382.

126. Cinotti A, Cinotti D, Grant W, et al. Levobunolol vs timolol for open-angle glaucoma and ocular hypertension. *Am J Ophthalmol.* 1985;99:11–17.

127. Levobunolol Study Group. Levobunolol: a four-year study of efficacy and safety in glaucoma treatment. *Ophthalmology.* 1989;96:642–645.

128. Krieglstein GK, Novack GD, Voepel E, et al. Levobunolol and metipranolol: comparative ocular hypotensive efficacy, safety, and comfort. *Br J Ophthalmol.* 1987;71: 250–253.

129. Dausch D, Brewitt H, Edelhoff R. Metipranolol eye drops: clinical suitability in the treatment of chronic open angle glaucoma. In: Merté H-J, ed. *Metipranolol: Pharmacology of Beta-Blocking Agents and Use of Metipranolol in Ophthalmology. Contributions to the First Metipranolol Symposium, Berlin, 1983.* New York: Springer-Verlag; 1984:132–147.

130. Feghali JG, Kaufman PL. Decreased intraocular pressure in the hypertensive human eye with betaxolol, beta-1 adrenergic antagonist. *Am J Ophthalmol.* 1985;100:777–782.

131. Caldwell DR, Salisbury CR, Guzek JP. Effects of topical betaxolol in ocular hypertensive patients. *Arch Ophthalmol.* 1984;102:539–540.

132. Berrospi AR, Leibowitz HM. Betaxolol: a new beta-adrenergic blocking agent for the treatment of glaucoma. *Arch Ophthalmol.* 1982;100:943–946.

133. Radius RL. Use of betaxolol in the reduction of elevated intraocular pressure. *Arch Ophthalmol.* 1983;101:898–900.

134. Stewart RH, Kimbrough RL, Ward RL. Betaxolol vs timolol: a six-month double-blind comparison. *Arch Ophthalmol.* 1986;104:46–48.

135. Feghali JG, Kaufman PL, Radius RL, Mandell AI. A comparison of betaxolol and timolol in open angle glaucoma and ocular hypertension. *Acta Ophthalmol.* 1988;66: 180–186.

136. Long DA, Johns GE, Mullen RS, et al. Levobunolol and betaxolol: a double-masked controlled comparison of efficacy and safety in patients with elevated intraocular pressure. *Ophthalmology.* 1988;95:735–741.

137. Messmer C, Flammer J, Stumpfig D. Influence of betaxolol and timolol on the visual fields of patients with glaucoma. *Am J Ophthalmol.* 1991;112:678–681.

138. Kaiser HJ, Flammer J, Stumpfig D, Hendrickson P. Longterm visual field follow-up of glaucoma patients treated with beta-blockers. *Surv Ophthalmol.* 1994;38(suppl): S156–S160.

139. Collignon-Brach J. Longterm effect of topical beta-blockers on intraocular pressure and visual field sensitivity in ocular hypertension and chronic open-angle glaucoma. *Surv Ophthalmol.* 1994;38(suppl):149–155.

140. Hoste AM, Sys SU. Ca^{2+} channel-blocking activity of propranolol and betaxolol in isolated bovine retinal microartery. *J Cardiovasc Pharmacol.* 1998;32:390–396.

141. Yu DY, Su EN, Cringle SJ, et al. Effect of betaxolol, timolol and nimodipine on human and pig retinal arterioles. *Exp Eye Res.* 1998;67:73–81.

142. Osborne NN, Cazevieille C, Carvalho AL, et al. In vivo and in vitro experiments show that betaxolol is a retinal neuroprotective agent. *Brain Res.* 1997;751:113–123.

143. Wood JP, DeSantis L, Chao HM, Osborne NN. Topically applied betaxolol attenuates ischaemia-induced effects to the rat retina and stimulates BDNF mRNA. *Exp Eye Res.* 2001;72(1):79–86.

144. Metoki T, Ohguro H, Ohguro I, Mamiya K, Ito T, Nakazawa M. Study of effects of antiglaucoma eye drops on N-methyl-D-aspartate-induced retinal damage. *Jpn J Ophthalmol.* 2005;49(6):453–461.

145. Cheon EW, Park CH, Kim YS, et al. Protective effects of betaxolol in eyes with kainic acid-induced neuronal death. *Brain Res.* 2006;1069(1):75–85. Epub 2006 Jan 4.

4

Adrenergic Agents

ELLIOTT M. KANNER AND HOWARD I. SAVAGE

T he nonselective adrenergic agonist epinephrine has been used for the treatment of chronic glaucoma for nearly a century. The discovery of distinct adrenergic receptor classes, termed *alpha-* and *beta-adrenergic receptors*, led to the development of potent new ocular hypotensive agents, principally the beta-adrenergic antagonists and the alpha-adrenergic agonists.[1] Beta blockers are discussed in chapter 3 of this monograph. Pharmacologic manipulation of alpha-adrenoreceptor subtypes (termed *alpha-1*, *alpha-2*, and *imidazole receptors*) has provided ophthalmologists with several potent ocular hypotensive agents, with varying local and systemic side effects. These alpha-adrenergic agents include clonidine and its two derivatives, apraclonidine and brimonidine.

4.1 ADRENERGIC PHYSIOLOGY IN THE EYE

The effects of adrenergic stimulation in the eye are mediated by cell-specific transmembrane receptors, which activate a regulatory guanine nucleotide–binding enzyme, or G-protein, and thereby activate various second-messenger systems in the cell. Three main adrenergic-receptor types are recognized: alpha-1, alpha-2, and beta. Each is associated with at least one unique regulatory G-protein: Gq, Gi, and Gs, respectively. Numerous additional receptor subtypes have been identified by a unique response to specific agonists and by the discovery of closely related genes (alpha-1A, -1B, and -1D; alpha-2A, -2B, -C, and -2D). However, the unique properties of these further subtypes are poorly delineated in the eye. An extensive review of adrenergic-receptor physiology as it relates to aqueous dynamics is available elsewhere.[2]

The cascade of events initiated by adrenoreceptor activation appears to regulate intraocular pressure (IOP) via the activity level of adenylate cyclase in the ciliary epithelium. While the final messengers are still uncertain, the net inhibition of adenylate cyclase and the reduction of intracellular cyclic adenosine monophosphate (cAMP) are implicated as necessary steps in the reduction in aqueous production by the ciliary epithelium. This unified hypothesis explains why both beta-receptor antagonists, which block endogenous stimulation of adenylate cyclase, and alpha-2 agonists, which actively inhibit adenylate cyclase, both effectively reduce IOP. Why, then, do both beta agonists such as epinephrine and beta blockers such as timolol reduce IOP in clinical practice? This apparent paradox may be due to adenylate cyclase down-regulation in response to chronic beta-agonist receptor occupancy.[3]

Prostaglandins appear to function as the intracellular second messenger for alpha-2 agonists in animal models,[4] but not in humans. Although the nonsteroidal anti-inflammatory drug flurbiprofen blocks apraclonidine's IOP-lowering effect in monkeys,[4] topical flurbiprofen pretreatment, at the 0.03% dosage used preoperatively in cataract surgery, does not block apraclonidine's effect on aqueous flow in humans.[5,6] The apparent species difference may be explained instead by the lower concentration of flurbiprofen tested clinically in human experiments than that used in animal trials.

Adrenergic agonists can occupy adrenergic and imidazole receptors in the brain and adrenergic receptors concentrated locally in the ciliary body, making the precise site of action unclear. Unilateral application of apraclonidine[7–10] or brimonidine[8,11] causes a 7% to 19% reduction of contralateral IOP, suggesting that a central mechanism may be responsible for at least part of the alpha-adrenergic drugs' efficacy. This central effect varies among different species. In the rabbit, the central effect of adrenergic drugs appears to be transmitted to the eye directly via the sympathetic nervous system,[12] but not, apparently, in humans[13] or monkeys.[8] Specific local and systemic side effects have been attributed to each receptor subtype (table 4.1).

Table 4.1 Receptor-Specific Side Effects of Adrenergic Agonists

Alpha-1 Receptor Effects	Electrolyte absorption in gut
	Miosis
Vasoconstriction	Reduced aqueous formation
Conjunctival blanching	Lipolysis
Dry nose and mouth	Inhibition of insulin release
Systemic hypertension	Renin release
Eyelid retraction	
Mydriasis	
	Beta Receptor Effects
Alpha-2 Receptor Effects	Vasodilation
	Tachycardia
Central nervous system depression	Bronchodilation
Sedation, confusion	Gluconeogenesis
Growth hormone release	Lipolysis
Peripheral vasodilation	Increased aqueous formation
Systemic hypotension	

Source: Information on alpha-2 receptor effects is from Coleman AL, Robin AL, Pollack IP, et al. Cardiovascular and intraocular pressure effects and plasma concentrations of apraclonidine. *Arch Ophthalmol.* 1990;108:1264–1267.

4.2 PHARMACOLOGY

Although many adrenergic drugs have been evaluated for their specificity for a particular receptor subtype, each adrenergic drug used in ophthalmology can occupy several different subreceptors. These receptors appear to differ in different animals. The level of specificity for a given receptor often defines certain clinical characteristics of a drug. Epinephrine is the least selective, activating alpha-1, alpha-2, and beta receptors. Among the alpha-2–selective agonists, brimonidine is the most alpha-2–selective in some animal models. The crossover activation of alpha-1 receptors by clonidine and apraclonidine accounts for their tendency to cause conjunctival blanching, eyelid retraction, and mydriasis. In contrast, brimonidine's more highly specific alpha-2 activation causes miosis, but still has enough residual alpha-1 activation to cause mild conjunctival blanching.

The ability of adrenergic drugs to penetrate the cornea is, in part, directly related to the lipophilicity of the compound. Intact corneal epithelial and endothelial membranes are a formidable barrier for hydrophilic drugs. That is why a 10-fold lower concentration of dipivefrin, 0.1%, the more lipophilic prodrug of epinephrine, can be used with efficacy equal to epinephrine 1%. Unfortunately, the lipophilic nature of clonidine and brimonidine, which permits rapid corneal penetration, also allows penetration of the blood–brain barrier, where stimulation of central alpha-2 receptors may cause sedation and systemic hypotension. Apraclonidine was made 25% more hydrophilic than clonidine by the addition of an amide group to the benzene ring, virtually eliminating potentially dangerous systemic side effects.[14]

4.3 NONSELECTIVE AGONISTS

Some brands of the nonselective agonists epinephrine and dipivefrin are listed in table 4.2.

4.3.1 *Epinephrine*. Epinephrine, a mixed alpha- and beta-adrenergic agonist, was the first topical adrenergic agent used to lower IOP in patients with open-angle glaucoma. Topical administration of epinephrine causes alpha-1–adrenoreceptor–induced conjunctival vasoconstriction, which manifests as blanching, and slight mydriasis. The mydriatic effect can be used to advantage during cataract surgery, where epinephrine added to the intraocular irrigating solution may retard the development of intraoperative miosis and enhance visualization. Epinephrine is employed routinely in ophthalmic plastic surgery to minimize bleeding and slow absorption of local anesthetics. However, it is strictly avoided in the correction of blepharoptosis, because epinephrine (like apraclonidine, clonidine, and brimonidine) induces upper eyelid retraction by stimulation of Müller's muscle and can lead to inadequate surgical correction. Similarly, epinephrine is not used in retrobulbar anesthesia because of the risk of vasospasm and occlusion of the ophthalmic or central retinal artery, along with systemic absorption resulting in tachyarrhythmias with reported fatalities.

Table 4.2 Nonselective Alpha- and
Beta-Adrenergic Agonists

Epinephrine

Glaucon, Epifrin 0.5%, 2% HCl salt
Eppy N, Epinal 0.5%, 1%, 2% borate
Epitrate, 2% bitartrate salt
E Pilo, P1E1, P2E1, P3E1, P4E1, P6E1
Mixtures of 1% epinephrine bitartrate and
    pilocarpine HCl 1%, 2%, 3%, 4%, 6%

Dipivefrin

Propine, 0.1%

The effect of epinephrine on IOP varies over time, initially raising IOP slightly, followed by reduction lasting 12 to 24 hours.[3] Epinephrine penetrates the cornea rather poorly; thus, while concentrations less than 0.5% lower IOP slightly, concentrations of 0.5% and 1% have greater efficacy. The effect of epinephrine is additive to long-term treatment with pilocarpine and oral acetazolamide.[15] Although awkward conceptually, the combination of epinephrine, a mixed alpha and beta agonist, with timolol, a nonselective beta blocker, has been common practice in the recent past. The additivity of these two agents, however, has been variable and short-lived,[16] and as medical options in glaucoma have expanded, the need to combine these agents has diminished.

Epinephrine may cause tachycardia, extra systoles, systemic hypertension, palpitation, and anxiety. Topical use can be uncomfortable, causing tearing and stinging. Long-term use leads to allergic blepharoconjunctivitis in a significant subset of patients, which resolves when the drug is discontinued. Epinephrine is contraindicated in patients with narrow anterior chamber angles, because the induced mydriasis can precipitate pupillary block, inciting a pupillary-block glaucoma attack. Epinephrine is also contraindicated in aphakic patients, because topical use is associated with symptomatic, usually reversible, cystoid macular edema (CME) in roughly 13% to 30%.[17,18] Of note, epinephrine-related CME has been described in aphakic, but not pseudophakic, patients. This may therefore be a problem seen only if the anterior hyaloid is disrupted following traumatic extracapsular cataract surgery. Finally, epinephrine can cause black adrenochrome deposits in the palpebral conjunctiva, on contact lenses, and on the cornea.

4.3.2 D*ipivefrin*. Dipivefrin is a derivative prodrug of epinephrine, made less hydrophilic by the diesterification of epinephrine and pivalic acid. Dipivefrin is converted to epinephrine inside the eye by esterases in the cornea, iris, and ciliary body, which cleave the pivalic acid moiety. Dipivefrin is less potent than most beta blockers, except perhaps for betaxolol 0.25%.[19]

Dipivefrin penetrates the corneal epithelium much more readily than epinephrine, allowing 10- to 20-fold lower concentrations to be used[20] with only slightly less efficacy.[21,22] While topical side effects, stinging and irritation, are less than those experienced with epinephrine, the intraocular effects are identical, including my-driasis and aphakic CME. Therefore, like epinephrine, dipivefrin is contraindicated in patients who are aphakic or have narrow anterior chamber angles. Also, like epinephrine, dipivefrin can cause a severe acute allergic blepharoconjunctivitis.

4.4 ALPHA-SELECTIVE AGONISTS

The alpha-selective agonists available clinically include clonidine, apraclonidine, and brimonidine. Key differences between these agents include therapeutic index, clinical safety, penetration, level of alpha-2 selectivity, and side effects. Clonidine was the first relatively selective alpha-2 agonist available; it lowers IOP well, but its narrow therapeutic index, particularly its propensity to cause sedation and systemic hypotension, has made it unpopular in glaucoma therapy. Apraclonidine was derived from clonidine in an attempt to obtain IOP lowering without the sedation and systemic hypotension of clonidine. Apraclonidine and brimonidine remain the most widely used alpha agonists in glaucoma therapy. To date, apraclonidine is the only agent approved by the FDA that is particularly well suited for acute prophylaxis of IOP elevation following argon laser trabeculoplasty, Nd:YAG and argon laser iridotomy, Nd:YAG capsulotomy, and cataract surgery. Brimonidine is the only alpha-2 agonist approved by the FDA for the long-term therapy of glaucoma and the most alpha-2 selective.

Some brands of the alpha-selective agonists clonidine, apraclonidine, and brimonidine are listed in table 4.3.

4.4.1 *Clonidine*. Synthesized in the early 1960s, clonidine was the first alpha agonist used systemically and topically for glaucoma. Because of its potent vasoconstriction effect, clonidine was originally tested as a topical nasal decongestant and shaving astringent, but clinical testing revealed its narrow therapeutic index. Moreover, the side effects of systemic hypotension and sedation have limited its widespread use in ophthalmology.[23] Among the three alpha agonists, clonidine is the most lipophilic, easily penetrating the corneal epithelium and endothelium and, unfortunately, the

Table 4.3 Alpha-Selective Agonists

Clonidine

Dichlorophenyl aminoimidazoline
Isoglaucon 0.125%, 0.2%, 0.5%

Apraclonidine

Apraclonidine
Iopidine 0.5%, 1%

Brimonidine tartrate

Alphagan-P 0.15%, 0.1%
Brimonidine 0.2%

blood–brain barrier.[24] Clonidine is a relatively selective alpha-2 agonist, having roughly 183 times more affinity for alpha-2 than for alpha-1 receptors. Nonetheless, clonidine causes mydriasis, an alpha-1 effect.[25] Tonographic investigations failed to demonstrate an effect on aqueous outflow, leading early researchers to conclude that clonidine reduces aqueous inflow.[26]

Clonidine was originally noted to lower IOP following intravenous administration.[27] Then, one-drop topical studies suggested that clonidine was a safe and effective ocular hypotensive agent;[28] however, long-term application of topical clonidine led to the discovery of the side effect of marked systemic hypotension. The German literature contains the first documentation of the ocular hypotensive effect of intravenous[27] and topical[28] clonidine. IOP reduction from topical clonidine 0.125% and 0.25% was equal to that of pilocarpine and lasted 8 hours, allowing three-times-daily usage.[29] These investigators found that long-term use of clonidine, even when applied topically, caused dramatic and dangerous shifts in systemic blood pressure. In half the subjects, systolic blood pressure fell 30 mm Hg, and in roughly one-third of subjects, diastolic pressure fell 30 mm Hg. The possible adverse effects of symptomatic hypotension, syncope, and sedation have limited the popularity of topical clonidine for glaucoma therapy.

4.4.2 Apraclonidine. The narrow therapeutic index of clonidine motivated the search for a compound that would retain clonidine's efficacy for lowering IOP but had a wider therapeutic index.

4.4.2.1 Pharmacology. Apraclonidine, a hydrophilic derivative of clonidine, achieves the substantial IOP reduction of clonidine without causing the centrally mediated side effects of systemic hypotension and drowsiness.[30] Hydrophilic molecules traverse the cornea and blood–brain barrier poorly. Apraclonidine is structurally similar to clonidine, except that it has a hydrophilic amide group at the C4 position of the imidazole (benzene) ring. This modification makes apraclonidine more hydrophilic, reducing systemic absorption and blood–brain barrier penetration, but it also makes the journey across the lipid-rich barrier of the corneal epithelium and endothelium more difficult. The corneal penetration coefficient of clonidine is 21.9 cm/s, nearly six times faster than apraclonidine, at 3.8 cm/s.[31] Given the poor penetration of apraclonidine, one group of investigators has even hypothesized that the route of ocular penetration for apraclonidine may be predominantly extracorneal.[24]

Apraclonidine retains moderate alpha-2–adrenoreceptor selectivity, having 72 times higher affinity for alpha-2 than for alpha-1 receptors.[24] Nonetheless, alpha-1 receptor activation by both 0.25% and 0.5% apraclonidine and its more alpha-2–selective cousin brimonidine 0.5% is sufficient to cause notable conjunctival blanching and eyelid retraction.[32,33]

4.4.2.2 Mechanism of action. Apraclonidine reduces IOP by reduced aqueous production, improved trabecular outflow, and reduced episcleral venous pressure. Modern techniques to determine a drug's mechanism of action rely heavily on the understanding of aqueous physiology modeled by the Goldmann equation:

$$IOP = P_{ev} + F - UC_{tm}$$

where

  IOP = intraocular pressure
  P_{ev} = episcleral venous pressure
  F = aqueous flow
  U = uveoscleral outflow
  C_{tm} = trabecular meshwork outflow facility

Each variable can be measured in humans directly or indirectly, except uveo-scleral outflow, which must be calculated from the others (table 4.4).

As should be clear from the equation, conclusive statements about mechanisms of action of glaucoma medications require precise measurement of at least three of the variables in the Goldmann equation—a formidable task. In studies that track only aqueous flow changes in response to a single drop of apraclonidine 1%, limited conclusions can be drawn, because two other independent variables (episcleral venous pressure and uveoscleral outflow) may not be constant after drug instillation. Authors of two such studies cautiously state that the observed IOP drop "could be explained" by an observed 30% to 45% decrease in aqueous flow in otherwise-untreated ocular hypertensive patients[34] and a 16% reduction in flow in glaucoma patients treated long term with timolol.[35] Based on the Goldmann equation, there may be some contribution from the unmeasured episcleral pressure or uveoscleral outflow. Similarly, a randomized, placebo-controlled, unilateral trial of apracloni-dine 1% found no significant change in tonographic outflow facility in treated eyes and concluded that decreased aqueous flow might be implicated.[36]

An elegant trial in ocular hypertensive patients challenges this theory and suggests that long-term use of apraclonidine lowers IOP through multiple mechanisms, principally by improving trabecular outflow facility.[10] The authors of this study endeavored to measure three of the four independent variables of the Goldmann equation, including IOP, P_{ev}, and C_{tm}. In agreement with prior work,[36] apracloni-dine had no effect on tonographic outflow facility. However, they did find that 1 week of unilateral apraclonidine 0.5% therapy lowered the IOP of the treated eye in ocular hypertensive patients primarily by increasing fluorophotometric outflow

Table 4.4 Techniques for Measuring Variables of Mechanism of Action

Variable	Measurement Technique
Episcleral venous pressure	Episcleral sphygmomanometry
Aqueous flow	Fluorophotometry: rate of reduction of aqueous fluorescein concentration gives rate of flow
Trabecular meshwork outflow facility	Dynamic fluorophotometry: changes in aqueous flow as intraocular pressure is lowered pharmacologically (old method: tonography)
Uveoscleral outflow	Cannot measure; must calculate from equation

facility (53%) and secondarily by reducing episcleral venous pressure (10%) and decreasing aqueous flow (12%). These researchers suggest that single-drop studies are affected by pseudofacility and that fluorophotometric techniques are more accurate when measuring flow parameters in a steady state.[10] Studies by Toris et al.[10,11] include measuring all three measurable variables in the Goldmann equation and testing patients who used apraclonidine long term. These design points raise the likelihood that their complex conclusions will stand the test of time.

4.4.2.3 *Safety*. Apraclonidine enjoys the widest therapeutic index for cardiovascular and central nervous system effects of the available alpha-2 agonists, with no or minimal effect on pulse, blood pressure, or alertness at approved dosages. The hydrophilic nature of apraclonidine may limit penetration of the blood–brain barrier, thereby reducing central hypotension and sedation. However, the contralateral ocular hypotensive effects of apraclonidine, similar to those of clonidine and brimonidine, suggest that the unilateral application of apraclonidine may reduce IOP through either central effects or contralateral peripheral action or both. Application of apraclonidine causes conjunctival, oral, and nasal vasoconstriction, leading to symptoms of dry nose and mouth and to a measurable reduction in conjunctival oxygen tension. One in vitro model of retinal circulation suggests that apraclonidine may constrict retinal arterioles; however, the existing evidence in humans suggests that apraclonidine probably does not induce retinal or optic nerve vasoconstriction in vivo. The principal use-limiting side effect of apraclonidine is allergy-like papillary conjunctivitis from long-term topical use.

Apraclonidine has little impact on human cardiovascular physiology when compared to clonidine. Examination of the safety of dosages approved by the FDA reveals little or no cardiovascular side effects of apraclonidine. In one double-masked, crossover study, normal female volunteers experienced no significant effects on blood pressure or exercise-induced tachycardia with either the 0.5% or the 0.25% apraclonidine concentration. By contrast, there was significant depression of heart rate in a group treated with timolol 0.5% who underwent treadmill testing.[9] In an uncontrolled, open-label investigation, a small, clinically insignificant reduction in diastolic blood pressure of 5 mm Hg was reported in normal volunteers using apraclonidine 0.5% or 1% twice daily for 1 month.[37]

The evidence suggests that apraclonidine does not cause sedation. While 10% of patients in the uncontrolled dose–response study complained of lethargy,[7] two prospective, placebo-controlled studies found no association between any dose of apraclonidine and fatigue in healthy volunteers[9] or glaucoma patients[16] using apraclonidine. These studies, however, had small enrollment and did not perform a rigorous symptom review with a validated survey instrument.

The most common acute symptom caused by apraclonidine is dosage-dependent dry nose or mouth, which affects 5% of subjects using 0.25% apraclonidine, 20% of those using 0.5% apraclonidine, and 57% of those using 1% apraclonidine.[7,36] Overall, these nasopharyngeal symptoms are mild and seem to diminish with time. Other detectable acute signs include transient eyelid retraction and subtle conjunctival blanching. Minimal mydriasis was measured, <0.5 mm in 45% of patients after treatment. The mydriasis is a sufficiently small effect that investigators have reported apraclonidine safe in patients with narrow-angle configuration. One case report has even described the use of apraclonidine to abort an attack of narrow-angle glaucoma.[38]

The known vasoactivity of alpha agonists has prompted evaluation of the vascular effects of ocular hypotensive agents on the optic nerve in glaucoma patients. Investigations described below suggest that topical apraclonidine therapy causes an acute reduction in blood flow in the anterior segment of the human eye,[39] but no vasoconstriction of the optic nerve or peripapillary retina has been identified in vivo. Unfortunately, optic nerve blood flow is difficult to measure directly in humans, and the vascular responses to alpha agonists can vary according to species, tissue, and even location within a given vascular bed,[40] making extrapolation from animal data uncertain.

Animal and human studies suggest that apraclonidine constricts anterior segment vasculature in rabbits and humans. Vascular casting studies of rabbit eyes show that treatment with apraclonidine causes constriction of the precapillary sphincters in the ciliary body,[41] but not of the anterior optic nerve vasculature.[42] In humans, apraclonidine causes a marked and prolonged reduction of conjunctival oxygen tension, lasting up to 5 hours.[39] Thus, apraclonidine would be a poor choice in patients with known ocular ischemic syndrome or advanced diabetic eye disease.

In certain animal models, apraclonidine can affect the retinal vasculature, but these effects have not been demonstrated in vivo. Human retinal xenografts in the cheek pouch of the newborn hamster offer a model for retinal vascular response to drugs. One such report found that, among the alpha agonists, clonidine induced the most retinal vasoconstriction, and brimonidine the least, with apraclonidine falling in between. Applied directly to the retina, apraclonidine produced a modest amount (15.9%) of retinal vascular constriction, after the lowest concentration (10^{-11} M), to a maximal 28% at the highest concentration (10^{-5} M). This in vitro finding is not supported by existing human studies: Doppler ultrasonography studies suggest that apraclonidine does not constrict retinal arterial or central ophthalmic artery flow.[43,44] Similarly, scanning laser Doppler flowmeter examinations in healthy human volunteers suggest that unilateral apraclonidine 0.5% does not reduce tissue perfusion in the neural rim or peripapillary retina of the treated eye compared to the contralateral eye.[45] Unfortunately, in these studies, investigators sought to demonstrate differences between the two eyes of an individual subject after unilateral application of apraclonidine. The known contralateral effects of apraclonidine would have minimized the apparent magnitude of a vasoactive effect in the treated eye. This raises the possibility that a small but deleterious effect on optic nerve or retinal blood flow due to apraclonidine may have been missed because of the study design.

No controlled investigation of an adrenergic agent suggests that these drugs cause vision loss. However, the concern that decreased blood flow might compromise vision led one group[46] to review the charts of apraclonidine users. Unfortunately, they did not include a control group or measure vision or blood flow in a validated fashion. This retrospective case series did find that 7% (14 of 185) patients lost two to four lines of vision over a mean of 7 weeks. Then, in a small subset of patients, the investigators measured the blood velocity within the short posterior ciliary arteries with color Doppler ultrasound. This technique is unable to determine flow without simultaneous measurement of the vessel diameter in question. Despite the lack of a control group to support the association or a validated technique for measuring blood flow, the researchers speculate that the vision loss might be due to reductions in perfusion of short posterior ciliary arteries. They qualify their conclusion by stating that "color Doppler as an estimate of optic nerve blood flow has not been established with certainty." No controlled investigation has suggested that apraclonidine, brimonidine, or clonidine promotes vision loss.

As with epinephrine and propine, the principal clinical side effect of apraclonidine 1% is a delayed allergy-like reaction, with prominent follicular conjunctivitis and periocular dermatitis in up to 48% of patients after a mean of 4.6 months.[47] The incidence of this reaction appears to be dose and time dependent. A 90-day, prospective, randomized trial yielded allergy rates of 9% (apraclonidine 0.25%) and 36% (apraclonidine 0.50%) versus none in the timolol 0.5% group.[48] Another 90-day trial found 13.8% incidence of allergy with apraclonidine 0.5% and 20.3% rate with apraclonidine 1%.[49] Other investigators report similar data.[46,50]

The cause of this delayed allergy-like reaction is unknown and may be either an increased susceptibility to external allergens or bioactivation and antigen formation of a specific part of the adrenergic molecule itself. Because epinephrine shrinks trabecular epithelial cells in vitro, Butler et al.[47] have hypothesized that adrenergically induced cell shrinkage may stress intercellular junctions, enabling the penetration of exogenous environmental allergens. Recent biochemical investigations suggest that apraclonidine allergy may be caused by oxidation of a hydroquinone-like subunit, which it shares chemically with its cousin epinephrine, but not with clonidine or brimonidine. This subunit is readily oxidized and may conjugate with thiol groups in ocular tissues, creating a potentially sensitizing hapten.[51] This theory requires further substantiation.

4.4.2.4 *Indications.* Apraclonidine indications include prophylaxis of acute IOP rise after ophthalmic anterior segment laser procedures:

4.4.2.4.1 *Argon laser trabeculoplasty.* Ironically, argon laser trabeculoplasty (ALT) was pioneered initially in part as a means of causing increased IOP and a novel primate model of open-angle glaucoma.[52] Thus, even after Wise and Witter[53] successfully demonstrated the IOP-lowering effect of lower energy ALT, the potential danger of IOP elevation following laser treatment remained.[54] And indeed, IOP elevations of at least 10 mm Hg were found in one-third of patients following 360° ALT.[55] The Glaucoma Laser Trial, a prospective, randomized, controlled trial, showed that treating half the trabecular meshwork led to some IOP rise in 54% of those treated. In 14% of the subjects, IOP rose 6 to 10 mm Hg, and in 7%, IOP rose 10 mm Hg above baseline.[56]

Several dramatic cases warn about the potential damage of post-ALT IOP spikes.[55] In an early randomized, double-masked study[55] comparing ALT of half versus the entire trabecular meshwork, investigators reported that one of the patients with exfoliative glaucoma and severe glaucomatous atrophy developed acute postlaser IOP elevation to a maximum of 62 mm Hg. This spike resulted in obliteration of the central island of vision and acuity loss within 24 hours. A similar case was reported in a series of 334 eyes with advanced glaucoma treated with ALT. In this study, one 83-year-old-man with phakic primary open-angle glaucoma who had a small central island lost vision after an ALT-induced IOP rise to 42 mm Hg, 3 days after ALT.[57]

While dramatic, the frequency of this type of dangerous field loss from a postlaser IOP spike in the average glaucoma patient is hard to gauge. These cases represent 2.5% of patients treated in the first study and 0.33% in the latter study. Because both cases noted above involved patients with end-stage glaucomatous optic neuropathy and only central islands of vision remaining, it is unclear whether the danger can be generalized to patients with mild or moderate glaucoma. Unfortunately, in the Glaucoma Laser Trial,[58] visual field results were not stratified by postlaser IOP response. Thus, it is not possible to evaluate whether those early glaucoma patients who participated in the Glaucoma Laser Trial and who had documented postlaser IOP rise suffered more rapid progression of visual field loss than did those whose IOP was not elevated transiently after the procedure.

The rationale for prophylaxis of post-ALT IOP spikes is as follows: At least 30% of axons in the optic nerve are irrevocably damaged in glaucoma patients before the first appearance of visual field defects.[59] And because the purpose of ALT is the reduction of IOP, any perioperative IOP elevation could be dangerous to the survival of retinal ganglion cell axons, even if immediate field loss is not apparent.

Robin et al.[60] found that apraclonidine 1% used perioperatively reduced the incidence of any IOP rise after ALT from 59% to 21%. More important, the percentage of eyes having a rise of 10 mm Hg fell from 18% to 0%. One randomized, multiple-treatment-arm study[61] compared the prophylactic efficacy of perioperative apraclonidine with pilocarpine 4%, timolol maleate 0.5%, dipivefrin 0.1%, and acetazolamide to reduce postoperative ocular hypertensive reactions following ALT. Apraclonidine proved superior to all of the other drugs, reducing IOP elevations above 5 mm Hg to 3% compared with 32% to 39% for all other tested medications. This finding was not entirely surprising, however, because apraclonidine was the only drop not used long term in any of the patients enrolled in the study. More than 90% of patients were already taking beta blockers long term: 72% to 86% epinephrine, 54% to 80% pilocarpine, and 16% to 25% carbonic anhydrase inhibitors. It may be that, if a drug is already in a patient's ciliary body from a morning application, use of the same drug may offer little additional benefit, unless sufficient time has elapsed for the drug to wash out. A subsequent study has shown that the long-term use of apraclonidine may reduce its efficacy in the prophylaxis of acute IOP elevation following ALT.[62] The investigators found that, among those patients naive to apraclonidine, only 3% experienced an IOP elevation of 5 mm Hg at 1 hour post-ALT. By contrast, those subjects who were long-term apraclonidine users at the time of ALT were four times more likely to experience an IOP elevation of at least 5 mm Hg at 1 hour after ALT. One trial compared the effect of using apraclonidine and pilocarpine together to the effect of using each agent alone.[63] The combination of apraclonidine and pilocarpine in patients naive to both appears slightly more effective than either drug alone. It appears that one drop of apraclonidine 1%, whether given 15 minutes or 60 minutes before ALT or just after ALT, is as effective as two drops in preventing IOP elevation.[64,65]

The FDA has approved the 1% concentration of apraclonidine for the prevention of postlaser IOP elevation, but the 0.5% apraclonidine solution has undergone limited testing, as well. One center has demonstrated equal efficacy between 0.5% and 1% apraclonidine when it is used both before and after ALT.[66] Another group found no difference between 0.5% and 1% apraclonidine when used just after ALT. This study, however, did not monitor IOP after 2 hours.[67]

The enhanced safety afforded by apraclonidine with ALT has enabled 360° treatment with apraclonidine 1% to be performed as safely as 180° ALT treatment without apraclonidine.[68] Apraclonidine's potency has led some clinicians to abandon the 24-hour postlaser IOP check.[69] While the case for apraclonidine's role in the prophylaxis of ALT-related IOP rise is well documented, the ultimate benefit to the average patient's visual field progression is uncertain. No prospective data are available on the benefit of prophylaxis, with clinical end points such as effect on visual acuity, visual field, color vision, vascular occlusions, progressive optic neuropathy, and glaucoma. The relatively low rate of documented field loss due to acute IOP rise after ALT[55,57] (between 0% and 2.5%) would make the numbers required to study in a prospective clinical trial rather large.

4.4.2.4.2 *Argon or Nd:YAG laser iridotomy.* The rationale for apraclonidine prophylaxis of laser iridotomy is similar to that for ALT. Roughly one-third of patients undergoing either argon or Nd:YAG laser iridotomy experience a marked IOP rise of 10 mm Hg or more.[70] Two drops of apraclonidine 1% have been proven to be highly effective in the prevention of IOP elevation following either argon or Nd:YAG laser iridotomy in white[71] and Hispanic American patients.[72]

4.4.2.4.3 *Nd:YAG laser capsulotomy.* The rationale for prophylaxis of IOP elevation after Nd:YAG laser capsulotomy is also similar to the rationale for prophylaxis after ALT. Numerous reports documenting IOP elevation in up to 59% of glaucomatous eyes undergoing Nd:YAG capsulotomy, combined with case reports of acute visual compromise in glaucoma patients after Nd:YAG laser capsulotomy, have generated understandable fears of this common phenomenon. Mechanisms of vision loss after Nd:YAG capsulotomy in one case included IOP-induced acute corneal edema and compromised chorioretinal perfusion, causing transient vision loss to light perception only.[73] In another case, a transient central retinal artery occlusion occurred, with transient loss of light perception.[74] In a third patient, with pre-existing field loss from primary open-angle glaucoma, Nd:YAG capsulotomy resulted in a prolonged (4- to 5-day) IOP elevation, peaking at 72 mm Hg. This patient developed progressive, permanent glaucomatous field loss just 4 weeks later.[75]

In pseudophakic eyes undergoing Nd:YAG laser capsulotomy, IOP increases to a maximum 31% higher than pretreatment levels, 41% having a rise of 5 mm Hg and 16% having a rise of 10 mm Hg or greater. Eyes of glaucoma patients undergo rises that are higher and longer lasting than do nonglaucomatous eyes, with 59% 5 mm Hg higher and 26% 10 mm Hg higher.[76] One multicentered, double-masked, placebo-controlled trial[77] found that apraclonidine 1% used 1 hour before and immediately after capsulotomy eliminated nearly all "clinically significant" IOP rise up to 3 hours. A cohort study using historical controls found that IOP rises exceeding 10 mm Hg were cut from 26% to 4% in glaucomatous eyes pretreated with apraclonidine.[76]

One investigation observed similar efficacy of apraclonidine 0.5% and 1% in the prophylaxis of IOP elevation after Nd:YAG laser capsulotomy, but IOP was monitored only 2 hours after the procedure.[67] Earlier dose–response data suggest a shorter duration of action for apraclonidine 0.5% versus the 1% concentration (8 hours vs. 12 hours, respectively). Thus, it is unlikely that the efficacy is truly equivalent over 24 hours.[7] One case report[78] warns of the limited protection that a single application of apraclonidine 1% affords. It points out that single-drop perioperative apraclonidine therapy may be insufficient to prevent marked IOP rise 24 to 48 hours following Nd:YAG capsulotomy, particularly when pigment is "polished" off the intraocular lens face. Therefore, while perioperative application of apraclonidine 1% has dramatically reduced the risk surrounding Nd:YAG laser capsulotomy, close follow-up is advised for patients undergoing secondary membrane discission or pigment "polishing," given the risk of late IOP rise.

Apraclonidine has been investigated in the treatment of ocular hypertension, as an adjunct to short- and long-term timolol use, as a surgery-sparing agent in patients with primary open-angle glaucoma failing maximum tolerable medical therapy, and in angle-closure glaucoma attacks.

1. Single-drop studies include one prospective, placebo-controlled trial of apraclonidine 0.5% and 1% in untreated ocular hypertensive patients that showed an acute 20% reduction in IOP compared to placebo within 2 hours and lasting up to 12 hours.[37] In a 1-week dose–response study of ocular hypertensive patients,[7] a 27% maximal IOP reduction was achieved compared to placebo, with either 0.25% or 0.5% apraclonidine at 2 to 5 hours. The peak hypotensive response with either concentration was equal in amplitude, but the duration of the response to apraclonidine 0.5% was longer than that of apraclonidine 0.25%. Longer term therapy with apraclonidine showed similar efficacy. A prospective comparison of apraclonidine or timolol in ocular hypertensive patients and mild glaucoma patients who completed 90 days of therapy showed that both groups achieved a similar IOP reduction of roughly 20% in the morning after a bedtime dose and again 20% reduction compared to baseline 8 hours after a morning dose. A rapid diminution of efficacy, or tachyphylaxis, was observed in only one patient (2%) treated with apraclonidine, and poor compliance was suspected.[48]

2. Several well-controlled studies have confirmed an additive IOP-lowering effect when apraclonidine is added to the regimen of open-angle glaucoma patients who use timolol long term. Morrison and Robin[16] demonstrated that a single drop of apraclonidine 1%, but not dipivefrin, given to patients with mild glaucoma treated long term with timolol resulted in an additional 15% to 18% reduction in IOP compared to placebo. A similar study demonstrated an average IOP reduction of 16.5% in the first 3 hours after a single drop of apraclonidine 1% was added to one eye of ocular hypertensive patients and early glaucoma patients treated long-term with either levobunolol 0.5% or timolol maleate 0.5%.[79] The authors suggest at least three-times-daily apraclonidine dosing in timolol users, because the additional effect lasted under 12 hours. A 3-month dose–response study of apraclonidine added to long-term timolol use in patients with mild glaucoma found equal efficacy of the 0.5% and 1% apraclonidine concentrations.[49]

3. Apraclonidine can also be used to lower IOP in patients failing maximum medical therapy.[50] Apraclonidine 0.5% three times daily added to one eye of patients with advanced glaucoma failing maximum medical therapy prevented or delayed by half the need for filtering surgery, compared to placebo alone. Of 174 patients randomized to apraclonidine or placebo, 60% of apraclonidine-treated patients, compared to 32% of placebo-treated patients, maintained adequate IOP control throughout the study and avoided surgery. Better responses were seen in patients with primary open-angle glaucoma not concurrently treated with beta blockers or carbonic anhydrase inhibitors. Since most patients requiring multiple agents for IOP control are usually taking brimonidine, the addition of apraclonidine is usually restricted to patients unable to tolerate such therapy.

4.4.3 *Brimonidine.* Initially investigated for the treatment of systemic hypertension, brimonidine is the latest alpha agonist to be approved by the FDA for the treatment of glaucoma and prophylaxis of laser-related IOP elevation. Despite similarities between apraclonidine and brimonidine, studies have shown limited cross-allergy, indicating that a reaction to one does not predict an allergy to the other.[80–82]

4.4.3.1 *Pharmacology.* In animal models, brimonidine is a highly alpha-2–selective agonist.[83] In the rabbit model, brimonidine is 7- to 12-fold more alpha-2 selective than clonidine and 23- to 32-fold more alpha-2 selective than apraclonidine. While initial studies with the first approved formulation of brominidine 0.5% had a fairly high rate of alpha-1–adrenergic side effects, such as conjunctival blanching and eyelid retraction,[84] more recent studies of the lower concentration 0.2% brominidine show a substantially improved side effect profile.[85–88] The newer formulation with Purite as the preservative agents and 0.15% brimonidine has been shown to be well tolerated and as effective in IOP lowering.[89] A lower concentration of brimonidine 0.1% has also been recently approved by the FDA as equally effective.

Brimonidine is less lipophilic than clonidine but more so than apraclonidine. Penetration of the cornea (and presumably the blood–brain barrier) is also intermediate between clonidine and apraclonidine.[24] While sedation and systemic hypotension were more common with 0.5% brimonidine, newer formulations have been better tolerated.[88,89]

4.4.3.2 *Mechanism of action.* Brimonidine reduces IOP in ocular hypertensive patients by reducing aqueous flow (20%) and possibly by increasing uveoscleral outflow.[90] Apraclonidine reduces aqueous flow and episcleral venous pressure but does not appear to improve uveoscleral outflow.[10,11] A central mechanism may account for part of the IOP reduction from brimonidine 0.2%, because a single-eye treatment trial for 1 week caused a statistically significant reduction of 1.2 mm Hg in the fellow eye.[11]

4.4.3.3 *Efficacy.* In the preclinical trial, a multicentered, double-masked, month-long, placebo-controlled trial[32] tested the efficacy of 0.08%, 0.2%, and 0.5% brimonidine in ocular hypertensive patients and patients with early glaucoma. All three concentrations reduced IOP throughout the month. A dose-dependent peak reduction of IOP of 16.1%, 22.4%, and 30.1%, respectively, was present in the first treatment week. At later time points, the dose effect was less direct, and the 0.2% brimonidine was as effective as the 0.5% brimonidine (and more effective at some averaged points). Over the later dates in the study, the reduction in IOP was in the 15.5% to 18.3% range. This is similar to the reduction in potency from 20% to 14% that was observed after 1 week of apraclonidine therapy.[7] Brimonidine's peak effect occurs at about 2 hours and, with the 0.2% and 0.5% concentrations, maintains significant albeit reduced effectiveness (14.5% and 12.0% reductions) after 8 hours. Several long-term studies have demonstrated IOP reductions comparable to timolol 0.5% with use of 0.2% brimonidine, with a mean peak reduction in IOP of 5.2 to 6.3 mm Hg (timolol) and 5.9 to 7.0 mm Hg (brimonidine), and similar side effect profiles, except for more reduction of heart rate in the timolol group.[86]

Brimonidine is also effective when added to other glaucoma mediations. When used as adjunctive therapy, a large retrospective study showed a 32.2% decrease in IOP by the addition of brimonidine to latanoprost and a 15.5% decrease in IOP when added to a beta blocker.[91] A direct comparison study with 24-hour diurnal measurements showed a 10.1% decrease in diurnal IOP when 0.15% brimonidine was added to latanoprost (which was equivalent to 2% dorzolamide in this study).[92] In another study of brimonidine added to combination timolol–dorzolamide treatment, more than 70% of the patients had a greater than 15% IOP reduction (the treatment goal in the study). This was equivalent to latanoprost added to fixed timolol–dorzolamide.[93] Another study compared a combination of brimonidine and latanoprost to timolol and dorzolamide and showed a decrease of 34.7% and 33.9% in two different arms of the study (which was greater than the timolol–dorzolamide reduction of 25.3% and 26.3%).[94]

4.4.3.4 *Safety*. As noted above, because the side effect profile of 0.5% brimonidine was less than ideal, lower concentration preparations are the only ones currently available in the United States and have a markedly reduced side effect profile.[85,86] Like apraclonidine, low-dose brimonidine 0.2% did not blunt exercise-induced tachycardia.[95]

A 1-year study[85] evaluated the safety and efficacy of long-term use of brimonidine 0.2% twice daily compared to timolol 0.5%. As with apraclonidine 0.25%, dry mouth and allergy were among the most common side effects in brimonidine-treated patients. Allergic blepharitis or conjunctivitis occurred in 9.6% of brimonidine-treated patients but in none of the timolol-treated patients. This is similar to the rate of allergy reported from low-dose apraclonidine 0.25% (9%) but less frequent than that found with the more common regimen for apraclonidine 0.5% (36%).[48] Fatigue and drowsiness were found to occur with similar frequency in the timolol and brimonidine groups. These long-term studies show allergy rates of 9%; dry mouth, 33%; fatigue, 19.9% (comparable to timolol at 17.9%); and hyperemia, 30.2%.[89]

Several studies have shown that patients that have had allergic reactions to apraclonidine could be safely treated with brimonidine, presumably due to the differences in chemical structure between the two molecules.[80–82]

4.4.3.5 *Indications.* Brimonidine indications include prophylaxis of postlaser IOP elevation (approved originally for 0.5%) and treatment of glaucoma and ocular hypertension (approved for 0.2%).

4.4.3.5.1 *Postlaser IOP rise.* Several placebo-controlled clinical trials of brimonidine have documented the efficacy of brimonidine 0.5% in the prevention of IOP elevation. Two peer-reviewed trials demonstrated that a single drop of brimonidine 0.5% given either 30 to 45 minutes before or just after ALT was effective in reducing the incidence of postlaser IOP elevation of 10 mm Hg from 23% among the placebo group to 2% or less in any brimonidine-treated patient. Table 4.5 shows the number of patients with IOP elevation of 5 and 10 mm Hg or greater following ALT when brimonidine 0.5% was used prophylactically before ALT, after ALT, and both before and after ALT.[84]

More recently, brimonidine 0.2% and 0.15% was compared to apraclonidine 0.5% and 1% for controlling IOP rise after anterior segment laser surgery and was found to be equally effective.[96,97] The unavailable 0.5% formulation is now not used for preventing IOP rise after laser procedures, but the 0.2% formulation (and others) is sometimes substituted for apraclonidine in allergic patients.

4.4.3.5.2 *Glaucoma and ocular hypertension.* Brimonidine may be used as primary or secondary treatment for open-angle glaucoma or ocular hypertension. Several long-term studies have demonstrated that brimonidine 0.2% has comparable peak IOP lowering, although slightly less trough IOP lowering, than timolol 0.5%. Both were equally effective at preventing visual field loss or visual acuity loss.[85,86] Since initial studies showed some decrease in effect over a 1-month study, the longer term data showing continued effectiveness is important.[88,98] Brimonidine is additive to timolol (4.4 mm Hg additional reduction), significantly better than dorzolamide 2% added to timolol.[99]

4.4.3.6 *Neuroprotection.* Medical or surgical reduction of IOP reduction is established as an effective treatment for open-angle glaucoma. Although investigational at this time, there is interest in the use of neuroprotective strategies for treatment of glaucoma. Ideally, treatments that directly prevent the loss of retinal ganglion cells

Table 4.5 Incidence of Intraocular Pressure Rise After Argon Laser Trabeculoplasty With Brimonidine 0.5%

Frequency of Administration	Number of Subjects	
	IOP >5 mm Hg	IOP >10 mm Hg
Before ALT ($n = 62$)	2	1
After ALT ($n = 61$)	3	0
Before and after ALT ($n = 60$)	2	0
Placebo ($n = 56$)	23	13

Source: David R, Spaeth GL, Clevenger, CE, et al. Brimonidine in the prevention of intraocular pressure elevation following argon laser trabeculoplasty. *Arch Ophthalmol.* 1993;111:1387–1390. See also Barnebey HS, Robin AL, Zimmerman TJ, et al. The efficacy of brimonidine in decreasing elevations in intraocular pressure after laser trabeculoplasty. *Ophthalmology.* 1993;100:1083–1088.

would be ideal, but since the exact mechanism of loss is not currently known, this has not been accomplished. Nevertheless, some agents have been suggested to have an effect on glaucoma that is independent of IOP. In animal models, brimonidine has been suggested to have a neuroprotective effect.[100,101] In the rat optic nerve crush system, intraperitoneal injection of 100 mg/kg preserved some optic nerve function.[102] In some human studies, brimonidine-treated patients were reported to have an improvement in their visual field testing.[103] In another human study, brimonidine and timolol were used to control IOP, and although the IOP control was the same, there was significant preservation of the retinal nerve fiber layer by scanning laser polarimetry in the brimonidine group.[104] While human studies have not conclusively shown neuroprotection, this is at least an encouraging area for further research.

4.5 CONCLUSION

Adrenergic agents lower IOP primarily through their alpha-2 stimulation, which lowers adenylate cyclase activity and reduces intracellular cAMP levels. Secondary mediators may include prostaglandins, but topical nonsteroidal anti-inflammatory drugs do not interfere with the efficacy of adrenergic agents in humans. Epinephrine, a nonspecific adrenergic agonist, increases aqueous flow and may raise IOP transiently, but long-term use lowers IOP and is additive to acetazolamide and pilocarpine. Dipivefrin is a more lipophilic prodrug of epinephrine that is converted by ciliary body esterases to epinephrine. Both dipivefrin and epinephrine are contraindicated in patients at risk for pupillary-block glaucoma and in patients with aphakia, hypertension, arrhythmia, or ischemic heart disease. Long-term therapy is discontinued in many patients because of a delayed allergy-like reaction.

Among alpha agonists, clonidine can lower IOP but is unpopular because of its side effects of severe systemic hypotension and sedation. Apraclonidine, a hydrophilic derivative of clonidine, lowers IOP by decreasing aqueous flow and reducing episcleral venous pressure. Apraclonidine 0.5% three times daily is safe and effective in the management of ocular hypertension and advanced glaucoma, although long-term use is hampered in many patients by a delayed allergy-like reaction. Apraclonidine 1% is indicated in the preoperative prophylaxis of acute IOP spikes associated with ALT, iridotomy, Nd:YAG laser capsulotomy, and cataract and glaucoma surgery. Apraclonidine reduces anterior segment blood flow and is therefore contraindicated in anterior segment ischemia and in advanced diabetic eye disease.

Brimonidine is an alpha-2–selective agonist. Brimonidine acts on alpha-2 and imidazole receptors and lowers IOP by decreasing aqueous flow and increasing uveoscleral outflow. The safety profile for long-term use of brimonidine 0.2% is similar to that for apraclonidine 0.5%, and the incidence of severe allergy-like reaction is somewhat lower. In very young children, it should be used with caution since the incidence of serious side effects increases (see chapter 13 for discussion of pediatric glaucoma). Lower concentrations of brimonidine available with newer preservative formulations have reduced the side effect profile further, without significantly reducing the IOP reducing effectiveness.

REFERENCES

1. Ahlquist RP. A study of the adrenotropic receptors. *Am J Physiol*. 1948;153:586–599.
2. Wax MB, Novack GD, Robin AL. Adrenergic agents. In: Albert DM, Jacobiec FA, eds. *Principles and Practice of Ophthalmology*. 2nd ed. Philadelphia: WB Saunders Co; 2000; Ch. 26, pp 267–300.
3. Brubaker RF, Gaasterland D. The effect of isoproterenol on aqueous humor formation in humans. *Invest Ophthalmol Vis Sci*. 1984;25:357–359.
4. Wang RF, Camras CB, Podos SM, et al. The role of prostaglandins in the para-aminoclonidine–induced reduction of intraocular pressure. *Trans Am Ophthalmol Soc*. 1989;87:94–104.
5. Sulewski ME, Robin AL, Cummings HL, Arkin LM. Effects of topical flurbiprofen on the intraocular pressure lowering of apraclonidine hydrochloride and timolol maleate. *Arch Ophthalmol*. 1991;109:807–809.
6. McCannel C, Koskela T, Brubaker RF. Topical flurbiprofen pretreatment does not block apraclonidine's effect on aqueous flow in humans. *Arch Ophthalmol*. 1991;109:810–811.
7. Jampel HD, Robin AL, Quigley HA, Pollack IP. Apraclonidine: a one-week dose–response study. *Arch Ophthalmol*. 1988;106:1069–1073.
8. Gabelt BT, Robinson JC, Hubbard WC, et al. Apraclonidine and brimonidine effects on anterior ocular and cardiovascular physiology in normal and sympathectomized monkeys. *Exp Eye Res*. 1994;59:633–644.
9. Coleman AL, Robin AL, Pollack IP, et al. Cardiovascular and intraocular pressure effects and plasma concentrations of apraclonidine. *Arch Ophthalmol*. 1990;108:1264–1267.
10. Toris CB, Tafoya ME, Camras CB, Yablonski ME. Effects of apraclonidine on aqueous humor dynamics in human eyes. *Ophthalmology*. 1995;102:456–461.
11. Toris CB, Gleason ML, Camras CB, Yablonski ME. Effects of brimonidine on aqueous humor dynamics in human eyes. *Arch Ophthalmol*. 1995;113:1514–1517.
12. Burke J, Crosson C, Potter D. Can UK-14,304–18 lower IOP in rabbits by a peripheral mechanism? *Curr Eye Res*. 1989;8:547–552.
13. Morales J, Ho P, Crosson CE. Effect of apraclonidine on intraocular pressure and pupil size in patients with unilateral Horner's syndrome. *Invest Ophthalmol Vis Sci*. 1992;34(suppl):929.
14. Robin A, Novack G. Alpha 2 agonist in the therapy of glaucoma. In: Drance SM, Neufeld AH, eds. *Glaucoma: Applied Pharmacology in Medical Treatment*. Orlando, FL: Grune & Stratton; 1991:103–124.
15. Becker B, Ley AP. Epinephrine and acetazolamide in the therapy of the chronic glaucomas. *Am J Ophthalmol*. 1958;45:639–643.
16. Morrison JC, Robin AL. Adjunctive glaucoma therapy: a comparison of apraclonidine to dipivefrin when added to timolol maleate. *Ophthalmology*. 1989;96:3–7.
17. Mackool RJ, Muldoon T, Fortier A, Nelson D. Epinephrine-induced cystoid macular edema in aphakic eyes. *Arch Ophthalmol*. 1977;95:791–793.
18. Kolker AE, Becker B. Epinephrine maculopathy. *Arch Ophthalmol*. 1968;79:552–562.
19. Albracht DC, LeBlanc RP, Cruz AM, et al. A double-masked comparison of betaxolol and dipivefrin for the treatment of increased intraocular pressure. *Am J Ophthalmol*. 1993;116:307–313.

20. Wei CP, Anderson JA, Leopold I. Ocular absorption and metabolism of topically applied epinephrine and a dipivalyl ester of epinephrine. *Invest Ophthalmol Vis Sci.* 1978;17:315–321.

21. Kass MA, Mandell AI, Goldberg I, et al. Dipivefrin and epinephrine treatment of elevated intraocular pressure: a comparative study. *Arch Ophthalmol.* 1979;97: 1865–1866.

22. Kohn AN, Moss AP, Hargett NA, et al. Clinical comparison of dipivalyl epinephrine and epinephrine in treatment of glaucoma. *Am J Ophthalmol.* 1979;87:196–201.

23. Hoffman BB, Lefkowitz RJ. Catecholamines and sympathomimetic drugs. In: Gilman AG, Rall TW, Nies AS, Taylor P, eds. *Goodman & Gilman's The Pharmacological Basis of Therapeutics.* 8th ed. New York: Pergamon Press; 1990:187–220.

24. Chien DS, Homsy JJ, Gluchowski C, Tang-Liu DD. Corneal and conjunctival/scleral penetration of *p*-aminoclonidine, AGN 190342, and clonidine in rabbit eyes. *Curr Eye Res.* 1990;9:1051–1059.

25. Krieglstein GK, Langham ME, Leydhecker W. The peripheral and central neural actions of clonidine in normal and glaucomatous eyes. *Invest Ophthalmol Vis Sci.* 1978;17:149–158.

26. Lee DA, Topper JE, Brubaker RF. Effect of clonidine on aqueous humor flow in normal human eyes. *Exp Eye Res.* 1984;38:239–246.

27. Makabe R. Ophthalmological studies with dichlorophenyl-aminoimidazoline with special regard to its effect on intraocular pressure. *Dtsch Med Wochenschr.* 1966;91: 1686–1688.

28. Hasslinger C. Catapresan (2-(2,6-dichlorphenylamino)-2-imidazoline-hydrochloride): a new intraocular pressure lowering agent. *Klin Monatsbl Augenheilkd.* 1969;154:95–105.

29. Hodapp E, Kolker A, Kass MA, et al. The effect of topical clonidine on intraocular pressure. *Arch Ophthalmol.* 1981;99:1208–1211.

30. Robin AL, Coleman A. Apraclonidine hydrochloride: an evaluation of plasma concentrations, and a comparison of its intraocular pressure lowering and cardiovascular effects to timolol maleate. *Trans Am Ophthalmol Soc.* 1990;88:149–162.

31. Coleman AL, Robin AL, Pollack IP. New ophthalmic drugs: apraclonidine hydrochloride. *Ophthalmol Clin North Am.* 1989;2:97–108.

32. Derick RJ, Robin AL, Walters TR, et al. Brimonidine tartrate: a one-month dose response study. *Ophthalmology.* 1997;104:131–136.

33. Brimonidine-ALT Study Group. Effect of brimonidine 0.5% on intraocular pressure spikes following 360° argon laser trabeculoplasty. *Ophthalmic Surg Lasers.* 1995;26: 404–409.

34. Gharagozloo NZ, Relf SJ, Brubaker RF. Aqueous flow is reduced by the alpha-adrenergic agonist, apraclonidine hydrochloride (ALO 2145). *Ophthalmology.* 1988: 95:1217–1220.

35. Gharagozloo NZ, Brubaker RF. Effect of apraclonidine in long-term timolol users. *Ophthalmology.* 1991;98:1543–1546.

36. Robin AL. Short-term effects of unilateral 1% apraclonidine therapy. *Arch Ophthalmol.* 1988;106:912–915.

37. Abrams DA, Robin AL, Pollack IP, et al. The safety and efficacy of topical 1% ALO 2145 (p-aminoclonidine hydrochloride) in normal volunteers. *Arch Ophthalmol.* 1987;105:1205–1207.

38. Krawitz PL, Podos SM. Use of apraclonidine in the treatment of acute angle closure glaucoma [letter]. *Arch Ophthalmol.* 1990;108:1208–1209.

39. Serdahl CL, Galustian J, Lewis RA. The effects of apraclonidine on conjunctival oxygen tension. *Arch Ophthalmol.* 1989;107:1777–1779.

40. Nichols AJ. Functions mediated by alpha-adrenoreceptors. In: Ruffolo RR, ed. *Alpha-Adrenoreceptors: Molecular Biology, Biochemistry, and Pharmacology.* New York: Karger; 1991:115–179.

41. Fahrenbach WH, Bacon DR, Van Buskirk EM. Vasoactive drug effects in the uveal vasculature of the rabbit: a corrosion casting study. *Invest Ophthalmol Vis Sci.* 1989;30(suppl):100.

42. Orgul S, Bacon DR, Van Buskirk EM, Cioffi GA. Optic nerve vasomotor effects of topical apraclonidine hydrochloride. *Br J Ophthalmol.* 1996;80:82–84.

43. Harris A, Caldemeyer KS, Mansberger SL, Martin BJ. α-Adrenergic agonists effects on ocular hemodynamics. *J Glaucoma.* 1995;4(suppl 1):S19–S23.

44. Celiker UO, Celibi S, Celiker H, Celibi H. Effect of topical apraclonidine on flow properties of central retinal and ophthalmic arteries. *Acta Ophthalmol.* 1996;74: 151–154.

45. Kim TW, Kim DM. Effects of 0.5% apraclonidine on optic nerve head and peripapillary retinal blood flow. *Br J Ophthalmol.* 1997;81:1070–1072.

46. Araujo SV, Bond JB, Wilson RP, et al. Long term effect of apraclonidine. *Br J Ophthalmol.* 1995;79:1098–1101.

47. Butler P, Mannschreck M, Lin S, et al. Clinical experience with the long-term use of 1% apraclonidine: incidence of allergic reactions. *Arch Ophthalmol.* 1995;113:293–296.

48. Nagasubramanian S, Hitchings RA, Demailly P, et al. Comparison of apraclonidine and timolol in chronic open-angle glaucoma: a three-month study. *Ophthalmology.* 1993;100:1318–1323.

49. Stewart WC, Ritch R, Shin DH, et al. The efficacy of apraclonidine as an adjunct to timolol therapy. Apraclonidine Adjunctive Therapy Study Group. *Arch Ophthalmol.* 1995;113:287–292.

50. Robin AL, Ritch R, Shin DH, et al. Short-term efficacy of apraclonidine hydrochloride added to maximum-tolerated medical therapy for glaucoma. Apraclonidine Maximum-Tolerated Medical Therapy Study Group. *Am J Ophthalmol.* 1995;120:423–432.

51. Thompson CD, Macdonald TL, Garst ME, et al. Mechanisms of adrenergic agonist induced allergy bioactivation and antigen formation. *Exp Eye Res.* 1997;64:767–773.

52. Gaasterland D, Kupfer C. Experimental glaucoma in the rhesus monkey. *Invest Ophthalmol.* 1974;13:455–457.

53. Wise JB, Witter SL. Argon laser therapy for open-angle glaucoma: a pilot study. *Arch Ophthalmol.* 1979;97:319–322.

54. Pollack IP, Patz A. Argon laser iridotomy: an experimental and clinical study. *Ophthalmic Surg.* 1976;7:22–30.

55. Weinreb RN, Ruderman J, Juster R, Zweig K. Immediate intraocular pressure response to argon laser trabeculoplasty. *Am J Ophthalmol.* 1983;95:279–286.

56. Glaucoma Laser Trial. I: acute effects of argon laser trabeculoplasty on intraocular pressure. Glaucoma Laser Trial Research Group. *Arch Ophthalmol.* 1989;107:1135–1142.

57. Thomas JV, Simmons RJ, Belcher D III. Argon laser trabeculoplasty in the presurgical glaucoma patient. *Ophthalmology.* 1982;89:187–197.

58. Glaucoma Laser Trial Research Group. The Glaucoma Laser Trial (GLT), 6: treatment group differences in visual field changes. *Am J Ophthalmol.* 1995;120:10–22.

59. Quigley HA, Addicks EM, Green WR. Optic nerve damage in human glaucoma, III: quantitative correlation of nerve fiber loss and visual field defect in glaucoma, ischemic neuropathy, papilledema, and toxic neuropathy. *Arch Ophthalmol*. 1982; 100:135–146.

60. Robin AL, Pollack IP, House B, Enger C. Effects of ALO 2145 on intraocular pressure following argon laser trabeculoplasty. *Arch Ophthalmol*. 1987;105:646–650.

61. Robin AL. Argon laser trabeculoplasty medical therapy to prevent the intraocular pressure rise associated with argon laser trabeculoplasty. *Ophthalmic Surg*. 1991;22: 31–37.

62. Chung HS, Shin DH, Birt CM, et al. Chronic use of apraclonidine decreases its moderation of post-laser intraocular pressure spikes. *Ophthalmology*. 1997;104: 1921–1925.

63. Dapling RB, Cunliffe IA, Longstaff S. Influence of apraclonidine and pilocarpine alone and in combination on post laser trabeculoplasty pressure rise. *Br J Ophthalmol*. 1994;78:30–32.

64. Birt CM, Shin DH, Reed SY, et al. One vs. two doses of 1.0% apraclonidine for prophylaxis of intraocular pressure spike after argon laser trabeculoplasty. *Can J Ophthalmol*. 1995;30:266–269.

65. Holmwood PC, Chase RD, Krupin T, et al. Apraclonidine and argon laser trabeculoplasty. *Am J Ophthalmol*. 1992;114:19–22.

66. Threlkeld AB, Assalian AA, Allingham RR, Shields MB. Apraclonidine 0.5% versus 1% for controlling intraocular pressure elevation after argon laser trabeculoplasty. *Ophthalmic Surg Lasers*. 1996;27:657–660.

67. Rosenberg LF, Krupin T, Ruderman J, et al. Apraclonidine and anterior segment laser surgery: comparison of 0.5% versus 1.0% apraclonidine for prevention of postoperative intraocular pressure rise. *Ophthalmology*. 1995;102:1312–1318.

68. Allf BE, Shields MB. Early intraocular pressure response to laser trabeculoplasty 180 degrees without apraclonidine versus 360 degrees with apraclonidine. *Ophthalmic Surg*. 1991;22:539–542.

69. Mittra RA, Allingham RR, Shields MB. Follow-up of argon laser trabeculoplasty: is a day-one postoperative IOP check necessary? *Ophthalmic Surg Lasers*. 1995;26:410–413.

70. Robin AL, Pollack IP. A comparison of neodymium:YAG and argon laser iridotomies. *Ophthalmology*. 1984;91:1011–1016.

71. Robin AL, Pollack IP, deFaller JM. Effects of topical ALO 2145 (*p*-aminoclonidine hydrochloride) on the acute intraocular pressure rise after argon laser iridotomy. *Arch Ophthalmol*. 1987;105:1208–1211.

72. Fernandez-Bahamonde JL, Alcaraz-Michelli V. The combined use of apraclonidine and pilocarpine during laser iridotomy in a Hispanic population. *Ann Ophthalmol*. 1990;22:446–449.

73. Blackwell C, Hirst LW, Kinnas SJ. Neodymium-YAG capsulotomy and potential blindness. *Am J Ophthalmol*. 1984;98:521–522.

74. Vine AK. Ocular hypertension following Nd:YAG laser capsulotomy: a potentially blinding complication. *Ophthalmic Surg*. 1984;15:283–284.

75. Kurata F, Krupin T, Sinclair S, Karp L. Progressive glaucomatous visual field loss after neodymium-YAG laser capsulotomy. *Am J Ophthalmol*. 1984;98:632–634.

76. Cullom RD Jr, Schwartz LW. The effect of apraclonidine on the intraocular pressure of glaucoma patients following Nd:YAG laser posterior capsulotomy. *Ophthalmic Surg Lasers*. 1993;24:623–626.

77. Pollack IP, Brown RH, Crandall AS, et al. Prevention of the rise in intraocular pressure following neodymium-YAG posterior capsulotomy using topical 1% apraclonidine. *Arch Ophthalmol.* 1988;106:754–757.

78. Nesher R, Kolker AE. Failure of apraclonidine to prevent delayed IOP elevation after Nd:YAG laser posterior capsulotomy. *Trans Am Ophthalmol Soc.* 1990;88: 229–236.

79. Yaldo MK, Shin DH, Parrow KA, et al. Additive effect of 1% apraclonidine hydrochloride to nonselective beta-blockers. *Ophthalmology.* 1991;98:1075–1078.

80. Gordon RN, Liebmann JM, Greenfield DS, Lama P, Ritch R. Lack of cross-reactive allergic response to brimonidine in patients with known apraclonidine allergy. *Eye.* 1998;12(pt 4):697–700.

81. Shin DH, Glover BK, Cha SC, et al. Long-term brimonidine therapy in glaucoma patients with apraclonidine allergy. *Am J Ophthalmol.* 1999;127:511–515.

82. Williams GC, Orengo-Nania S, Gross RL. Incidence of brimonidine allergy in patients previously allergic to apraclonidine. *J Glaucoma.* 2000;9:235–238.

83. Burke JA, Potter DE. Ocular effects of a relatively selective alpha 2 agonist (UK-14,304-18) in cats, rabbits and monkeys. *Curr Eye Res.* 1986;5:665–676.

84. David R, Spaeth GL, Clevenger CE, et al. Brimonidine in the prevention of intraocular pressure elevation following argon laser trabeculoplasty. *Arch Ophthalmol.* 1993;111:1387–1390.

85. Schuman JS. Clinical experience with brimonidine 0.2% and timolol 0.5% in glaucoma and ocular hypertension. *Surv Ophthalmol.* 1996;41(suppl 1):S27–S37.

86. Schuman JS, Horwitz B, Choplin NT, et al. A 1-year study of brimonidine twice daily in glaucoma and ocular hypertension. A controlled, randomized, multicenter clinical trial. Chronic Brimonidine Study Group. *Arch Ophthalmol.* 1997;115: 847–852.

87. LeBlanc RP. Twelve-month results of an ongoing randomized trial comparing brimonidine tartrate 0.2% and timolol 0.5% given twice daily in patients with glaucoma or ocular hypertension. Brimonidine Study Group 2. *Ophthalmology.* 1998; 105:1960–1967.

88. Katz LJ. Brimonidine tartrate 0.2% twice daily vs timolol 0.5% twice daily. 1-year results in glaucoma patients. Brimonidine Study Group. *Am J Ophthalmol.* 1999; 127:20–26.

89. Katz LJ. Twelve-month evaluation of brimonidine-Purite versus brimonidine in patients with glaucoma or ocular hypertension. *J Glaucoma.* 2002;11:119–126.

90. Toris CB, Camras CB, Yablonski ME. Acute versus chronic effects of brimonidine on aqueous humor dynamics in ocular hypertensive patients. *Am J Ophthalmol.* 1999; 128:8–14.

91. Lee DA, Gornbein JA. Effectiveness and safety of brimonidine as adjunctive therapy for patients with elevated intraocular pressure in a large, open-label community trial. *J Glaucoma.* 2001;10:220–226.

92. Konstas AG, Karabatsas CH, Lallos N, et al. 24-hour intraocular pressures with brimonidine Purite versus dorzolamide added to latanoprost in primary open-angle glaucoma subjects. *Ophthalmology.* 2005;112:603–608.

93. Akman A, Cetinkaya A, Akova YA, Ertan A. Comparison of additional intraocular pressure-lowering effects of latanoprost vs brimonidine in primary open-angle glaucoma patients with intraocular pressure uncontrolled by timolol-dorzolamide combination. *Eye.* 2005;19:145–151.

94. Zabriskie N, Netland PA. Comparison of brimonidine/latanoprost and timolol/dorzolamide: two randomized, double-masked, parallel clinical trials. *Adv Ther.* 2003;20:92–100.

95. Nordlund JR, Pasquale LR, Robin AL, et al. The cardiovascular, pulmonary, and ocular hypotensive effects of 0.2% brimonidine. *Arch Ophthalmol.* 1995;113:77–83.

96. Yuen NS, Cheung P, Hui SP. Comparing brimonidine 0.2% to apraclonidine 1.0% in the prevention of intraocular pressure elevation and their pupillary effects following laser peripheral iridotomy. *Jpn J Ophthalmol.* 2005;49:89–92.

97. Chen TC. Brimonidine 0.15% versus apraclonidine 0.5% for prevention of intraocular pressure elevation after anterior segment laser surgery. *Cataract Refract Surg.* 2005;31:1707–1712.

98. Derick RJ, Robin AL, Walters TR, et al. Brimonidine tartrate: a one-month dose response study. *Ophthalmology.* 1997;104:131–136.

99. Simmons ST. Efficacy of brimonidine 0.2% and dorzolamide 2% as adjunctive therapy to beta-blockers in adult patients with glaucoma or ocular hypertension. *Clin Ther.* 2001;23:604–619.

100. Wheeler LA, Gil DW, WoldeMussie E. Role of alpha-2 adrenergic receptors in neuroprotection and glaucoma. *Surv Ophthalmol.* 2001;45(suppl 3):S290–S294.

101. WoldeMussie E, Ruiz G, Wijono M, Wheeler LA. Neuroprotection of retinal ganglion cells by brimonidine in rats with laser-induced chronic ocular hypertension. *Invest Ophthalmol Vis Sci.* 2001;42:2849–2855.

102. Yoles E, Wheeler LA, Schwartz M. α2-Adrenoreceptor agonists are neuroprotective in a rat model of optic nerve degeneration. *Invest Ophthalmol Vis Sci.* 1999;40:65–73.

103. Ruiz LC, Ruiz LA, Link B. Influence of topical brimonidine on visual field in glaucoma. *Eur J Ophthalmol.* 2001;11(suppl 2):S67–S71.

104. Tsai JC, Chang HW. Comparison of the effects of brimonidine 0.2% and timolol 0.5% on retinal nerve fiber layer thickness in ocular hypertensive patients: a prospective, unmasked study. *J Ocul Pharmacol Ther.* 2005;21:475–482.

Cholinergic Drugs

B'ANN TRUE GABELT AND PAUL L. KAUFMAN

Cholinomimetics are the senior citizens of glaucoma therapy, and the mechanism underlying their efficacy has been considered to be the most straightforward of all the drug classes used. Although they have been supplanted by newer medications over the past three decades, they are still useful in carefully selected patients, such as open-angle glaucoma patients who are presbyopes with clear lenses or pseudophakes, and angle-closure glaucoma patients.

5.1 MECHANISM OF ACTION

Cholinergic drugs mimic the effects of acetylcholine (ACh), which is a transmitter at postganglionic parasympathetic junctions, as well as at other autonomic, somatic, and central synapses. ACh is synthesized by the enzyme choline acetyltransferase and produces its effects by binding to cholinergic receptors at the effector site.[1]

ACh, released from vesicles in nerve terminals, is then hydrolyzed within a few milliseconds by acetylcholinesterase (AChE). This rapid destruction of ACh frees the cholinergic receptors in preparation for the next stimulation. Cholinergic drugs act either directly by stimulating cholinergic receptors or indirectly by inhibiting the enzyme cholinesterase, thereby protecting endogenous ACh.[1]

The modified Goldmann equation can be used to describe the hydraulics of aqueous humor dynamics as follows:

$$F = C_{trab} (IOP - P_e) + U$$

where

> F = aqueous humor flow
>
> C_{trab} = facility of outflow from the anterior chamber via the trabecular meshwork (TM) and Schlemm's canal
>
> IOP = intraocular pressure
>
> P_e = episcleral venous pressure (the pressure against which fluid leaving the anterior chamber via the trabecular–canalicular route must drain)
>
> U = uveoscleral outflow

If we rearrange the equation to isolate IOP, it is apparent that for a modality (e.g., a drug) to lower IOP, it must either decrease F or P_e, or increase C_{trab} or U.[2]

Cholinergic drugs have been used in glaucoma therapy for more than a century.[3] They have a minimal effect on aqueous humor formation and episcleral venous pressure.[1] Rather, their effect on IOP is the result of various actions on aqueous humor outflow, which have been thought consequent to agonist-induced, muscarinic receptor–mediated contraction of the ciliary muscle.

Ciliary muscle contraction can affect aqueous outflow in two ways. Because there is no epithelial or endothelial barrier separating the spaces between the trabecular lamellae from those between the ciliary muscle bundles, in the absence of cholinergic stimulation, aqueous humor is free to flow down a pressure gradient from the former to the latter, and then into the suprachoroidal space, through the sclera, and into the orbit (figure 5.1).[1] This posterior, unconventional, or uveoscleral route can account for nearly one-third of aqueous drainage in normal young monkeys[4] but less in older primates.[5] Ciliary muscle contraction obliterates the intermuscular spaces (figure 5.2),[6,7] obstructing uveoscleral outflow.[8]

The other way in which ciliary muscle contraction can affect IOP is by increasing conventional outflow facility. There is an intimate anatomic relationship between the anterior tendons of the ciliary muscle bundles and the scleral spur, peripheral cornea, TM, and inner wall of Schlemm's canal.[9,10] One function of some of these tendons is to anchor the muscle to the spur and the cornea. Other tendons splay out and intermingle with the elastic network within the TM (figure 5.3), ultimately inserting onto specialized regions on the surface of the inner wall endothelial cells via connecting fibrils. Muscle contraction results in an unfolding of the meshwork and widening of the canal, facilitating aqueous outflow from the anterior chamber through the mesh into the canal lumen and thence into the venous collector channels and the general venous circulation.[1,11] Facilitation of outflow via the conventional route more than compensates for the obstruction of the uveoscleral route; thus, the net effect of ciliary muscle contraction is to decrease IOP.[12]

Cholinomimetic drug effects on IOP have been presumed to be due to these biomechanical consequences of ciliary muscle contraction, with little or no effect due to iris sphincter constriction[13] (except in angle closure, e.g., pupillary block and plateau iris, where sphincter contraction pulls the iris root away from the TM). Total removal of the iris from the monkey eye does not alter the facility response to pilocarpine, indicating that neither miosis nor even the presence of the iris is necessary for the response.[14] The pilocarpine effect on outflow facility is abolished if the anterior tendons of the ciliary muscle are severed (figure 5.4),[15]

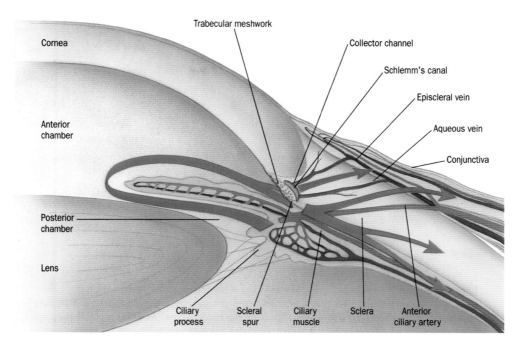

Figure 5.1. Primate anterior ocular segment. Arrows indicate aqueous flow pathways. Aqueous is formed by the ciliary processes, enters the posterior chamber, flows through the pupil into the anterior chamber, and exits at the chamber angle via trabecular and uveoscleral routes. Redrawn with permission from figure 4 (p. 160) of Kaufman PL, Wiedman, T, Robinson JR. Cholinergics. In: Sears ML, ed. *Pharmacology of the Eye.* New York: Springer-Verlag; 1984:149–191. *Handbook of Experimental Pharmacology*; Vol 69. Copyright 1984 Springer-Verlag GmbH & Co KG.

indicating the necessity of the muscle–meshwork attachment and the absence of a facility-relevant effect directly on the cells of the TM or of Schlemm's canal.

Pilocarpine is only a partial agonist[16,17] and is atypical in other ways. Uncertainty remains as to whether there is also some effect of cholinergic agonists on the TM itself. The cholinomimetic agonist aceclidine increases outflow facility in monkey eyes after ciliary muscle disinsertion, although the disinsertion may not have been complete.[18] Cultured TM cells produce second messengers in response to physiologic concentrations of carbachol.[19] Perfused organ cultured human eyes devoid of the ciliary muscle exhibit an increase in outflow facility in response to very low doses of cholinergic agonist, but not to higher doses.[20] However, this effect of low doses of pilocarpine on outflow facility could not be reproduced in intact monkey eyes in vivo.[21] The TM itself may have a contractile biology, possibly mediated via a muscarinic mechanism and with relevance to aqueous outflow.[22–24] Muscarinic receptors, primarily of the M3 subtype, have been identified in cultured human TM cells.[19] Excised bovine TM strips exhibit contractile responses to the muscarinic agonist carbachol, aceclidine, and pilocarpine.[25] However, in vivo contractility of the TM, possibly mediated by muscarinic mechanisms, may be overshadowed by the

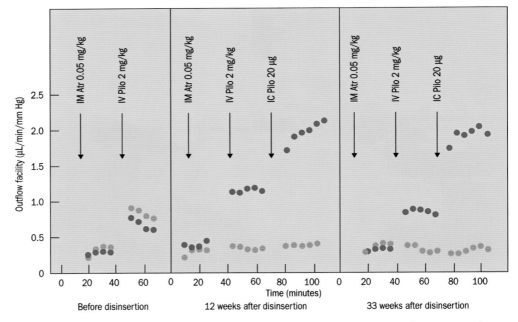

Figure 5.4. Outflow facility and facility responses to intravenous (IV) and intracameral (IC) pilocarpine hydrochloride (Pilo) before and after unilateral ciliary muscle disinsertion in a typical bilaterally iridectomized cynomolgus monkey. Intramuscular (IM) atropine sulfate (Atr) was given before each perfusion to minimize systemic effects of intravenous pilocarpine. Note the absence of facility increase following intravenous and intracameral pilocarpine in the iridectomized and disinserted eye (orange circles), as opposed to large facility increases in opposite iridectomized-only eye (blue circles). Redrawn with permission from Kaufman PL, Bárány EH. Loss of acute pilocarpine effect on outflow facility following surgical disinsertion and retrodisplacement of the ciliary muscle from the scleral spur in the cynomolgus monkey. *Invest Ophthalmol.* 1976;15:793–807. Copyright 1976 Association for Research in Vision and Ophthalmology.

5. Intraocular surgery: may be complicated by severe uveitis
6. Marked vagotonia

Echothiophate and demecarium may decrease plasma concentrations or activity of pseudocholinesterase, the enzyme that metabolizes succinylcholine, thereby enhancing the neuromuscular blockade effect of depolarizing muscle relaxants, such as succinylcholine, when they are used concurrently. In this case, cardiovascular collapse, increased or prolonged respiratory depression, or paralysis may occur. The effects of this interaction may persist for weeks or months after echothiophate has been discontinued.

Caution is recommended in administering edrophonium to patients with symptoms of myasthenic weakness who are also using echothiophate. Symptoms of cholinergic overdosage crisis—sweating, salivation, nausea, tremors, slowing of the pulse, and decrease in blood pressure—may be similar to those occurring with myasthenic crisis (underdosage), and the patient's condition may be worsened by use of edrophonium.

5.3 INDICATIONS AND TREATMENT

Pilocarpine is used in the long-term treatment of glaucoma; it is generally administered as a 0.5% to 4.0% aqueous solution four times per day. It is the standard cholinergic agent for treatment of open-angle glaucoma. During episodes of acute primary angle-closure glaucoma with pupillary block, 1% or 2% pilocarpine is administered two or three times over a 30-minute period to produce miosis once IOP has been lowered by secretory supressants and hyperosmotic agents to the point where iridial blood flow has been restored. Miosis pulls the peripheral iris away from the TM, thereby allowing aqueous humor to leave the eye. The miotic action of pilocarpine is also occasionally utilized to overcome the mydriasis produced by anticholinergics or sympathomimetics. Alternated with mydriatics, pilocarpine is employed to break adhesions between the iris and the lens. Pilocarpine has been used in the treatment of Adie's syndrome.[27] Prolonged drug delivery may be accomplished through the use of polymer emulsions[28] or gels.[29,30]

Carbachol in 0.75% to 3.0% solution is used three times daily to decrease IOP in open-angle glaucoma. The 0.01% solution (0.5 mL) is given intracamerally at the conclusion of cataract surgery to prevent postsurgical IOP elevation or to produce miosis during ocular surgery.

Because of its toxicity, echothiophate should be reserved for patients with one of the following conditions:

1. Open-angle glaucoma not satisfactorily controlled with short-acting miotics and other agents
2. Primary open-angle or nonuveitic secondary open angle glaucoma
3. Angle-closure glaucoma after iridectomy
4. Accommodative esotropia, because echothiophate enhances the cyclotonic effect of parasympathetic neuronal input to the ciliary muscle, necessitating less input to achieve accommodation and thus stimulating less accommodation-linked convergence

Echothiophate iodide is marketed as a powder accompanied by a separately packaged diluent; the two are mixed for clinical use. The 0.03% solution is the most commonly employed strength for treatment of open-angle glaucoma and accommodative esotropia. Demecarium bromide is available as 0.125% or 0.25% solutions and is applied once or twice a day.

Table 5.1 summarizes the cholinergic drugs used to treat glaucoma.

5.4 SIDE EFFECTS

As with any topical agent, transient symptoms of stinging and burning may occur with cholinomimetic therapy. Conjunctival vascular congestion and true allergy

Table 5.1 Cholinergic Drugs Available for Glaucoma Therapy[a]

Drug	Concentration	Dosing
Aceclidine[b]	0.5% to 4%	qid
Carbachol		
Isopto carbachol	0.75% to 3%	up to tid
Miostat	0.01% (1.5 mL vial)	Intracameral
Demecarium		
Humorsol	0.125% to 0.25%	q 12 or 24 h
Echothiophate iodide		
Phospholine Iodide	0.03 to 0.25%	q 12–48 h
Isoflurophate[b]		
DFP, Floropryl	0.025% ointment	q 8–72 h
Physostigmine		
Eserine sulfate	0.25% ung	up to tid
Isopto Eserine	0.25% to 0.5%	qid
Pilocarpine HCl (most available and commonly used cholinergic)		
Adsorbocarpine	2%	qid
Akarpine[b]	1, 2, 4 %	qid
Isopto Carpine	0.5% to 6%	qid[c]
Ocu-Carpine	0.5% to 6%	qid
Miocarpine[b]	1% to 6%	qid
Mistura P[b]	0.5% to 4%	qid
Pilocar	0.5% to 6%	bid to qid
Pilocarpine HCl	0.5% to 6%	qid
Pilogel[b]	40 mg/g	qhs
Pilopine HS	4% gel	qhs
Piloptic	1% to 6%	qid
Pilostat	1% to 4%	qid
Betoptic Pilo[b]	1.75% (+0.25% betaxolol)	bid
E-Pilo-1–6	1% to 6% (+1% ephedrine bitartrate)	qid
Isopto P-ES[b]	2% (+0.25% physostigmine)	qid
P1E1	1% (+1% epinephrine bitartrate)	qid
Pilocarpine–timolol combinations[b]		
Timpilo	2, 4% (+0.5% timolol)	qid
Fotil	2, 4% (+0.5% timolol)	qid
Pilocarpine nitrate		
Pilagan	1%, 2%, 4%	qid
Pilofrin	0.5% (+0.12% phenylephrine HCl)	qid

[a]If available in the United States, then only those brands are listed.

[b]Not used in the United States.

[c]Twice-daily application may suffice for light eyes.

Source: Red Book. Thomson Micromedix Healthcare Series. Greenwood Village, CO: Thomson Micromedix; 2006.

may occur but are unusual. Recent evidence suggests that prolonged use of topical glaucoma drug therapy, including pilocarpine, may increase inflammatory cells in the conjunctival tissues, making subsequent glaucoma filtration surgery more likely to fail.[31,32] Intraocular vascular congestion may occur in, and aggravate, uveitic conditions. Following long-term use of the strongest indirect-acting cholinomimetics, dilation of blood vessels and resulting greater permeability can increase postoperative inflammation ad may increase the risk of hyphema during ophthalmic surgery.[33] Ciliary spasm, temporal or supraorbital headache, and induced myopia may occur, all consequent to drug-induced contraction of the ciliary muscle; this is most common in young, prepresbyopic patients. Reduced visual acuity in poor illumination is frequently experienced by older individuals and those with lens opacities, consequent to miosis reducing the amount of light reaching the retina through an already partly opaque lens. Young individuals with clear lenses are rarely bothered by the miosis. A few cases of retinal detachment have been attributed to pilocarpine in certain susceptible individuals. Some evidence suggests that long-term use of pilocarpine may accelerate the development of lens opacities, but this is not proven conclusively. Intense miosis and cyclotonia produced at the higher doses may, respectively, increase pupillary block or induce ciliary block sufficiently to induce angle-closure glaucoma in susceptible individuals.

The primate ciliary muscle is structurally unique, exhibiting three distinct morphologic regions: an outer, longitudinal portion; an inner, apical circular portion; and an intermediate, obliquely oriented reticular region. The appearance, relative sagittal section area, and topographic interrelationship of the three regions differ in the relaxed versus cholinergic-agonist–contracted muscle (figure 5.5).[34] Histochemical and ultrastructural differences exist between different regions of the ciliary muscle,[35] more than one subtype of muscarinic receptor may be present, and the receptor subtypes may differ between regions.[36–39] In monkeys, topical or intracameral pilocarpine induces a greater facility response per diopter of accommodation than does systemic pilocarpine,[40] and in humans topical pilocarpine increases facility more per diopter of accommodation than does voluntary near focus.[41] This finding suggests selective cholinomimetic stimulation of receptor subtypes may permit separation of desirable and undesirable ocular side effects. However, in monkeys, one subtype (the M3 subtype) appears to modulate the outflow facility and the accommodative and miotic responses to pilocarpine and aceclidine. The concentrations of these agonists required to produce an effective outflow facility response also induce miosis.[42,43] More recently, a muscarinic agonist with no activity at the M3 subtype was able to lower IOP in a monkey glaucoma model.[44]

Some glaucoma patients become refractory to the IOP-lowering effects of pilocarpine during long-term therapy, even when successively higher doses are given. The mechanism underlying this phenomenon is unclear. It could be consequent to worsening of the outflow disease or to desensitization. Responsiveness to cholinergic drugs may be mediated in part by muscarinic receptor content of the smooth muscle (figure 5.6).[45–49] Topical treatment of the monkey eye with echothiophate drops, sustained-release pilocarpine delivery systems, or a single dose of carbachol under a contact lens causes decreased responsiveness to cholinergic agonists in the accommodative and aqueous outflow mechanisms, attributed to agonist-induced cholinergic

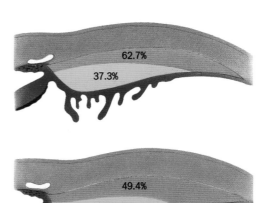

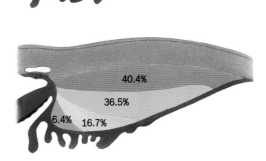

Figure 5.5. Results of morphometric analysis of ciliary muscle of vervet monkeys during relaxation (A) and during moderate (B) and strong (C) contraction induced by pilocarpine: area of longitudinal (dark orange), reticular (light orange), reticular plus circular (yellow), and purely circular (green) muscle portions as percentages of the entire muscle area. Modified with permission from figures 4 and 5 (pp. 127 and 128) of Lütjen E. Histometrische Untersuchungen über den Ziliarmuskel der Primaten. [Histometric studies on the ciliary muscle in primates.] *Graefes Arch Klin Exp Ophthalmol.* 1966;171:121–133. Copyright 1966 Springer-Verlag GmbH & Co KG.

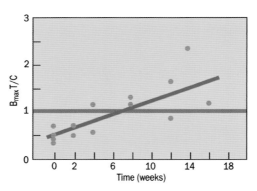

Figure 5.6. Ciliary muscle muscarinic receptor content at various times after discontinuing 2 weeks of twice-daily unilateral topical echothiophate iodide. B_{max} for each animal is expressed as the ratio of treated (T) eye to control (C) eye; B = binding; blue line represents least-squares linear regression; R (correlation coefficient) = 0.76; P (probability that R = 0) = 0.002. Green line represents T/C = 1.0, that is, equal B_{max} values in treated eye and control eye. Redrawn with permission from Croft MA, Kaufman PL, Erickson-Lamy K, Polansky JR. Accommodation and ciliary muscle muscarinic receptors after echothiophate. Invest Ophthalmol Vis Sci. 1991;32:3288–3297.

subsensitivity in the ciliary muscle. Functional recovery occurs when agonist treatment is discontinued,[50–53] even in the face of permanent anatomic abnormalities in the ciliary muscle and TM.[54,55]

Corneal toxicity, conjunctival and intraocular vascular congestion, fibrinous iritis (especially in predisposed individuals or following intraocular surgery), retinal detachment (in predisposed individuals), lacrimal canalicular stenosis, posterior synechiae, iris cysts, angle closure, and, most important, cataracts may occur especially with cholinesterase inhibitors.

Systemic toxicity following appropriate topical ocular administration is extremely rare. Theoretically, sensitive individuals may develop sweating and gastrointestinal overactivity following suggested dosage and administration, but this is much more likely to occur with inappropriate dosing and/or in children because of their lower body weight. Overdosage can produce sweating, salivation, nausea, tremors, slowing of the pulse, and a decrease in blood pressure. In moderate overdosage, spontaneous recovery is to be expected and is aided by intravenous fluids to compensate for dehydration. For severe poisoning, atropine is the pharmacologic antagonist to pilocarpine.

Frequency of dosage is an important factor in systemic toxicity. Pure echothiophate powder should never be applied directly to the eye, because serious systemic poisoning will result.

5.5 DRUG INTERACTIONS

A combination of outflow-enhancing with inflow-suppressing compounds can be used to decrease IOP further than with maximal doses of either compound alone. Combining different classes within the outflow-enhancing or inflow-suppressing groups may also lead to a greater IOP reduction than with either alone. However, the IOP response to a combination of drugs is usually less than the sum of the individual effects.

The IOP reduction caused by cholinergics may be partially additive to that of the uveoscleral outflow-enhancing prostaglandin (PG) derivative latanoprost. This finding has caused some confusion in the ophthalmologic community, given pilocarpine's ability to contract the ciliary muscle and thereby reduce uveoscleral outflow and the ability of high pilocarpine doses to inhibit the IOP-lowering effect of $PGF_{2\alpha}$ in monkeys. Ciliary muscle contraction is probably not maximal at the concentrations of miotics used clinically; therefore, some PG most likely can still penetrate the spaces between ciliary muscle bundles to initiate changes that enhance uveoscleral outflow.[56] Latanoprost is indeed less additive to stronger miotic therapies, where spaces between ciliary muscle bundles presumably would be more completely obliterated.[57] One study noted that latanoprost and eserine were partially additive, but that neither the eserine dosing regimen nor clinically employed pilocarpine dosing contracts the ciliary muscle in the living human maximally for very long, if at all.[58] Furthermore, even massive doses of cholinomimetics do not completely eliminate uveoscleral outflow in monkeys,[59] and $PGF_{2\alpha}$ can partly relax even a maximally cholinergically precontracted ciliary muscle.[60] Thus, some PG can be expected to reach the relevant parts of the ciliary muscle even if the only access is via the anterior chamber, and even more so if a transconjunctival–transscleral penetration pathway is operative. The net result, assuming no other factors, is partial but not complete attenuation and partial but not complete additivity of cholinomimetics to PG-induced ocular hypotension.

Conversely, because $PGF_{2\alpha}$ relaxes the cholinomimetically precontracted ciliary muscle,[60] latanoprost and $PGF_{2\alpha}$ may actually enhance the IOP-lowering effect of cholinomimetics by inhibiting their obstruction of uveoscleral outflow, in addition to enhancing uveoscleral outflow themselves. However, PG-induced relaxation of the ciliary muscle might also reduce cholinomimetic enhancement of facility via the TM route, which depends upon contraction of the muscle.[2] Furthermore, a small PG enhancement of facility via the TM cannot be entirely excluded in humans.[61] The apparent effect of the eicosanoids on cholinomimetic-induced IOP lowering will be the net resultant of these processes.

Pilocarpine may also be used to control IOP in combination with beta-adrenergic antagonists, carbonic anhydrase inhibitors, alpha-2– or beta-2–adrenergic agonists, or hyperosmotic agents. Concurrent local use of anticholinergic drugs will interfere with the action of pilocarpine; appropriate doses of systemic anticholinergics usually will not, because of insufficient ocular drug levels. Use of ophthalmic physostigmine prior to echothiophate may partially attenuate the magnitude and duration of the effects of the latter, because the short-acting physostigmine binds to and protects the cholinesterase enzyme until the echothiophate has diffused.[33]

Concurrent use of echothiophate with ester-derived local mucosal or parenteral anesthetics may inhibit the metabolism of these anesthetics, leading to prolonged anesthetic effect and increased risk of toxicity.

Exposure of patients using echothiophate to carbamate (e.g., aldicarb, methomyl, carbofuran) or organophosphate-type insecticides or pesticides (e.g., malathion, parathion, fenitrothion, mevinphos) may increase the possibility of systemic effects because the insecticide or pesticide is absorbed through the respiratory tract or skin.

Inhibition of cholinesterase activity by echothiophate reduces or slows cocaine metabolism, thereby increasing and/or prolonging cocaine's effects and increasing the risk of toxicity.

5.6 RESULTS OF CLINICAL TRIALS

Major clinical trials of cholinomimetics have not been undertaken, because the compounds were already in use before the methodology for clinical trials was standardized. However, numerous smaller studies have documented their safety, efficacy, and mode of action.

5.7 DIRECT, SHORT-ACTING DRUGS

Muscarine, pilocarpine, aceclidine (3-acetoxyquinuclidine), arecoline, and acetyl-beta-methylcholine (methacholine) are examples of direct-acting muscarinic drugs;

they directly stimulate muscarinic receptors to initiate a response.[1,3,27,33,62,63] Carbachol (carbamylcholine) is both a direct-acting muscarinic agonist and a direct-acting nicotinic agonist, in addition to having indirect agonist activities (i.e., it increases drug activity by inhibiting the degradative enzyme cholinesterase). Aceclidine is also slightly cholinesterase resistant and has weak anticholinesterase activity.

5.7.1 Pilocarpine

Chemical Structure	
Composition	$C_{11}H_{16}N_2O_2$

5.7.1.1 Formulations. The official drug name for pilocarpine is (3S-*cis*)-3-ethyldihydro-4-[(1-methyl-1H-imidazol-5-yl)methyl]-2(3H)-furanone] Brand names are listed in table 5.1. Pilocarpine hydrochloride solutions usually contain methylcellulose or a similar polymer and range in concentrations from 0.5% to 6%. Pilocarpine nitrate solutions range from 0.5% to 4%. The usual vehicles for pilocarpine are hydroxypropyl methylcellulose and polyvinyl alcohol. Benzalkonium chloride and sodium EDTA are added to prevent microbial growth. When maintained in a buffered, slightly acid solution, pilocarpine is indefinitely stable, retaining full activity at 6 months. Its effectiveness is maintained across a broad temperature range.

Pilocarpine is also formulated in a high-viscosity gel. In one study of adults with elevated IOP, a single dose of pilocarpine 4% gel applied at bedtime was approximately equal in effect to pilocarpine 2% or 4% eye drops applied four times daily, although the effect waned somewhat near the end of the 24-hour period.

Pilocarpine polymer is an aqueous emulsion consisting of a polymeric material to which pilocarpine base is chemically bound. The drug is released over a period of hours as the polymer is hydrolyzed.

Pilocarpine has also been combined in solution with other glaucoma therapeutics such as betaxolol, epinephrine, and physostigmine (table 5.1).

While pilocarpine is an inexpensive and effective IOP-lowering agent, it is not as commonly used today as in previous years because of its local adverse effects and multiple daily dosage requirements.

5.7.1.2 Pharmacokinetics, concentration–effect relationship, and metabolism. Pilocarpine penetrates the cornea well and produces a low incidence of allergic reactions. Animal studies indicate that the cornea absorbs pilocarpine rapidly and then releases it slowly to the aqueous humor. However, degradation and complexing in the cornea result in only a small percentage (<3%) reaching the anterior chamber.

The onset of miosis with a 1% solution is 10 to 30 minutes. The maximum reduction in IOP occurs within 75 minutes with a solution, depending on its strength. The duration of action for miosis is about 4 to 8 hours following administration with a solution. The reduction in IOP lasts for 4 to 14 hours with a solution, varying with the strength used. In light-eyed individuals, 2% solution is at the top of the dose–response curve for lowering IOP. In brown-eyed white individuals, 4% solution may be required for maximum effect, while extremely dark-eyed individuals (African, Hispanic, and Asian Americans) may require a 6% solution. These differences relate to binding of the drug by pigment within the eye, making it unavailable to the relevant muscarinic receptors. In light-eyed individuals, the higher concentrations have been used to extend the duration of action, thereby reducing the frequency of administration to twice daily.

Pilocarpine is inactivated by tissues of the anterior segment of the eye, partly by reversible binding of the drug to tissues, but also by appreciable enzymatic hydrolysis to the primary metabolite, pilocarpic acid. Human serum contains a heat-labile component capable of inactivating pilocarpine. Incubation of 500 mg of pilocarpine with 0.5 mL human serum at 37°C for 1 hour will inactivate 40% of the pilocarpine. The amount of pilocarpine-hydrolyzing enzyme is not changed by prolonged pilocarpine use by glaucoma patients.

Cholinergic sensitivity varies inversely with local ACh concentration,[45,48] the negative feedback putatively mediated by down- and up-regulation of muscarinic receptors without change in rate of receptor degradation.[48,49] Resistance to the IOP-lowering effect of miotics may occur after prolonged use. Responsiveness may be restored by substituting another miotic, timolol, epinephrine, or a carbonic anhydrase inhibitor for a for a short period of time, then resuming treatment with the original drug,[33] although this seems inconsistent with our present understanding of the receptors and mechanisms controlling cholinergic responsiveness.

5.7.2 *Carbachol.* Carbachol is the carbamyl ester of choline and was synthesized in the early 1930s. It is no longer commonly used in current medical practice.

Chemical Structure	NH_2C—O—CH_2—CH_2—$\overset{+}{N}$—$CH_3 \cdot Cl^-$ with O (double bond) above first C and CH_3 above and below the N
Composition	$C_6H_{15}N_2O_2Cl$

5.7.2.1 *Formulations.* The official drug name for carbachol (carbamylcholine chloride) is ethanaminium, 2-[(aminocarbonyl)oxy]-N,N,N-trimethyl-, chloride. Brand names are listed in table 5.1.

Carbachol occurs as white or faintly yellow hygroscopic crystals or crystalline powder, is freely soluble in water, and is sparingly soluble in alcohol. The drug is odorless or has a slight amine-like odor. Commercially available ophthalmic solutions contain benzalkonium chloride as a preservative and wetting agent. The commercially available ophthalmic solution of 0.75% to 3% carbachol has a pH of 5 to 7. The commercially available intraocular injection of 100 µg/mL has a pH of 5 to 7.5. Carbachol intraocular injection should be stored at 15°C to 30°C and protected from freezing and excessive heat. The commercially available carbachol intraocular injection is stable for 18 months after the date of manufacture.

5.7.2.2 *Pharmacokinetics, concentration–effect relationship, and metabolism.* Carbachol is not destroyed by cholinesterase; therefore, its action is not enhanced by anticholinesterase drugs. Carbachol is stable in solution. It is not lipid soluble at any pH; hence, it penetrates the intact corneal epithelium poorly.

To be clinically useful, carbachol must be dispensed in combination with a wetting agent, such as benzalkonium chloride 0.03%, which increases corneal penetration.

A 1.5% solution of carbachol used three times daily has been reported to be more effective than a 2% solution of pilocarpine given four times daily in the control of IOP in primary open-angle glaucoma.

When administered as a solution, the onset of miosis is within 10 to 20 minutes and lasts 4 to 8 hours. The maximum reduction in IOP occurs within 4 hours and lasts about 8 hours.

When used intracamerally, carbachol (Miostat 0.01%) is an intensely powerful miotic. It is 100 times more effective and longer lasting than ACh similarly instilled intracamerally (which is rapidly hydrolyzed by endogenous cholinesterase) and 200 times more effective than pilocarpine. Maximal miosis is achieved within 5 minutes and lasts about 24 hours.

5.8 INDIRECT, LONG-ACTING DRUGS

Some of these indirect, long-acting drugs are still available in the United States but are more commonly used for the treatment of glaucomas in aphakia or pseudophakia across much of Europe and Latin America. This group of drugs (physostigmine, demecarium, echothiophate, isoflurophate) blocks AChE, thus preventing metabolic inactivation of ACh released from parasympathetic nerve endings. [1,27,33,62,63] None of these drugs has any affinity for muscarinic ACh receptors; instead, they act by either carbamylating or phosphorylating AChE. For the carbamyl enzyme, the half-life is hours; for the phosphoryl enzyme, it is days. Thus, these drugs are suicide substrates of AChE, and some of their effects can last for days or weeks.

5.8.1 *Echothiophate.* Cholinesterase inhibitors other than echothiophate that have been or are still available for clinical ocular use include eserine, isofluorophate, and demecarium. However, echothiophate is most commonly employed by far and is discussed as the paradigm for this drug class.

Chemical Structure	C_2H_5O $\diagdown$ $\overset{O}{\overset{\|}{P}}$ $\diagup$ $\diagdown$ $SCH_2CH_2\overset{+}{N}(CH_3)_3$ $\quad I^-$ C_2H_5O $\diagup$
Composition	$C_9H_{23}INO_3PS$

5.8.1.1 *Formulations.* The official drug name for echothiophate (echothiophate iodide) is ethanaminium, 2-[(diethoxyphosphinyl)-thio]-*N,N,N*-trimethyl-, iodide, or (2-mercaptoethyl)trimethylammonium iodide *S*-ester with *O,O*-diethylphosphorothioate]. It is sold under the brand name Phospholine Iodide, available in the following concentrations: 0.03%, 0.06%, 0.125%, and 0.25%.

Indefinitely stable when dry, echothiophate must be kept in a tightly sealed container because the powdered form is hygroscopic. Assays of refrigerated aqueous solutions show a drop to 90% of the original potency within 4 weeks. At room temperature, this drop is to 83% of the original potency within 4 weeks and to 76% in 8 weeks. Benzalkonium is incompatible, so chlorobutanol is used instead as a preservative.

5.8.1.2 *Pharmacokinetics, concentration-effect relationship, and metabolism.* Dose–response analysis of echothiophate with respect to IOP[64] and outflow facility indicates that, often, little additional pharmacologic response is obtained by increasing the drug concentration to more than 0.06%.[65] Occasionally, concentrations as high as 0.125% or, very occasionally, 0.25% are required, although the potential for ocular side effects increases substantially at these higher concentrations. A 0.03% concentration of echothiophate iodide has an effect similar to pilocarpine 1% to 2%, while 0.06% is approximately equivalent to pilocarpine 4%. Echothiophate has a duration of ocular hypotensive action significantly longer than pilocarpine, with a maximal effect in 4 to 6 hours and a substantial effect maintained after 24 hours. Miosis begins within 1 hour and is maximal within 2 hours. Miosis and IOP reduction can, in some cases, last for several weeks, but usually lasts at least 24 to 48 hours. Thus, drug administration is often needed only once daily.

ACKNOWLEDGMENT

This work was supported by National Institutes of Health grant EY02698, Research to Prevent Blindness, and the Ocular Physiology Research and Education Foundation.

REFERENCES

1. Mindel JS. Cholinergic pharmacology. In: Tasman W, Jaeger EA, eds. *Duane's Foundations of Clinical Ophthalmology on CD-ROM.* Philadelphia, PA: Lippincott Williams & Wilkins; 2006.

2. Gabelt BT, Kiland JA, Tian B, et al. Aqueous humor: secretion and dynamics. In: Tasman W, Jaeger EA, eds. *Duane's Foundation of Clinical Ophthalmology on CD-ROM*. Philadelphia, PA: Lippincott Williams & Wilkins; 2006.

3. Shields MB. Cholinergic agents. In: *Shields' Textbook of Glaucoma*. Philadelphia, PA: Lippincott Williams & Wilkins; 2005;501–508.

4. Bill A. Aqueous humor dynamics in monkeys (Macaca irus and Cercopithecus ethiops). *Exp Eye Res*. 1971;11:195–206.

5. Gabelt BT, Gottanka J, Lütjen-Drecoll E, et al. Aqueous humor dynamics and trabecular meshwork and anterior ciliary muscle morphologic changes with age in rhesus monkeys. *Invest Ophthalmol Vis Sci*. 2003;44:2118–2125.

6. Bárány EH, Rohen JW. Localized contraction and relaxation within the ciliary muscle of the vervet monkey (Cercopithecus ethiops). In: Rohen JW, ed. *The Structure of the Eye, Second Symposium*. Stuttgart: FK Schattauer Verlag; 1965;287–311.

7. Rohen JW, Lütjen E, Bárány E. The relation between the ciliary muscle and the trabecular meshwork and its importance for the effect of miotics on aqueous outflow resistance. *Albrecht von Graefes Arch Klin Exp Ophthalmol*. 1967;172:23–47.

8. Bill A. Effects of atropine and pilocarpine on aqueous humour dynamics in cynomolgus monkeys (Macaca irus). *Exp Eye Res*. 1967;6:120–125.

9. Rohen JW, Futa R, Lütjen-Drecoll E. The fine structure of the cribriform meshwork in normal and glaucomatous eyes as seen in tangential sections. *Invest Ophthalmol Vis Sci*. 1981;21:574–585.

10. Lütjen-Drecoll E, Futa R, Rohen JW. Ultrahistochemical studies on tangential sections of the trabecular meshwork in normal and glaucomatous eyes. *Invest Ophthalmol Vis Sci*. 1981;21:563–573.

11. Bárány EH. The immediate effect on outflow resistance of intravenous pilocarpine in the vervet monkey. *Invest Ophthalmol*. 1967;6:373–380.

12. Hart WM. Intraocular pressure. In: Hart WM, ed. *Adler's Physiology of the Eye*. 9th ed. St Louis, MO: Mosby; 1992;248–267.

13. Kaufman PL. Total iridectomy does not alter outflow facility responses to cyclic AMP in cynomolgus monkeys. *Exp Eye Res*. 1986;43:441–447.

14. Kaufman PL. Aqueous humor dynamics following total iridectomy in the cynomolgus monkey. *Invest Ophthalmol Vis Sci*. 1979;18:870–875.

15. Kaufman PL, Bárány EH. Loss of acute pilocarpine effect on outflow facility following surgical disinsertion and retrodisplacement of the ciliary muscle from the scleral spur in the cynomolgus monkey. *Invest Ophthalmol*. 1976;15:793–807.

16. Bárány E, Berrie CP, Birdsall NJM, et al. The binding properties of the muscarinic receptors of the cynomolgus monkey ciliary body and the response to the induction of agonist subsensitivity. *Br J Pharmacol*. 1982;77:731–739.

17. Erickson-Lamy KA, Polansky JR, Kaufman PL, et al. Cholinergic drugs alter ciliary muscle response and receptor content. *Invest Ophthalmol Vis Sci*. 1987;28:375–383.

18. Hubbard WC, Kee C, Kaufman PL. Aceclidine effects on outflow facility after ciliary muscle disinsertion. *Ophthalmologica*. 1996;210:303–307.

19. Shade DL, Clark AF, Pang IH. Effects of muscarinic agents on cultured human trabecular meshwork cells. *Exp Eye Res*. 1996;62:201–210.

20. Erickson KA, Schreoder A. Direct effects of muscarinic agents on the outflow pathways in human eyes. *Invest Ophthalmol Vis Sci*. 2000;41:1743–1748.

21. Kiland JA, Hubbard WC, Kaufman PL. Low doses of pilocarpine do not significantly increase outflow facility in the cynomolgus monkey. *Exp Eye Res*. 2000;70: 603–609.

22. de Kater AW, Spurr-Michaud SJ, Gipson IK. Localization of smooth muscle myosin-containing cells in the aqueous outflow pathway. *Invest Ophthalmol Vis Sci.* 1990; 31:347–353.

23. de Kater AW, Shahsafaei A, Epstein DL. Localization of smooth muscle and non-muscle actin isoforms in the human aqueous outflow pathway. *Invest Ophthalmol Vis Sci.* 1992;33:424–429.

24. Flügel C, Tamm E, Lütjen-Drecoll E, et al. Age-related loss of a smooth muscle actin in normal and glaucomatous human trabecular meshwork of different age groups. *J Glaucoma.* 1992;1:165–173.

25. Lepple-Wienhues A, Stahl F, Wiederholt M. Differential smooth muscle-like contractile properties of trabecular meshwork and ciliary muscle. *Exp Eye Res.* 1991;53: 33–38.

26. Bershadsky AD, Balaban NQ, Geiger B. Adhesion-dependent cell mechanosensitivity. *Ann Rev Cell Dev Biol.* 2003;19:677–695.

27. Miotics. In: *American Hospital Formulary Service Drug Information.* Bethesda, MD: American Society of Health-System Pharmacists; 1998;2318–2328.

28. Klein HZ, Lugo M, Shields MB, et al. A dose-response study of piloplex for duration of action. *Am J Ophthalmol.* 1985;99:23–26.

29. Goldberg I, Ashburn FS, Kass MA, et al. Efficacy and patient acceptance of pilocarpine gel. *Am J Ophthalmol.* 1979;88:843–846.

30. Johnson DH, Epstein DL, Allen RC, et al. A one-year multicenter clinical trial of pilocarpine gel. *Am J Ophthalmol.* 1984;97:723–729.

31. Lavin MJ, Wormald RP, Migdal CS, et al. The influence of prior therapy on the success of trabeculectomy. *Arch Ophthalmol.* 1990;108:1543–1548.

32. Sherwood MB, Grierson I, Millar L, et al. Long-term morphologic effects of anti-glaucoma drugs on the conjunctiva and Tenon's capsule in glaucomatous patients. *Ophthalmology.* 1989;96:327–335.

33. ntiglaucoma agents, cholinergic, long-acting. In: *Drug Information for the Health Care Professional.* Englewood, CO: Micromedix Inc; 1999;315–319.

34. Lütjen E. Histometrische Untersuchungen über den Ziliarmuskel der Primaten. *Albrecht von Graefes Arch Klin Exp Ophthalmol.* 1966;171:121–133.

35. Flügel C, Bárány EH, Lütjen-Drecoll E. Histochemical differences within the ciliary muscle and its function in accommodation. *Exp Eye Res.* 1990;50:219–226.

36. Zhang X, Hernandez MR, Yang H, et al. Expression of muscarinic receptor subtype mRNA in the human ciliary muscle. *Invest Ophthalmol Vis Sci.* 1995;36:1645–1657.

37. Gupta N, Drance SM, McAllister R, et al. Localization of M3 muscarinic receptor subtype and mRNA in the human eye. *Ophthalmic Res.* 1994;26:207–213.

38. Gupta N, McAllister R, Drance SM, et al. Muscarinic receptor M1 and M2 subtypes in the human eye: QNB, pirenzipine, oxotremorine, and AFDX-116 in vitro autoradiography. *Br J Ophthalmol.* 1994;78:555–559.

39. Gil DW, Krauss HA, Bogardus AM, et al. Muscarinic receptor subtypes in human iris-ciliary body measured by immunoprecipitation. *Invest Ophthalmol Vis Sci.* 1997;38: 1434–1442.

40. Bárány EH. Dissociation of accommodation effects from outflow effects of pilocarpine. In: Paterson G, Miller SJH, Paterson GH, eds. *Drug Mechanisms in Glaucoma.* London: Churchill Ltd; 1966;275–282.

41. Croft MA, Oyen MJ, Gange SJ, et al. Aging effects on accommodation and outflow facility responses to pilocarpine in humans. *Arch Ophthalmol.* 1996;114:586–592.

42. Gabelt BT, Kaufman PL. Inhibition of outflow facility, accommodative, and miotic responses to pilocarpine in rhesus monkeys by muscarinic receptor subtype antagonists. *J Pharmacol Exp Ther*. 1992;263:1133–1139.

43. Gabelt BT, Kaufman PL. Inhibition of aceclidine-stimulated outflow facility, accommodation and miosis by muscarinic receptor subtype antagonists in rhesus monkeys. *Exp. Eye Res*. 1994;58:623–630.

44. Gil D, Spalding T, Kharlamb A, et al. Exploring the potential for subtype-selective muscarinic agonists in glaucoma. *Life Sci*. 2001;68:2601–2604.

45. Bito LZ, Dawson MJ, Petrinovic L. Cholinergic sensitivity: normal variability as a function of stimulus background. *Science*. 1971;172:583–585.

46. Bito LZ, Hyslop A, Hyndman J. Antiparasympathomimetic effects of cholinesterase inhibitor treatment. *J Pharmacol Exp Ther*. 1967;157:159–169.

47. Bito LZ, Banks N. Effects of chronic cholinesterase inhibitor treatment. I. The pharmacological and physiological behavior of the anti-ChE-treated (Macaca mulatta) iris. *Arch Ophthalmol*. 1969;82:681–686.

48. Bito LZ, Dawson MJ. The site and mechanism of the control of cholinergic sensitivity. *J Pharmacol Exp Ther*. 1970;175:673–684.

49. Claesson H, Bárány E. Time course of light-induced changes in pilocarpine sensitivity of rat iris. *Acta Physiol Scand*. 1978;102:394–398.

50. Kaufman PL, Bárány EH. Subsensitivity to pilocarpine of the aqueous outflow system in monkey eyes after topical anticholinesterase treatment. *Am J Ophthalmol*. 1976;82:883–891.

51. Bárány E. Pilocarpine-induced subsensitivity to carbachol and pilocarpine of ciliary muscle in vervet and cynomolgus monkeys. *Acta Ophthalmol*. 1977;55:141–163.

52. Kaufman PL. Anticholinesterase-induced cholinergic subsensitivity in primate accommodative mechanism. *Am J Ophthalmol*. 1978;85:622–631.

53. Kaufman PL, Bárány EH. Subsensitivity to pilocarpine in primate ciliary muscle following topical anticholinesterase treatment. *Invest Ophthalmol*. 1975;14:302–306.

54. Lütjen-Drecoll E, Kaufman PL. Echothiophate-induced structural alterations in the anterior chamber angle of the cynomolgus monkey. *Invest Ophthalmol Vis Sci*. 1979;18:918–929.

55. Lütjen-Drecoll E, Kaufman P. Biomechanics of echothiophate-induced anatomic changes in monkey aqueous outflow system. *Graefes Arch Clin Exp Ophthalmol*. 1986;224:564–575.

56. Lindsey JD, Kashiwagi K, Kashiwagi F, et al. Prostaglandin action on ciliary smooth muscle extracellular matrix metabolism—implications for uveoscleral outflow. *Surv Ophthalmol*. 1997;41(suppl 2):S53–S59.

57. Patelska B, Greenfield DS, Liebmann JM, et al. Latanoprost for uncontrolled glaucoma in a compassionate case protocol. *Am J Ophthalmol*. 1997;124:279–286.

58. Lindén C, Alm A. Latanoprost and physostigmine have mostly additive ocular hypotensive effects in human eyes. *Arch Ophthalmol*. 1997;115:857–861.

59. Bill A, Wålinder P-E. The effects of pilocarpine on the dynamics of aqueous humor in a primate (Macaca irus). *Invest Ophthalmol*. 1966;5:170–175.

60. Poyer JF, Millar C, Kaufman PL. Prostaglandin F_{2a} effects on isolated rhesus monkey ciliary muscle. *Invest Ophthalmol Vis Sci*. 1995;36:2461–2465.

61. Anthony TL, Pierce KL, Stamer WD, et al. Prostaglandin F_{2a} receptors in the human trabecular meshwork. *Invest Ophthalmol Vis Sci*. 1998;39:315–321.

62. Brown JH, Taylor P. Muscarinic receptor agonists and antagonists. In: Brunton LL, Lazo JS, Parker KL, eds. *Goodman & Gilman's The Pharmacological Basis of Therapeutics*. New York: McGraw-Hill; 2006;183–200.

63. Taylor P. Anticholinesterase agents. In: Brunton LL, Lazo JS, Parker KL, eds. *Goodman & Gilman's The Pharmacological Basis of Therapeutics*. New York: McGraw-Hill; 2006;201–216.

64. Stockdill P, Drance SM. Dose response of human intraocular pressure to various concentrations of echothiophate iodide. *Trans Ophthalmol Soc U K*. 1965;85:537–543.

65. Harris L. Dose-response analysis of echothiophate iodide. *Arch Ophthalmol*. 1971;86:503–505.

6

Carbonic Anhydrase Inhibitors

EVE J. HIGGINBOTHAM AND ROBERT C. ALLEN

*F*or more than 50 years, carbonic anhydrase inhibitors (CAIs) have remained consistent and critical components in the armamentarium of the clinician. Despite systemic toxicity observed in some glaucoma patients, this category of medication has emerged as an important option for those patients who remain resistant to alternative intervention. Although beyond the reach of those individuals who have demonstrated a legitimate allergy to sulfa drugs in the past, CAIs have exhibited versatility in use across a broad range of ages and coexistent systemic comorbidities. It is the only category that can be administered as either a topical or a systemic agent, and patients rarely present with complaints of ocular hyperemia, shortness of breath, fatigue, or loss of libido when the topical agents are administered. This chapter provides an updated evidence-based review of the efficacy and safety of CAIs in an effort to provide the clinician a suitable guide for determining when best to use CAIs given the availability of more effective treatment alternatives.

The history of CAIs dates back to 1954 when oral acetazolamide was first introduced for the treatment of glaucoma. Investigators proposed minor modifications in the original acetazolamide molecule, and thus created methazolamide, which had clear pharmacologic and clinical advantages. Although this molecular innovation led to better gastric absorption, less serum protein binding, and longer duration of action, systemic side effects still prompted uneven compliance. Continued research efforts led to two effective topical agents that are now available to glaucoma patients. Although the availability of topical CAIs has significantly diminished the use of oral agents, a brief discussion of the oral agents is warranted given their continued importance in the medical armamentarium of the clinician.

6.1 SYSTEMIC CARBONIC ANHYDRASE INHIBITORS

6.1.1 *General Pharmacology.* Per Wistrand was the first to discover carbonic anhydrase in the anterior uvea of the rabbit. His initial studies were later confirmed by Ballintine and Maren. Richard Roblin, the director of the Chemotherapy Division of Cyanamid, has been credited for the synthesis of acetazolamide (2-acetyl-amino-1,3,4-thiadizole-5-sulfonamide). In 1954, Thomas Maren further developed the molecule, which was soon followed by the administration of the drug to 19 patients by Dr. Bernard Becker in 1955.[1]

Two oral CAIs are currently available (table 6.1, figure 6.1), all of which are members of the sulfonamide family. A free sulfonamide group ($-SO_2NH_2$) coupled with an aromatic ring is the common feature of these compounds. Studies suggest that the inhibitor occupies the active site of the enzyme, rendering it inactive. Other CAIs that are currently no longer available include ethoxzolamide and dichlorophenamide. In therapeutic doses, they are able to reduce production of aqueous by a maximum of 50%, with a corresponding decrease in intraocular pressure (IOP).

6.1.2 *Mechanism of Action.* After several years of controversy, there seems to be agreement that IOP reduction is caused by a reduction in the accumulation of bicarbonate in the posterior chamber, with a decrease in sodium and associated fluid movement linked to the bicarbonate ion (figure 6.2).[2,3] With high doses of acetazolamide, it appears that an additional decrease in IOP may be caused by relative metabolic acidosis. However, the two effects of IOP lowering, shifts in bicarbonate ion and changes related to acidosis, appear to be independent of one another, because other causes of metabolic acidosis also reduce IOP.[4]

Although a 50-mg oral dose of the CAI methazolamide produces a slightly smaller reduction in IOP than does a 250-mg oral dose of acetazolamide, the

Table 6.1 Pharmacologic Properties of Carbonic Anhydrase Inhibitors

Name	K_{a1} $(2\times10^9 M)^a$	pK_{a1}	Partition Coefficient to Buffer pH 7.4 Ether	CHCl$_3$	Solubility in H$_2$O (mM)	Human %[b] Bound to Plasma	$t_{1/2}$[c] Plasma (hr)	$k_m/h\times10^3$ RBC[d]	Aqueous Humor
Acetazolamide	6	7.4	0.14	10^{-3}	3	95	4	27	2
Methazolamide	8	7.2	0.62	0.06	5	55	15	195	8

[a]Against pure carbonic anhydrase C, in hydration.

[b]At concentrations of 4 to 40 μM.

[c]After oral dose in humans.

[d]From free concentration in plasma to human red blood cells.Source: Reprinted with permission from Maren TM. A general view of HCO$_3^-$ transport processes in relation to the physiology and biochemistry of carbonic anhydrase. In: Case RM, Lingard JM, Young J, eds. *Secretion: Mechanisms and Control.* Manchester, UK: Manchester University Press; 1984:47–66.

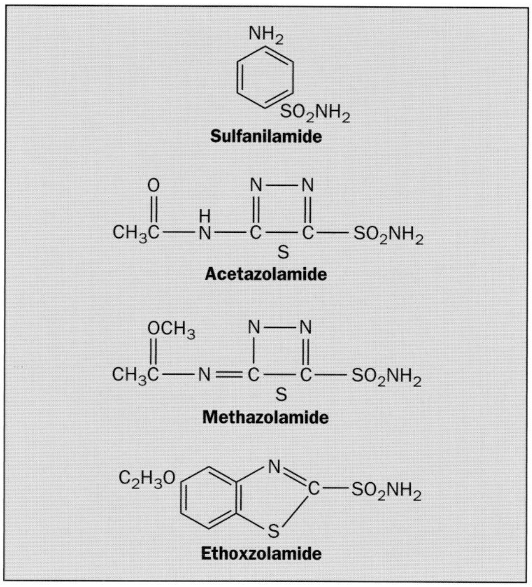

Figure 6.1. Chemical structure of carbonic anhydrase inhibitors compared with sulfanilamide "parent."

pharmacology of the former compound has several advantages.[5–8] The slight difference in the drugs' IOP-lowering effects at these doses is probably due to the metabolic acidosis caused by acetazolamide, which can be deleterious in many clinical situations. Methazolamide has a more favorable partition coefficient, which allows enhanced systemic absorption and easier access into ocular tissues. In addition, methazolamide is only 55% bound to plasma protein, whereas acetazolamide is 95% bound. In practical terms, this means that a far smaller quantity of oral methazolamide is needed to produce therapeutic levels in target tissue (presumably the ciliary processes), compared with acetazolamide. Because of this difference in dose, the renal effects of carbonic anhydrase inhibition can be avoided with administration of methazolamide at doses of less than 2 mg/kg/day.

Another advantage is methazolamide's serum half-life of 15 hours, compared with the 4-hour half-life of acetazolamide (see table 6.1). It is therefore unnecessary to give methazolamide more often than every 12 hours; this twice-a-day dosage schedule is much more convenient than that required for acetazolamide tablets. Methazolamide also undergoes predominantly hepatic, rather than renal, metabolism, so dosages do not have to be adjusted in the large patient population with renal dysfunction secondary to diabetes or other diseases.

6.1.3 *Indications*. Given the current availability of topical CAIs, the use of systemic CAIs has dropped significantly in the last decade. However, there are instances when systemic CAIs may be very useful. Considering the rapidity of the effect of this class on IOP, in those instances where pressure reduction is needed on an urgent basis, the administration of acetazolamide 250 mg four times daily is recommended. In other circumstances, such as the very young who are awaiting surgery and when the administration of drops may be problematic for elderly patients who may be hampered by arthritis or cognitive difficulties, systemic CAIs may be the best option.

Figure 6.2. Hypothetical diagram of aqueous production in nonpigmented ciliary process epithelium (NPE). Note linkage of Na^+,K^+-ATPase with carbonic anhydrase–linked bicarbonate production, as well as questionable role of Cl^- and ultrafiltration. $Cl^- = $ chloride ion, $Na^+ = $ potassium ion, PC = posterior chamber. Redrawn with permission from Caprioli J. The ciliary epithelia and aqueous humor. In: Hart WM Jr, ed. *Adler's Physiology of the Eye: Clinical Application.* 9th ed. St Louis, Mo: CV Mosby Co; 1992:234.

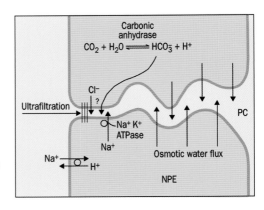

6.1.4 *Contraindications.* Patient groups in whom metabolic acidosis related to CAI therapy may be a serious risk include the following:[9–11]

1. Diabetic patients susceptible to ketoacidosis
2. Patients who have hepatic insufficiency and cannot tolerate the obligatory increase in serum ammonia
3. Patients with chronic obstructive pulmonary disease, in whom increased retention of carbon dioxide can cause potentially fatal narcosis from a combination of both renal and respiratory acidosis

6.1.5 *Treatment Regimen.* A starting dose of 25 to 50 mg methazolamide twice a day is very easily tolerated by many patients (table 6.2). The maximum dose of 150 mg methazolamide twice a day or 250 mg acetazolamide four times a day may be less well tolerated, but sustained-release capsules of 500 mg acetazolamide used twice daily may improve compliance and have been reported to give an unexplained advantage in IOP reduction.[12] It is advisable to administer methazolamide and acetazolamide after meals to decrease gastrointestinal side effects.

6.1.6 *Side Effects.* Many well-known ocular and systemic side effects occur with administration of all the CAIs. These include numbness, paresthesias, malaise, anorexia, nausea, flatulence, diarrhea, depression, decreased libido, poor tolerance of carbonated beverages, myopia, hirsutism, increased serum urate, and, rarely, thrombocytopenia and idiosyncratic aplastic anemia (table 6.3).[13] Some investigators believe that the malaise-anorexia-depression syndrome may be related to concomitant acidosis and have found some success in reducing the incidence of these complaints with the coadministration of sodium bicarbonate.[14]

An early, mild hypokalemia usually follows the initiation of most CAIs but does not progress unless patients are taking diuretics concomitantly. The exception is the drug dichlorphenamide, which has a unique chloruretic effect that may cause chronic and potentially dangerous loss of potassium. A deformity of the forelimb

Table 6.2 Carbonic Anhydrase Inhibitors

Drug	Concentration	Route	Dosage
Acetazolamide[a]			
Diamox[a]	125-mg and 250-mg tablets	Oral	qid
Diamox Sequels	500-mg capsules	Oral	bid
Methazolamide[a]			
Neptazane[a]	25, 50, 100 mg	Oral	bid, tid
Dorzolamide HCl[a]			
Trusopt	2.0%	Topical	bid, tid
Brinzolamide[a]			
Azopt	1%	Topical	bid, tid

[a]Generic available.

has been seen in the offspring of animals given acetazolamide, and the drug should definitely be avoided by women of child-bearing age.[15]

Urolithiasis is believed to be much more common in patients taking CAIs, most likely because of the depressed excretion of renal citrate and the higher urine levels of calcium available to form urate stones. In a case study with controls, the incidence of renal stones was 15 times higher after treatment with acetazolamide than before its administration.[16] The incidence was 11 times higher than in the age-matched control group. The incidence of stones in this study did not seem to increase after 15 months, suggesting that susceptible persons ordinarily experience this side effect during the first or second year of treatment, if at all. Although methazolamide has been linked to the formation of kidney stones in several patients on high doses (> 200 mg/day),[17] the lack of a significant renal effect with low-dose therapy seems to suggest a potentially lower risk of urolithiasis with regimens such as 50 mg twice a day.

Because blood dyscrasias have been reported after the use of both agents,[18] there has been considerable debate about whether surveillance of blood count is justified. Despite the poor outcome in patients who develop idiosyncratic aplastic anemia,[19,20] some patients also develop isolated neutropenia, thrombocytopenia, and pancytopenia but have an uneventful recovery if the condition is discovered and the drug discontinued.[21] Because such reactions are rare, with an incidence of about 1 in 14,000, it would not seem justified to continue obtaining blood counts during the entire course of therapy. It is reasonable and relatively inexpensive to obtain a pretreatment "complete blood count" and one or two follow-up studies during the first 6 months of treatment, when most of the serious hematologic events were noted to occur. Although some ophthalmologists believe that oral therapy with CAIs should be abandoned, oral CAIs may still be useful in some patients who show a documented efficacy advantage or who have difficulty instilling topical CAI eye drops.

Table 6.3 Side Effects of Oral Carbonic Anhydrase Inhibitors

Ocular	Systemic
Decreased intraocular pressure	Paresthesia
Decreased vision	Malaise syndrome
Myopia	Acidosis
Decreased accommodation	Asthenia
Forward displacement of lens	Anorexia
Eyelid or conjunctival disorder	Weight loss
Allergic reactions	Depression
Erythema	Somnolence
Photosensitivity	Confusion
Urticaria	Impotence
Purpura	Decreased libido
Erythema multiforme	Gastrointestinal disorder
Stevens-Johnson syndrome	Nausea
Lyell's syndrome	Vomiting
Loss of eyelashes or eyebrows	Renal disorder
Retinal or macular edema	Urolithiasis
Iritis	Polyuria
Ocular signs of gout	Hematuria
Globus hystericus	Glycosuria
Subconjunctival or retinal hemorrhages	Blood dyscrasia
secondary to drug-induced anemia	Aplastic anemia
Color vision disorder (with methazolamide)	Thrombocytopenia
Color vision defect	Agranulocytosis
Objects have yellow tinge	Hypochromic anemia
	Convulsion

Source: Reprinted with permission from Fraunfelder FT, Grove JA, eds. *Drug-Induced Ocular Side Effects.* Baltimore, MD: Williams & Wilkins; 1996:439–441.

6.2 TOPICAL AGENTS

In 1955, a year after the introduction of oral acetazolamide as an effective ocular hypotensive agent, an unsuccessful attempt to solubilize it for topical treatment was reported.[22] The effort to develop a topical agent was revisited in the late 1970s and led to the introduction of several prototype molecules that preceded the approval of dorzolamide in 1995 and brinzolamide in 1998. The availability of these agents has not only dramatically reduced the justification for using oral CAIs but has greatly reduced the side effects associated with the oral agents and has reminded ophthalmologists of the long-term advantage of low pharmacologic tolerance with these nonadrenergic drugs.

6.2.1 *Pharmacology.* Two topical CAIs that are currently available are dorzolamide and brinzolamide. Dorzolamide ($C_{10}H_{16}N_2O_4S_3$ HCl) and brinzolamide ($C_{12}H_{21} \cdot N_3O_5S_3$) are water-soluble CAIs. Dorzolamide has a substituted amino group ($-NHCH_2CH_3$) and thus differs in that respect from the systemic CAIs previously discussed. Both compounds specifically inhibit carbonic anhydrase II, which is found primarily in red blood cells but is also found in ocular tissue such as ciliary processes, corneal endothelium, and Müller cells in the retina.[1]

6.2.2 *Mechanism of Action*. The mechanism of action is similar to systemic CAIs. By inhibiting the formation of bicarbonate, the influx of sodium and fluid is reduced, thus reducing IOP. Ingram and Brubaker[23] measured the effects of dorzolamide 2% and brinzolamide 1% on aqueous humor formation in a series of 25 normal subjects using fluorophotometry. Compared to the placebo-treated eyes, brinzolamide 1% reduced aqueous production by 0.47 ± 0.20 µL/min ($19\% \pm 10\%$) during the day and 0.16 ± 0.12 µL/min ($16\% \pm 14\%$) during the evening. Similarly, dorzolamide 2% reduced aqueous production by 0.34 ± 0.20 µL/min ($12\% \pm 12\%$) during the day and 0.10 ± 0.13 µL/min ($8\% \pm 14\%$) at night. As suppressors of aqueous production, the researchers considered the two drugs equivalent.

6.2.3 *Indications*. The indications for topical CAIs are broader than the indications for systemic agents. In most instances, topical CAIs work well as adjunctive agents rather than first-line agents. However, in special instances when first-line agents may not be well tolerated, particularly in the very young and the elderly, topical CAIs may be considered as first-line agents.

6.2.4 *Dorzolamide*. Rudimentary attempts at developing a topical CAI included use of acetazolamide-soaked contact lenses,[24] as well as new derivatives such as ethoxzolamide gel,[25] trifluoro methazolamide,[26] and a 6-amino compound.[27] Some of these showed transient reductions in IOP in animal models, but there was difficulty achieving adequate ocular penetration to allow the 99% of carbonic anhydrase enzymatic inhibition in ciliary processes required for a sustained IOP effect. Finally, one of the many screened compounds, dorzolamide, was found to be 10 times more effective than acetazolamide at inhibiting carbonic anhydrase isoenzyme II, which is the predominant form in both nonpigmented and pigmented ciliary process epithelium (figure 6.3). Dorzolamide was also twice as effective as acetazolamide in inhibiting isoenzyme II in an in vitro lung preparation.[28] Starting in 1990, this compound was tested in glaucomatous monkey and rabbit models,[29,30] followed by clinical trials in both normal volunteers and glaucoma patients. At the 2% concentration, the compound was very effective in lowering IOP in both primates and humans. Aqueous dynamics in glaucomatous monkeys showed a 38% reduction in aqueous secretion with no change in outflow facility following single-drop therapy.[31] Dorzolamide administered three times daily was compared with twice-daily timolol and twice-daily betaxolol over 12 months in a large, multicenter, prospective, masked trial.[32] At peak effect (2 hours), the sustained IOP-lowering effect of dorzolamide was 1 to 2 mm Hg less than timolol solution, but approximately 1 mm Hg better than betaxolol 0.5%. The IOP effect was maintained for the 12 months of the study, but the difference between the treatment groups at peak disappeared. The trough IOPs, or IOPs measured before the morning dose of medication, while initially very similar, actually increased at 12 months, and again, dorzolamide was intermediate in efficacy between timolol and betaxolol by a small magnitude.

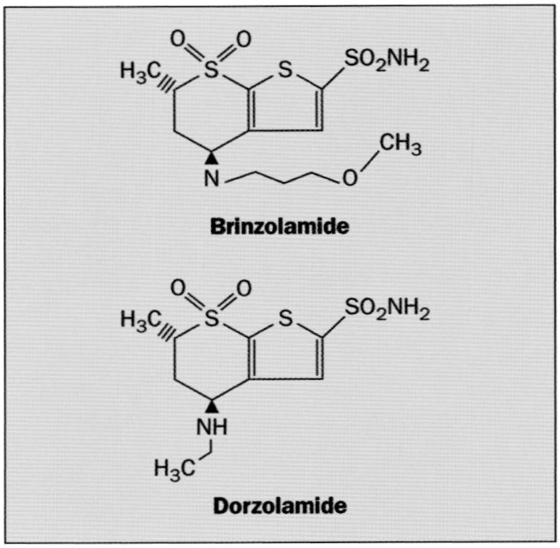

Figure 6.3. Chemical structure of topical carbonic anhydrase inhibitors.

Additional clinical investigations were carried out on use of dorzolamide as an adjunctive agent to timolol. At peak, there was an additional IOP drop of 4 mm Hg, which decreased to 3.5 mm Hg at 8 hours.[33] Another study, examining different alternatives for adjunctive therapy, found comparable efficacy between dorzolamide and pilocarpine 2% when added to timolol. Patients tolerated dorzolamide much better and had considerably fewer complaints of decreased vision and induced myopia.[34]

Considerable attention has been paid to whether three-times-daily application of dorzolamide is significantly better than twice-daily application. Because of the 8- to 10-hour duration of dorzolamide, it does seem that there is a small but definite increase in efficacy with three-times-daily monotherapy compared to twice daily. A prospective clinical trial showed lack of a statistically significant difference in three-times-daily versus twice-daily dorzolamide treatment, but three-times-daily treatment gave approximately 1 mm Hg better IOP lowering at 8 to 12 hours (figure 6.4).[35] Many ophthalmologists use dorzolamide twice daily as both monotherapy and adjunctive therapy, but there is an occasional patient who benefits from monotherapy administered three times daily. The efficacy of dorzolamide 2% was evaluated in a series of patients who were younger than 6 years of age in a 3-month, controlled, randomized trial. Of the 66 patients who were 2 or more years of age and randomized to dorzolamide 2%, only two patients discontinued treatment due to ocular symptoms. After 3 months of treatment, the mean reduction in IOP compared to baseline was −20.6% among those younger than 2 years of age, and −23.3% among those 2 or more years of age. Thus, when considering patients younger than 6 years of age, dorzolamide is generally effective and well tolerated.[36]

Careful attempts have been made to document potential ocular and systemic side effects of dorzolamide (table 6.4).[37] The ocular effects seem to be principally confined to a 33% incidence of stinging on instillation and a 10% to 15% incidence of punctate keratitis. Incidences of blurred vision, tearing, dryness, and photophobia were all less than 5%. Some of the stinging on instillation is most likely related to

Figure 6.4. Mean IOP for dorzolamide 2% twice daily (7:00 A.M. and 7:00 P.M.) for 5 days, followed by three-times-daily dosing (7:00 A.M., 3:00 P.M., and 11:00 P.M.) for 7 days. Orange circles, prestudy; green circles, day 1; blue circles, day 5; red circles, day 12. Redrawn with permission from Lippa EA. Carbonic anhydrase inhibitors. In: Ritch R, Shields MB, Krupin T, eds. *The Glaucomas.* 2nd ed. St Louis, Mo: CV: Mosby Co; 1996:1463–1481.

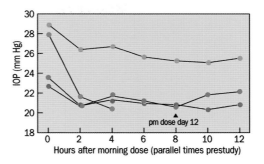

the molecule itself, but there is also a potential factor of the slightly low pH (5.8) required to keep the relatively insoluble compound in solution. Periorbital dermatitis has been described in a small case series of patients who were treated with dorzolamide for a mean period of 20.4 weeks. In 8 of the 14 patients described, the dermatitis resolved once the dorzolamide was discontinued.[38] After long-term dorzolamide treatment, analysis of both serum and urine chemistries revealed no changes in a group of healthy volunteers.[39] There was a decrease in red blood cell carbonic anhydrase II activity, substantiating some systemic absorption, and previous reports have noted that this red blood cell binding is present in detectable amounts for at least 4 months.[40] An initial concern during preapproval trials was a small increase in corneal thickness in a dorzolamide-treated group. However, an extensive three-armed, masked, postapproval, phase IV study using endothelial

Table 6.4 Side Effects of Topical Carbonic Anhydrase Inhibitors

Ocular

Burning/stinging eye
Punctate keratitis
Blurred vision
Blepharitis
Conjunctivitis
Eye discharge
Tearing
Foreign-body sensation
Corneal erosion
Visual disturbance

Systemic

Taste perversion

Source: Reprinted with permission from Adamsons I, Clineschmidt C, Polis A, et al. The efficacy and safety of dorzolamide as adjunctive therapy to timolol maleate gellan solution in patients with elevated intraocular pressure. Additivity Study Group. *J Glaucoma.* 1998;7:253–260.

videokeratography in patients with normal corneas failed to find any increased corneal thickness or significant change in endothelial morphology. It is interesting that, in both the dorzolamide-treated groups and the two beta blocker–treated control groups, there was a trend toward a decrease in overall endothelial cell count.[41] However, in patients with severe corneal disease, topical dorzolamide 2% may be problematic. In a series of nine patients with corneal pathology such as Fuch's endothelial dystrophy or surgical trauma, administration of topical dorzo-lamide for period of 3 to 20 weeks resulted in irreversible corneal decompensation. Seven of the nine eyes subsequently underwent penetrating keratoplasties.[42] Some patients have developed urolithiasis during dorzolamide treatment, but the preva-lence is low enough to suggest no relationship to the topical medication. Ad-ditionally, there have been no reports of Stevens-Johnson syndrome or blood dys-crasias following dorzolamide use, but because of the observed systemic absorption of this drug, continued clinical surveillance is appropriate. The one consistent sys-temic effect that occurs frequently is a bitter taste following administration, which approximately 25% of patients notice, but which seldom complicates long-term therapy. This side effect is easily reduced by use of punctal occlusion.

Most clinicians have had a positive experience with both the tolerance and the efficacy of dorzolamide, but questions continue to linger regarding equivalence of topical and oral compounds. Although fluorophotometric investigation showed a 17% reduction in aqueous flow following dorzolamide application to nine glau-comatous volunteers, compared with a 30% reduction following acetazolamide,[43] most of the long-term dosing trials show equivalence in observed IOP lowering. A 12-week study on 31 patients showed good maintenance of IOP reduction when topical dorzolamide was substituted for oral acetazolamide.[44] A larger prospective study has also shown that the oral and topical forms are essentially interchangeable when used as adjunctive therapy (figure 6.5).[45] The comparative efficacy of topical CAIs versus the systemic agents may differ on an individual patient basis, and thus clinicians may wish the try various formulations of the drug prior to abandoning this class. The question of whether dorzolamide used topically offers additional IOP lowering when added to oral treatment with acetazolamide was answered by a recent clinical trial that showed lack of such an additive effect. Because it was a three-armed design, the study was also able to substantiate that the group using dorzolamide alone was comparable to the group using acetazolamide alone in IOP reduction.[46]

Perhaps because of early impressions that oral CAIs may have an advantageous effect on ocular blood flow, considerable attention has been paid to the effect of dorzolamide on blood flow as measured by several contemporary methodologies. Both optic nerve head blood flow in animals, measured by a laser Doppler flow-meter, and arteriovenous passage time, measured with a scanning laser ophthal-moscope, seemed to be improved following use of topical dorzolamide.[47] Recently, Nagel et al.[48] assessed the effects of dorzolamide on the autoregulation of major retinal vessels in a series of glaucoma patients. The IOP was elevated to 38 mm Hg for 100 seconds. Changes in the diameter of the retinal vessels were measured before, during, and after IOP elevation at baseline, and the measurements were repeated

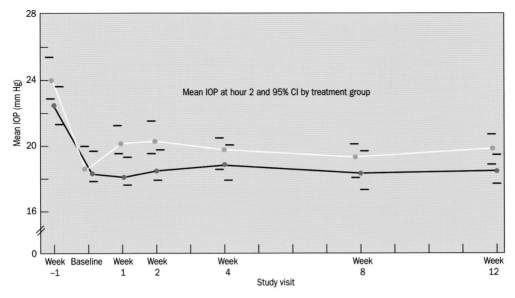

Figure 6.5. Mean IOP at hour 2 (with 95% confidence intervals) by treatment group. At peak, both dorzolamide and acetazolamide provided additional IOP lowering when added to timolol. At week 12, IOP level at hour 2 in patients receiving acetazolamide was slightly lower (about 1 mm Hg) compared to patients receiving dorzolamide. Orange circles, dorzolamide ($n = 53$); blue circles, acetazolamide ($n = 49$). Redrawn with permission from Hutzelmann JE, Polis AB, Michael AJ, Adamsons IA. A comparison of the efficacy and tolerability of dorzolamide and acetazolamide as adjunctive therapy to timolol. *Acta Ophthalmol Scand.* 1998;76:717–722.

4 weeks later following treatment with dorzolamide three times daily. The arterial diameter was greater following treatment with dorzolamide, before and during the elevation of IOP. In the posttreated eyes, the vessel diameter decreased by −1.7% ± 3.0. The researchers concluded that the dilation of the vessels during the IOP elevation may be an indication that dorzolamide may influence the vascular response due to changes in IOP. Whether research such as this small study can show any impact of treatment on the long-term effect on the glaucomatous process remains to be seen. Nevertheless, it seems encouraging that dorzolamide has not been shown to reduce flow in all studies published thus far.

The efficacy and safety of using dorzolamide to prevent the conversion from ocular hypertension to glaucoma were explored in the European Glaucoma Prevention Study (EGPS), a multicenter, randomized, prospective study.[49] A total of 1,081 patients 30 or more years of age with IOP at baseline that measured 22 to 29 mm Hg were randomized to either treatment with dorzolamide 2% three times daily or placebo three times daily. Although dorzolamide reduced IOP by 15% to 22% throughout the 5-year follow-up period, there was no statistically significant difference between the two groups of patients. In fact, within the placebo group, the mean IOP reduction ranged from 9% at 6 months to 19% at 5 years. Significant numbers of patients dropped out of both groups by the end of the study. Other factors such as the use of a single agent rather than multiple agents may have contributed to the findings of this study versus the Ocular Hypertension Treatment Study (OHTS),[50] which did find a significant difference among those participants who received topical antiglaucoma therapy versus a group of patients who were simply observed. It should be noted that more than one-third of the patients in the treated group in OHTS required more than one medication to achieve of an IOP reduction goal of at least 20% compared to baseline. No such goal was set in the EGPS prior to the initiation of the study. Topical CAIs were among the choices of drugs available to clinicians to achieve the study goal of 20% in OHTS. Thus, clinicians are urged to examine the differences in study design and the demographics of the population before drawing conclusions regarding the role of topical CAIs in the treatment of ocular hypertension.

6.2.5 *Brinzolamide*. Brinzolamide is available in a 1% concentration (see figure 6.3). Using a formulation similar to that previously employed with betaxolol, brinzolamide is a suspension that allows buffering to a more neutral pH than does dorzolamide. This difference in formulation may be the reason why patients demonstrate less ocular irritation with brinzolamide versus dorzolamide.[51] Multicenter studies have been completed comparing both twice-daily brinzolamide and three-times-daily brinzolamide 1% to timolol 0.5%. These results show efficacy similar to that of dorzolamide, but with IOP lowering slightly less than timolol use with either dosing regimen of brinzolamide. Differences between twice-daily and three-times-daily dosing were less than 1mm Hg (figure 6.6).[52] A meta-analysis of the IOP-lowering effects of commonly used glaucoma drugs was conducted by van der Valk et al.[53] These investigators based their analysis on 27 articles that described 28 randomized clinical trials involving move than 6,000 individuals. Moreover, the analysis was based on 1-month data. When considering the reduction of IOP from baseline, the investigators noted that a peak reduction for dorzolamide of –22% (range, –24% to –20%) and trough of –17% (–19% to –15%) versus brinzolamide, with peak reduction of –17% (range –19% to –15%) and trough of –17% (–19% to –15%). This range is similar to the response of patients to topical dorzolamide in the EGPS and underscores the role of these topical agents as adjunctive therapy rather than monotherapy. In another study, topical and systemic side effects were minimal, with a 2.7% incidence of keratitis and a 0.7% incidence of corneal edema. Systemic plasma levels were detectable in red blood cells at 5 months.[54]

The most striking difference between brinzolamide and dorzolamide seems to be tolerance. In a 1997 preliminary study involving more than 200 patients, there were significantly more complaints of severe and moderately severe discomfort following masked dorzolamide use compared with masked brinzolamide use.[55] Ocular hyperemia and tearing were also less in the brinzolamide group, but foreign-body sensation and blurred vision were significantly greater in the brinzolamide group. The early clinical use of brinzolamide suggests that patients do occasionally have blurred vision, which is most likely related to the nature of the suspension. Overall, brinzolamide 1% seems to be a safe and effective option with a slightly different tolerance profile compared with dorzolamide for the treatment of glaucoma.

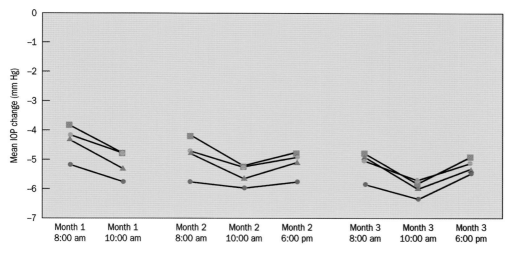

Figure 6.6. Mean change in IOP for each treatment group by visit and time of day during 3-month treatment period. Values reported are least-squares means of change from corresponding baseline diurnal IOP. All changes from baseline were statistically significant (P < .0001). Green squares, brinzolamide 1% twice daily; orange circles, brinzolamide 1% three times daily; blue triangles, dorzolamide 2% three times daily; red circles, timolol 0; 5% twice daily. Redrawn from Silver LH. Clinical efficacy and safety of brinzolamide (Azopt), a new topical carbonic anhydrase inhibitor for primary open-angle glaucoma and ocular hypertension. Brinzolamide Primary Therapy Study Group. *Am J Ophthalmol.* 1998;126:400–408. Copyright 1998, with permission from Elsevier Science.

6.3 CONCLUSIONS

The mechanism of action of CAIs is the suppression of aqueous production by inhibiting the isoenzyme carbonic anhydrase II. Systemic side effects such as fatigue, malaise, and weight loss may prevent the use of oral agents in many patients. Since the introduction of topical CAIs dorzolamide and brinzolamide, side effects related to this class of medications have markedly diminished. Either agent can be administered either twice daily or three times daily; the efficacy is similar when comparing the two agents; however, brinzolamide may be better tolerated due to its more neutral pH compared to dorzolamide.

REFERENCES
1. Higginbotham EJ. Topical Carbonic anhydrase inhibitors. New ophthalmic drugs. *Ophthalmol Clin North Am.* 1989;2:113–130.
2. Maren TH. The rates of movement of Na$^+$, Cl$^-$ and HCO3$^-$ from plasma to posterior chamber: effect of acetazolamide and relation to the treatment of glaucoma. *Invest Ophthalmol.* 1976;15:356–364.

3. Caprioli J. The ciliary epithelia and aqueous humor. In: Hart WM Jr, ed. *Adler's Physiology of the Eye: Clinical Application*. 9th ed. St Louis, MO: CV Mosby Co; 1992:234.

4. Friedman Z, Krupin T, Becker B. Ocular and systemic effects of acetazolamide in nephrectomized rabbits. *Invest Ophthalmol Vis Sci*. 1982;23:209–213.

5. Maren TH, Haywood JR, Chapman SK, Zimmerman TJ. The pharmacology of methazolamide in relation to the treatment of glaucoma. *Invest Ophthalmol Vis Sci*. 1977;16:730–742.

6. Stone RA, Zimmerman TJ, Shin DH, et al. Low-dose methazolamide and intraocular pressure. *Am J Ophthalmol*. 1977;83:674–679.

7. Dahlen K, Epstein DL, Grant WM, et al. A repeated dose–response study of methazolamide in glaucoma. *Arch Ophthalmol*. 1978;96:2214–2218.

8. Merkle W. Effect of methazolamide on the intraocular pressure of patients with open-angle glaucoma. *Klin Monatsbl Augenheilkd*. 1980;176:181–185.

9. Heller I, Halevy J, Cohen S, Theodor E. Significant metabolic acidosis induced by acetazolamide: not a rare complication. *Arch Intern Med*. 1985;145:1815–1817.

10. Margo CE. Acetazolamide and advanced liver disease. *Am J Ophthalmol*. 1986;101:611–612.

11. Block ER, Rostand RA. Carbonic anhydrase inhibition in glaucoma: hazard or benefit for the chronic lunger? *Surv Ophthalmol*. 1978;23:169–172.

12. Lichter PR, Musch DC, Medzihradsky F, Standardi CL. Intraocular pressure effects of carbonic anhydrase inhibitors in primary open-angle glaucoma. *Am J Ophthalmol*. 1989;107:11–17.

13. Fraunfelder FT, Grove JA, eds. *Drug-Induced Ocular Side Effects*. Baltimore, MD: Williams & Wilkins; 1996:439–441.

14. Arrigg CA, Epstein DL, Giovanoni R, Grant WM. The influence of supplemental sodium acetate on carbonic anhydrase inhibitor–induced side effects. *Arch Ophthalmol*. 1981;99:1969–1972.

15. Maren TH, Ellison AC. The teratological effect of certain thiadiazoles related to acetazolamide, with a note on sulfanilamide and thiazide diuretics. *Johns Hopkins Med J*. 1972;130:95–104.

16. Kass MA, Kolker AE, Gordon M, et al. Acetazolamide and urolithiasis. *Ophthalmology*. 1981;88:261–265.

17. Shields MB, Simmons RJ. Urinary calculus during methazolamide therapy. *Am J Ophthalmol*. 1976;81:622–624.

18. Werblin TP, Pollack IP, Liss RA. Blood dyscrasias in patients using methazolamide (Neptazane) for glaucoma. *Ophthalmology*. 1980;87:350–354.

19. Wisch N, Fischbein FI, Siegel R, et al. Aplastic anemia resulting from the use of carbonic anhydrase inhibitors. *Am J Ophthalmol*. 1973;75:130–132.

20. Zimran A, Beutler E. Can the risk of acetazolamide-induced aplastic anemia be decreased by periodic monitoring of blood cell counts? *Am J Ophthalmol*. 1987;104:654–658.

21. Fraunfelder FT, Meyer SM, Bagby CG Jr, Dreis MW. Hematologic reactions to carbonic anhydrase inhibitors. *Am J Ophthalmol*. 1985;100:79–81.

22. Foss RH. Local application of Diamox: an experimental study of its effect on the intraocular pressure. *Am J Ophthalmol*. 1955;39:336.

23. Ingram C, Brubaker RF. Effect of brinzolamide and dorzolamide on aqueous humor flow in human eyes. *Am J Ophthalmol*. 1999;128:292–296.

24. Friedman Z, Allen RC, Raph SM. Topical acetazolamide and methazolamide delivered by contact lenses. *Arch Ophthalmol.* 1985;103:963–966.
25. Lewis RA, Schoenwald RD, Eller MG, et al. Ethoxzolamide analogue gel: a topical carbonic anhydrase inhibitor. *Arch Ophthalmol.* 1984;102:1821–1824.
26. Stein A, Pinke R, Krupin T, et al. The effect of topically administered carbonic anhydrase inhibitors on aqueous humor dynamics in rabbits. *Am J Ophthalmol.* 1983;95: 222–228.
27. Kalina PH, Shetlar DJ, Lewis RA, et al. 6-Amino-2-benzothiazole-sulfonamide: the effect of a topical carbonic anhydrase inhibitor on aqueous humor formation in the normal human eye. *Ophthalmology.* 1988;95:772–777.
28. Hageman GS, Zhu XL, Waheed A, Sly WS. Localization of carbonic anhydrase IV in a specific capillary bed of the human eye. *Proc Natl Acad Sci U S A.* 1991;88:2716–2720.
29. Sugrue MF, Mallorga P, Schwam H, et al. A comparison of L-671,152 and MK-927, two topically effective ocular hypotensive carbonic anhydrase inhibitors, in experimental animals. *Curr Eye Res.* 1990;9:607–615.
30. Wang RF, Serle JB, Podos SM, Sugrue MF. The ocular hypotensive effect of the topical carbonic anhydrase inhibitor L-671,152 in glaucomatous monkeys. *Arch Ophthalmol.* 1990;108:511–513.
31. Wang RF, Serle JB, Podos SM, Sugrue MF. MK-507 (L-671,152), a topically active carbonic anhydrase inhibitor, reduces aqueous humor production in monkeys. *Arch Ophthalmol.* 1991;109:1297–1299.
32. Strahlman E, Tipping R, Vogel R. A double-masked, randomized 1-year study comparing dorzolamide (Trusopt), timolol, and betaxolol. International Dorzolamide Study Group. *Arch Ophthalmol.* 1995;113:1009–1016.
33. Nardin G, Lewis R, Lippa EA, et al. Activity of the topical CAI MK-507 bid when added to timolol bid. *Invest Ophthalmol Vis Sci.* 1991;32(suppl):989.
34. Strahlman EL, Tipping RW, Clineschmidt CM. A controlled clinical trial comparing dorzolamide (MK-507) and pilocarpine as adjunctive therapy to timolol. *Ophthalmology.* 1994;101(suppl):129.
35. Lippa EA, Schuman JS, Higginbotham EJ, et al. Dose response and duration of action of dorzolamide, a topical carbonic anhydrase inhibitor. *Ophthalmology.* 1992;110: 495–499.
36. Ott EZ, Mills MD, Arango S, et al. A randomized trial assessing dorzolamide in patients with glaucoma who are younger than 6 years. *Arch Ophthalmol.* 2005;123(9): 1177–1186.
37. Adamsons I, Clineschmidt C, Polis A, et al. The efficacy and safety of dorzolamide as adjunctive therapy to timolol maleate gellan solution in patients with elevated intraocular pressure. Additivity Study Group. *J Glaucoma.* 1998;7:253–260.
38. Delaney YM, Salmon JF, Mossa F, et al. Periorbital dermatitis as a side effect of topical dorzolamide. *Br J Ophthalmol.* 2002;86(4):378–380.
39. Wilkerson M, Cyrlin M, Lippa EA, et al. Four-week safety and efficacy study of dorzolamide, a novel, active topical carbonic anhydrase inhibitor. *Arch Ophthalmol.* 1993;111:1343–1350.
40. Kitazawa Y, Shimizu U, Ido T. MK-417 and MK-507, topical CAIs: the effect of lowering intraocular pressure and the pharmacokinetics in normal volunteers. Presented at: International Glaucoma Symposium; August 20, 1991; Jerusalem, Israel.
41. Lass JH, Khosrof SA, Laurence JT, et al. A double-masked, randomized, 1-year study comparing the corneal effects of dorzolamide, timolol, and betaxolol. Dorzolamide Corneal Effects Study Group. *Arch Ophthalmol.* 1998;116:1003–1010.

42. Konowal A, Morrison JC, Brown SVL, et al. Irreversible corneal decompensation in patients treated with topical dorzolamide. *Am J Ophthalmol.* 1999;127:403–406.

43. Maus TL, Larsson LI, McLaren JW, Brubaker RF. Comparison of dorzolamide and acetazolamide as suppressors of aqueous humor flow in humans. *Arch Ophthalmol.* 1997;115:45–49.

44. Kitazawa Y, Azuma I, Araie M, et al. Topical dorzolamide hydrochloride can be a substitute for oral CAIs [abstract]. *Invest Ophthalmol Vis Sci.* 1994;35(suppl):2177.

45. Hutzelmann JE, Polis AB, Michael AJ, Adamsons IA. A comparison of the efficacy and tolerability of dorzolamide and acetazolamide as adjunctive therapy to timolol. *Acta Ophthalmol Scand.* 1998;76:717–722.

46. Rosenberg LF, Krupin T, Tang LQ, et al. Combination of systemic acetazolamide and topical dorzolamide in reducing intraocular pressure and aqueous humor formation. *Ophthalmology.* 1998;105:88–93.

47. Harris A, Arend O, Arend S, Martin B. Effect of topical dorzolamide on retinal and retrobulbar hemodynamics. *Acta Ophthalmol Scand.* 1996;74:569–574.

48. Nagel E, Vilser W, Lanzl I. Dorzolamide influences the autoregulation of major retinal vessels caused by artificial intraocular pressure elevation in patients with POAG: a clinical study. *Curr Eye Res.* 2005;30(2):129–137.

49. The European Glaucoma Prevention Study Group. Results of the European Glaucoma Prevention Study. *Ophthalmology.* 2005;112:366–375.

50. Kass MA, Heuer DK, Higginbotham EJ, et al. Ocular Hypertension Treatment Study Group. The Ocular Hypertension Treatment Study. A randomized trial determines that topical hypotensive medication delays or prevents the onset of primary open angle glaucoma. *Arch Ophthalmol.* 2002;120:701–713.

51. Tsukamot H, Noma H, Mukai S, et al. The efficacy and ocular discomfort of substituting brinzolamide for dorzolamide in combination therapy with latanoprost, timolol, and dorzolamide. *J Ocul Pharmacol Ther.* 2005;21(5):395–399.

52. Silver LH. Clinical efficacy and safety of brinzolamide (Azopt), a new topical carbonic anhydrase inhibitor for primary open-angle glaucoma and ocular hypertension. Brinzolamide Primary Therapy Study Group. *Am J Ophthalmol.* 1998;126:400–408.

53. van der Valk R, Webers CA, Schouten JS, et al. Intraocular pressure-lowering effects of all commonly used glaucoma drugs. a meta-analysis of randomized clinical trials. *Ophthalmology.* 2005;112(7):1177–1185.

54. McCarty GR, Dahlin D, Curtis M, et al. A double-masked, parallel group, placebo-controlled, multiple-dose pharmacokinetic study of brinzolamide following oral administration in normal volunteers [abstract 3246]. *Invest Ophthalmol Vis Sci.* 1998;39:707.

55. Stewart R; Brinzolamide Comfort Study Group. The ocular comfort of TID-dosed brinzolamide 1.0% compared to tid-dosed dorzolamide 2.0% in patients with primary open-angle glaucoma or ocular hypertension. *Invest Ophthalmol Vis Sci.* 1997;38:559.

7

Fixed-Combination Drugs

ALBERT S. KHOURI, TONY REALINI, AND ROBERT D. FECHTNER

*I*nitial therapy for glaucoma typically consists of topical medications that lower intraocular pressure (IOP), and frequently more than one agent is required to achieve adequate control of IOP. For example, initial monotherapy failed to control IOP within the first 2 years of treatment in up to 50% of glaucoma patients in the United States.[1] The recent Ocular Hypertension Treatment Study randomized patients to observation or treatment in which the therapeutic goal was a relatively modest 20% IOP reduction; in that study, 40% of patients randomized to treatment required more than one medication to achieve the therapeutic goal.[2]

The importance of making therapy convenient for glaucoma patients cannot be overemphasized. Consider the burdens of treatment from the patient's perspective: Early and even moderate glaucoma is often symptom-free, which tends to reduce adherence to medical regimens. Unlike chronic therapy for some medical ailments where a clear therapeutic benefit is evident to patients, no such benefit is evident to treated glaucoma patients. In fact, there often exist treatment disincentives: Medicines are costly and time-consuming to instill and may have side effects that are often perceived by the patient as being worse than the glaucoma prior to treatment.

These observations underscore the potential benefits of fixed-combination medications compared with using multiple medication bottles, thus reducing the burdens of therapy. Among the advantages of fixed combinations for patients are cost savings and a reduction in the total number of drops instilled per day. This also reduces the amount of preservative applied to the eye, which may improve tolerability and may favorably influence eventual surgical outcomes in patients who ultimately require filtering procedures.[3,4] A frequent occurrence in patients using multiple medication bottles is the established washout effect resulting from rapid-sequence instillation of multiple drops. Although it is recommended that patients wait approximately 5 minutes between eye drops,[5] the inconvenience of this recommendation may affect adherence.

Attempts to develop effective fixed combinations of glaucoma medications date back several decades. Few such combinations have emerged, due in part to limitations such as differences between the component optimal dosing frequency, indications and contraindications, additive side effects, and drug interactions of the components (table 7.1).

The evaluation of a potential fixed combination of topical IOP-lowering drugs should include, at a minimum, studies comparing the combination to the individual components and to the components administered as concomitant therapy. One would expect the fixed combination to provide greater IOP reduction than either of the components administered as monotherapy, and safety and efficacy comparable to concomitant dosing. A fixed combination may show slightly less efficacy at some time points if there are dosing differences (e.g., component administered three times daily versus twice-daily administration of a fixed combination), but if small enough, such a difference may be a worthwhile trade-off to gain the advantages of combination therapy.

7.1 PRODUCTS OF HISTORICAL INTEREST

7.1.1 *Pilocarpine–Epinephrine.* Adrenergic and cholinergic combinations were reported as early as the 1960s.[6,7] The first available combination of IOP-lowering agents was a mixture of pilocarpine and epinephrine. This product evolved during the period when these two classes represented available glaucoma medications, and with additive properties in combination.[8,9] Many patients were receiving both in separate bottles, and combining them in a single bottle offered dosing convenience. Some patients may have been better off with concomitant therapy because the combination was approved for use four times daily, posing a significant overdosage of the epinephrine component.

7.1.2 *Timolol–Pilocarpine and Timolol–Epinephrine.* As the topical beta blocker timolol became first-line treatment, its combination with other topical agents such as epinephrine[10] and pilocarpine[11] was studied. These combinations arose due in large part to a paucity of available medications. The fixed timolol–pilocarpine[12,13] and timolol–epinephrine[10] combinations offered dosing convenience to glaucoma

Table 7.1 Fixed Combinations of Glaucoma Medications

Brand Name	Components	Manufacturer
Cosopt	Timolol 0.5% and dorzolamide 2.0%	Merck and Co., Inc.
Xalacom	Timolol 0.5% and latanoprost 0.005%	Pfizer, Inc.
DuoTrav, Extravan	Timolol 0.5% and travoprost 0.004%	Alcon Laboratories, Inc.
Ganfort	Timolol 0.5% and bimatoprost 0.03%	Allergan, Inc.
Combigan	Timolol 0.5% and brimonidine 0.2%	Allergan, Inc.

patients at the time. Like the pilocarpine–epinephrine combination, a dosing mis-match existed, with timolol requiring one to two drops per day and pilocarpine up to four drops daily to reach maximal efficacy. The timolol–pilocarpine combination was never approved for use in the United States.

7.1.3 Betaxolol–Pilocarpine.

Although never released into the market, the fixed combination of betaxolol and pilocarpine[14] was studied and approved by the FDA in April 1997.

7.2 MODERN FIXED COMBINATION APPROVED IN THE UNITED STATES: TIMOLOL–DORZOLAMIDE

Timolol maleate 0.5%–dorzolamide hydrochloride 2.0% fixed combination (Cosopt; Merck and Co., Inc., Whitehouse Station, N.J.) was approved by the FDA in 1998. It is the only fixed combination drug available in the United States. At present, prostaglandins are first-line choice medications for most patients; however, in the mid-1990s, beta blockers were the drugs of choice for first-line IOP reduction. The choices besides beta blockers, prior to the approval of dorzolamide in 1994, included pilocarpine and dipivefrin. Because of its safety, efficacy, and convenience of dosing, dorzolamide quickly became a popular second-line choice until the introduction of latanoprost in 1996. Thus, as with the older combination products, the development of the timolol–dorzolamide fixed-combination product reflected common clinical usage at the time. The labeled indication reflects treatment practice at that time: The fixed combination is indicated for patients with primary open-angle glaucoma or ocular hypertension who are insufficiently responsive to beta blockers.

Comparison studies confirmed that the timolol–dorzolamide fixed combination was more efficacious than either of its constituents in monotherapy.[15,16] In the first study, 335 subjects underwent a washout period and were randomized into three groups (timolol, 112 subjects; dorzolamide, 109; fixed-combination timolol–dorzolamide, 114). At three months, the combination twice daily provided a 2-hour peak IOP reduction of 32.7% versus 19.8% and 22.6% for dorzolamide three times daily and timolol twice daily, respectively; and the morning trough IOP reduction of 27.4% for the combination twice daily versus 15.5% and 22.2% for the dorzolamide three times daily and timolol twice daily (figure 7.1).[16]

Another study of 242 patients randomized to receive the fixed combination (121 subjects) or the concomitant administration of its components (121 subjects), after a 2-week timolol run-in, also demonstrated equivalence to concomitant therapy with components in separate bottles,[17] with a nonsignificant difference of only 0.73 mm Hg favoring concomitant therapy at the 4 P.M. time point attributable to the three-times-daily dosing of dorzolamide in the concomitant group versus only twice daily in the fixed-combination group. In these studies, the fixed combination yielded peak and trough IOP reductions from untreated baseline of 9 mm Hg and 7.7 mm Hg, respectively.[16] Following a 3-week timolol run-in, switching to the fixed combination of timolol and dorzolamide further reduced IOP at peak and trough by 15.8% to 17.3% and 10.6% and 11.3%, respectively.[15]

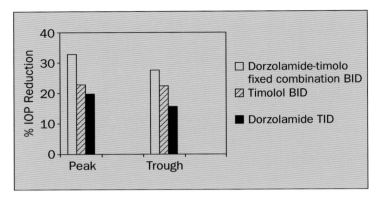

Figure 7.1. Dorzolamide–timolol fixed combination versus components at 3 months. Adapted from Boyle JE, et al. A randomized trial comparing the dorzolamide-timolol combination given twice daily to monotherapy with timolol and dorzolamide. Dorzolamide-Timolol Study Group. *Ophthalmology.* 1998;105(10):1945–1951. Adapted from reference 16.

Three published studies have demonstrated a potentially greater IOP-lowering effect from the fixed combination compared to concomitant therapy.[18–20] In these studies, patients receiving concomitant therapy with dorzolamide and a beta blocker were switched to the fixed combination. Each of the three studies showed a statistically significant IOP reduction after the switch to the fixed combination, ranging from 1.3 to 1.5 mm Hg. This likely represents improved compliance associated with reduction in both bottles and drops per day, as well as elimination of the washout effect.

In head-to-head comparisons with contemporary drugs, the timolol–dorzolamide fixed combination has been shown to be equal in efficacy to latanoprost monotherapy,[21–25] timolol and unoprostone concomitant therapy,[26] and timolol and brimonidine concomitant therapy.[27] Concomitant therapy with latanoprost and brimonidine has been shown to provide greater IOP reduction than the fixed combination of timolol and dorzolamide.[28]

7.3 MODERN FIXED COMBINATIONS APPROVED OUTSIDE THE UNITED STATES

In recent years, fixed combinations of commonly paired drugs have not received FDA approval due to insufficient additional demonstrated efficacy when compared to their components, despite such potential benefits as improved convenience and compliance and reduced cost to patients. Although the additive effects of prostaglandins to beta blockers have been demonstrated in several studies,[29–31] fewer data exist about the efficacy of adding beta blockers for subjects already on prostaglandins.

7.3.1 *Timolol–Latanoprost.* The fixed combination timolol maleate 0.5%–latanoprost 0.005% (Xalacom; Pfizer, Inc., New York, N.Y.) was the first beta blocker–prostaglandin combination released in 2001 after gaining regulatory approval in many regions of the world. Latanoprost was the first approved prostaglandin (in 1996) and quickly became a first-line agent of choice in the United States and around the world. Because timolol remains a popular and effective choice for adjunctive therapy, development of a fixed combination of these two agents once again reflects common clinical use. This fixed combination is approved in several countries for the reduction of IOP in patients with open-angle glaucoma and ocular hypertension.

Several studies have compared the fixed combination to monotherapy with the component medications. Higginbotham et al.,[32] in a 6-month, double-blind study, enrolled 418 patients that were randomized to receive either the fixed combination at 8 A.M. and placebo at 8 P.M. (138 subjects), timolol twice daily at 8 A.M. and 8 P.M. (140 subjects), or latanoprost at 8 A.M. and placebo at 8 P.M. (140 subjects), after a run-in treatment of timolol twice daily for 2 to 4 weeks. They demonstrated a 1 mm Hg greater diurnal IOP reduction among patients receiving the fixed combination compared to latanoprost monotherapy; this difference, although small, did reach the level of statistical significance.[32] Pfeiffer[33] performed a similar study on 436 patients after a 2 to 4 week timolol run-in period. Subjects were randomized similarly into three groups: 140 subjects received the fixed combination at 8 A.M., 147 received latanoprost at 8 A.M., and 149 received timolol at 8 A.M. and 8 P.M. Patients receiving the fixed combination showed a 1.2 mm Hg greater difference in mean diurnal IOP reduction compared to latanoprost monotherapy.[33] This result was also statistically significant.

The concomitant use of latanoprost and timolol did not demonstrate a statistically significant benefit over latanoprost monotherapy.[34] After a 2 to 4 week run-in on timolol twice daily, 148 patients were randomized to receive either latanoprost alone once daily (50 subjects) or concomitant therapy with latanoprost once daily and timolol (49 subjects), or pilocarpine 2% three times daily and timolol (49 subjects). After 6 months of treatment, latanoprost lowered mean diurnal IOP 5.5 mm Hg, while the combination of latanoprost and timolol achieved a mean diurnal reduction of 6.1 mm Hg. This 0.6 mm Hg difference in mean diurnal IOP was not statistically significant compared to latanoprost monotherapy (figure 7.2).

In a second concomitant use study, Konstas et al.[35] randomized 36 patients, after an 8-week timolol run-in, to receive either morning (8:00 A.M. and 8:15 A.M.) or evening (8:00 P.M. and 8:15 P.M.) dosing of latanoprost and timolol. The dosing regimen was continued for 7 weeks, after which the subjects were crossed over to the second dosing regimen for a minimum of 7 weeks. In-hospital diurnal IOP testing was performed every 4 hours for 24 hours. There were no statistical differences at individual time points or in mean diurnal IOP between the two dosing regimens.[35]

While it remains unclear whether the fixed combination of latanoprost and timolol offers clinically significant diurnal IOP reduction over latanoprost monotherapy, both the Higginbotham et al. and Pfeiffer studies demonstrated larger

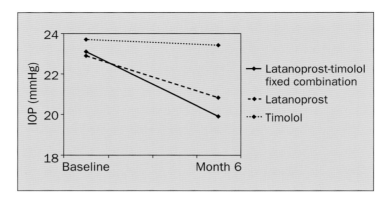

Figure 7-2. Latanoprost–timolol fixed combination versus components after timolol run-in. Adapted from Bucci MG. Intraocular pressure-lowering effects of latano-prost monotherapy versus latanoprost or pilocarpine in combination with timolol: a randomized, observer-masked multicenter study in patients with open-angle glaucoma. Italian Latanoprost Study Group. *J Glaucoma.* 1999;8(1):24–30. Adapted from reference 34.

diurnal IOP reductions with the fixed combination compared to timolol mono-therapy; Pfeiffer reported a 1.9 mm Hg advantage with the fixed combination,[33] and in Higginbotham et al.'s study, the advantage was 2.9 mm Hg.[32]

Several other smaller studies have compared the fixed combination timolol–latanoprost with concomitant therapy with timolol and brimonidine[36] and with the fixed combination timolol–dorzolamide.[37,38] Comparisons of the timolol-dorzolamide fixed combination to the latanoprost–timolol fixed combination have produced mixed results, with one study showing no difference in mean diurnal IOP between the two combinations[37] and another study finding a mean diurnal IOP approximately 1 mm Hg lower with the latanoprost–timolol combination.[38]

7.3.2 *Timolol–Travoprost.* The timolol 0.5%–travoprost 0.004% fixed combination (DuoTrav; Alcon Laboratories, Inc., Fort Worth, Tex.) was first approved in Australia in 2005 and is available in the European Union, Canada, Chili, Iceland, and Norway.

When compared to its individual components as monotherapy, the timolol–travoprost fixed combination produced greater IOP reductions than either of its components administered separately in a 3-month study of 263 subjects. The fixed combination produced a mean IOP reduction from baseline of 1.9 to 3.3 mm Hg greater than timolol that was statistically significant at 2-week, 6-week, and 3-month 8 A.M., 10 A.M., and 4 P.M. time points. Compared with travoprost, the fixed combination produced 0.9 to 2.4 mm Hg greater IOP reduction. This was statistically significant at all time points at week 2 and at all except the 4 P.M. time point at week 6 and month 3 (vs. travoprost).[39]

Two double-masked studies comparing timolol–travoprost fixed combination to the concomitant use of its components were conducted. In the first, 316 patients with open angle glaucoma or ocular hypertension were randomized, after a therapeutic washout, to receive either the timolol–travoprost fixed combination dosed in the morning, or concomitant therapy with timolol dosed in the morning and travoprost dosed in the evening. Measurements of IOP were performed at 8 A.M., 10 A.M., and 4 P.M. Significant IOP reductions from baseline at 3 months were achieved by both the fixed combination (15.2 to 16.5 mm Hg) and the concomitant use of timolol and travoprost (14.7 to 16.1 mm Hg). Although reductions were similar at the 8 A.M. time point, the concomitant use of the components was slightly superior at the 10 A.M. and 4 P.M. time points by almost 1 mm Hg.[40] This may be due to different dosing times for the components versus the fixed combination. The second study was of similar design and randomized 403 subjects into three groups: the fixed combination administered in the morning, concomitant administration of timolol in the morning and travoprost in the evening, or timolol twice daily. The fixed combination produced statistically significant IOP reductions of 7.0 to 8.2 mm Hg from baseline that lasted approximately 24 hours, with only slight increases in pressure between 4 P.M. and 8 A.M. The concomitant administration of the components produced slightly greater IOP reductions than the fixed combination at the 10 A.M. and 4 P.M. time points (mean differences from the fixed combination ranged from 0.4 to 1.1 mm Hg). Timolol twice daily was less effective than the two regimens containing timolol and travoprost in combination.[41]

7.3.3 *Timolol–Bimatoprost*. A bimatoprost 0.03%–timolol maleate 0.5% fixed combination (Ganfort; Allergan, Inc., Irvine, Calif.) has been recently approved in the European Union. Unpublished data (A. Hommer and colleagues) from a multicenter, double-blind, randomized study have been presented. In this trial, patients at 35 sites were randomized to one of three treatment arms. Each received the fixed combination dosed in the morning (178 subjects), or the concomitant use of timolol twice daily and bimatoprost once in the evening (177 subjects), or bimatoprost once in the evening (99 subjects). All subjects were naive to pharmacotherapy and returned 3 weeks after randomization for IOP measurements at 8 A.M., 10 A.M., and 4 P.M. The mean diurnal IOPs for the fixed-combination and concomitant-use groups were within 1.5 mm Hg (95% confidence interval) at all three time points. This met the defined criterion for noninferiority. The fixed combination decreased mean diurnal IOP from baseline by 8.8 mm Hg and was statistically significantly more effective than bimatoprost alone (0.8 mm Hg difference).

7.3.4 *Timolol–Brimonidine*. The timolol 0.5%–brimonidine tartrate 0.2% fixed-combination product (Combigan; Allergan, Inc., Irvine, Calif.), first approved in 2006, is a recent addition to the fixed-combination group of glaucoma treatments. It is indicated for the reduction of IOP in patients with primary open-angle glaucoma or ocular hypertension who are insufficiently responsive to topical beta blockers. The fixed combination of timolol and brimonidine is approved in Europe and several other countries worldwide.

The fixed combination provided significantly better IOP control compared to monotherapy with either brimonidine or timolol used alone. Craven et al.[42] reported 3-month results from a study of patients with treated glaucoma or ocular hypertension who underwent a washout period and were randomized to receive the fixed brimonidine–timolol combination twice daily or the individual components (brimonidine three times daily, or timolol twice daily). A total of 999 patients completed 3 months of assigned therapy. The mean decrease in IOP from baseline ranged from 4.9 to 7.6 mm Hg with the brimonidine–timolol combination. This was greater than reductions with the single components at all follow-up points at 8 A.M., 10 A.M., and 3 P.M. At the 5 P.M. measurements, when the brimonidine three-times-daily monotherapy group was at peak, and the fixed combination was approaching trough, there was no statistical difference between the brimonidine monotherapy and fixed combination groups. Sherwood et al.[43] reported the 12-month results combined from two identical trials. A total of 1,159 patients were randomized, and 833 completed the study. The mean decrease in IOP from baseline for the fixed combination was 4.4 to 7.6 mm Hg. Similar to previous observations, the fixed combination had greater IOP reductions than its individual components at the 8 A.M., 10 A.M., and 3 P.M. time points, but not the 5 P.M. time point, compared to brimonidine monotherapy (when dosed three times daily and at peak effect).

A study by Goni[44] of 355 patients included in a double-masked 12-week trial compared the fixed combination to the concomitant use of its individual components. Mean IOP reduction from baseline was significant and ranged from 4.4 to 5.7 mm Hg in the combination group. The combination was as effective as concomitant therapy at all time points and visits.

7.4 CONCLUSION

Existing fixed-combination glaucoma products, and those under development, reflect common concomitant usage in clinical practice. With so many new drugs to choose from, the optimal order in which to utilize drug classes in the traditional stepped treatment algorithm is less obvious than ever before. And with emerging evidence that lower and less variable IOP best prevents the progression of glaucoma, the tradition of adding only one drug at a time may no longer be universally applicable.

In an era of many drug choices and the ability to individualize patient care as never before,[45] the fixed combinations limit clinicians' ability to customize dosing regimens. Unless prescribed with caution, fixed-combination drugs may result in overtreatment for patients who may be controlled with a single agent or fewer doses of combined medications if dosed concomitantly. Fixed combinations offer advantages over concomitant therapy in terms of reduced cost, increased compliance, and reduction of the washout effect and exposure to preservatives.

In the face of so many choices, the challenge is to keep medical therapy reasonable. The current concept of reasonable medical therapy probably consists of two bottles, one of which is a fixed-combination product.

REFERENCES

1. Kobelt-Nguyen G, Gerdtham UG, Alm A. Costs of treating primary open-angle glaucoma and ocular hypertension: a retrospective, observational two-year chart review of newly diagnosed patients in Sweden and the United States. *J Glaucoma.* 1998;7(2): 95–104.

2. Kass MA, et al. The Ocular Hypertension Treatment Study: a randomized trial determines that topical ocular hypotensive medication delays or prevents the onset of primary open-angle glaucoma. *Arch Ophthalmol.* 2002;120(6):701–713, 829–830.

3. Lavin MJ, et al. The influence of prior therapy on the success of trabeculectomy. *Arch Ophthalmol.* 1990;108(11):1543–1548.

4. Broadway DC, et al. Adverse effects of topical antiglaucoma medication. II. The outcome of filtration surgery. *Arch Ophthalmol.* 1994;112(11):1446–1454.

5. Chrai SS, et al. Drop size and initial dosing frequency problems of topically applied ophthalmic drugs. *J Pharm Sci.* 1974;63(3):333–338.

6. Kronfeld PC. The efficacy of combinations of ocular hypotensive drugs. A tonographic approach. *Arch Ophthalmol.* 1967;78(2):140–146.

7. Demailly P, Kerisel JB. [Combination of 2 percent pilocarpine—5 percent neosynephrine in the treatment of chronic and aphakic glaucoma]. *Arch Ophthalmol Rev Gen Ophthalmol.* 1967;27(7):683–696.

8. Krieglstein GK, Leydhecker W. [The pressure reducing effects of pilocarpin in combination with dipivalyl-epinephrine in glaucoma simplex]. *Klin Monatsbl Augenheilkd.* 1979;175(1):86–90.

9. Trotta N, O'Connor R. Efficacy of a combination solution of epinephrine and pilocarpine. *Eye Ear Nose Throat Mon.* 1971;50(9):350–352.

10. Knupp JA, et al. Combined timolol and epinephrine therapy for open angle glaucoma. *Surv Ophthalmol.* 1983;28(suppl):280–285.

11. Hovding G, Aasved H. Timolol/pilocarpine combination eye drops in open angle glaucoma and in ocular hypertension. A controlled randomized study. *Acta Ophthalmol (Copenh).* 1987;65(5):594–601.

12. Maclure GM, et al. Effect on the 24-hour diurnal curve of intraocular pressure of a fixed ratio combination of timolol 0.5% and pilocarpine 2% in patients with COAG not controlled on timolol 0.5%. *Br J Ophthalmol.* 1989;73(10):827–831.

13. Moriarty AP, Dowd TC, Trimble RB. Clinical experience with a fixed dose combination therapy of timolol and pilocarpine used twice daily in the management of chronic open angle glaucoma. *Eye.* 1994;8(pt 4):410–413.

14. Robin AL. Ocular hypotensive efficacy and safety of a combined formulation of betaxolol and pilocarpine. *Trans Am Ophthalmol Soc.* 1996;94:89–103.

15. Clineschmidt CM, et al. A randomized trial in patients inadequately controlled with timolol alone comparing the dorzolamide-timolol combination to monotherapy with timolol or dorzolamide. Dorzolamide-Timolol Combination Study Group. *Ophthalmology.* 1998;105(10):1952–1959.

16. Boyle JE, et al. A randomized trial comparing the dorzolamide-timolol combination given twice daily to monotherapy with timolol and dorzolamide. Dorzolamide-Timolol Study Group. *Ophthalmology.* 1998;105(10):1945–1951.

17. Strohmaier K, et al. The efficacy and safety of the dorzolamide-timolol combination versus the concomitant administration of its components. Dorzolamide-Timolol Study Group. *Ophthalmology.* 1998;105(10):1936–1944.

18. Choudhri S, Wand M, Shields MB. A comparison of dorzolamide-timolol combination versus the concomitant drugs. *Am J Ophthalmol.* 2000;130(6):832–833.

19. Gugleta K, Orgul S, Flammer J. Experience with Cosopt, the fixed combination of timolol and dorzolamide, after switch from free combination of timolol and dorzolamide, in Swiss ophthalmologists' offices. *Curr Med Res Opin.* 2003;19(4):330–335.

20. Bacharach J, Delgado MF, Iwach AG. Comparison of the efficacy of the fixed-combination timolol/dorzolamide versus concomitant administration of timolol and dorzolamide. *J Ocul Pharmacol Ther.* 2003;19(2):93–96.

21. Honrubia FM, Larsson LI, Spiegel D. A comparison of the effects on intraocular pressure of latanoprost 0.005% and the fixed combination of dorzolamide 2% and timolol 0.5% in patients with open-angle glaucoma. *Acta Ophthalmol Scand.* 2002; 80(6):635–641.

22. Konstas AG, et al. Twenty-four-hour diurnal curve comparison of commercially available latanoprost 0.005% versus the timolol and dorzolamide fixed combination. *Ophthalmology.* 2003;110(7):1357–1360.

23. Orzalesi N, et al. Comparison of latanoprost, brimonidine and a fixed combination of timolol and dorzolamide on circadian intraocular pressure in patients with primary open-angle glaucoma and ocular hypertension. *Acta Ophthalmol Scand.* 2002; 236(suppl):55.

24. Fechtner RD, et al. Efficacy of the dorzolamide/timolol fixed combination versus latanoprost in the treatment of ocular hypertension or glaucoma: combined analysis of pooled data from two large randomized observer and patient-masked studies. *J Ocul Pharmacol Ther.* 2005;21(3):242–249.

25. Fechtner RD, et al. Efficacy and tolerability of the dorzolamide 2%/timolol 0.5% combination (Cosopt) versus 0.005% (Xalatan) in the treatment of ocular hypertension or glaucoma: results from two randomized clinical trials. *Acta Ophthalmol Scand.* 2004;82(1):42–48.

26. Day DG, et al. Timolol 0.5%/dorzolamide 2% fixed combination vs timolol maleate 0.5% and unoprostone 0.15% given twice daily to patients with primary open-angle glaucoma or ocular hypertension. *Am J Ophthalmol.* 2003;135(2):138–143.

27. Sall KN, et al. Dorzolamide/timolol combination versus concomitant administration of brimonidine and timolol: six-month comparison of efficacy and tolerability. *Ophthalmology.* 2003;110(3):615–624.

28. Zabriskie N, Netland PA. Comparison of brimonidine/latanoprost and timolol/dorzolamide: two randomized, double-masked, parallel clinical trials. *Adv Ther.* 2003; 20(2):92–100.

29. Alm A, et al. Latanoprost administered once daily caused a maintained reduction of intraocular pressure in glaucoma patients treated concomitantly with timolol. *Br J Ophthalmol.* 1995;79(1):12–16.

30. Rulo AH, Greve EL, Hoyng PF. Additive effect of latanoprost, a prostaglandin F2 alpha analogue, and timolol in patients with elevated intraocular pressure. *Br J Ophthalmol.* 1994;78(12):899–902.

31. Orengo-Nania S, et al. Evaluation of travoprost as adjunctive therapy in patients with uncontrolled intraocular pressure while using timolol 0.5%. *Am J Ophthalmol.* 2001; 132(6):860–868.

32. Higginbotham EJ, et al. Latanoprost and timolol combination therapy vs monotherapy: one-year randomized trial. *Arch Ophthalmol.* 2002;120(7):915–922.

33. Pfeiffer N. A comparison of the fixed combination of latanoprost and timolol with its individual components. *Graefes Arch Clin Exp Ophthalmol.* 2002;240(11):893–899.

34. Bucci MG. Intraocular pressure-lowering effects of latanoprost monotherapy versus latanoprost or pilocarpine in combination with timolol: a randomized, observer-masked multicenter study in patients with open-angle glaucoma. Italian Latanoprost Study Group. *J Glaucoma.* 1999;8(1):24–30.

35. Konstas AG, et al. A comparison of once-daily morning vs evening dosing of concomitant latanoprost/timolol. *Am J Ophthalmol.* 2002;133(6):753–757.

36. Stewart WC, et al. Efficacy and safety of timolol maleate/latanoprost fixed combination versus timolol maleate and brimonidine given twice daily. *Acta Ophthalmol Scand.* 2003;81(3):242–246.

37. Konstas AG, et al. Daytime diurnal curve comparison between the fixed combinations of latanoprost 0.005%/timolol maleate 0.5% and dorzolamide 2%/timolol maleate 0.5%. *Eye.* 2004;18(12):1264–1269.

38. Shin DH, Feldman RM, Sheu WP. Efficacy and safety of the fixed combinations latanoprost/timolol versus dorzolamide/timolol in patients with elevated intraocular pressure. *Ophthalmology.* 2004;111(2):276–282.

39. Barnebey HS, et al. The safety and efficacy of travoprost 0.004%/timolol 0.5% fixed combination ophthalmic solution. *Am J Ophthalmol.* 2005;140(1):1–7.

40. Hughes BA, et al. A three-month, multicenter, double-masked study of the safety and efficacy of travoprost 0.004%/timolol 0.5% ophthalmic solution compared to travoprost 0.004% ophthalmic solution and timolol 0.5% dosed concomitantly in subjects with open angle glaucoma or ocular hypertension. *J Glaucoma.* 2005;14(5):392–399.

41. Schuman JS, et al. Efficacy and safety of a fixed combination of travoprost 0.004%/timolol 0.5% ophthalmic solution once daily for open-angle glaucoma or ocular hypertension. *Am J Ophthalmol.* 2005;140(2):242–250.

42. Craven ER, et al. Brimonidine and timolol fixed-combination therapy versus monotherapy: a 3-month randomized trial in patients with glaucoma or ocular hypertension. *J Ocul Pharmacol Ther.* 2005;21(4):337–348.

43. Sherwood MB, et al. Twice-daily 0.2% brimonidine-0.5% timolol fixed-combination therapy vs monotherapy with timolol or brimonidine in patients with glaucoma or ocular hypertension: a 12-month randomized trial. *Arch Ophthalmol.* 2006;124(9):1230–1238.

44. Goni FJ. 12-Week study comparing the fixed combination of brimonidine and timolol with concomitant use of the individual components in patients with glaucoma and ocular hypertension. *Eur J Ophthalmol.* 2005;15(5):581–590.

45. Realini T, Fechtner RD. 56,000 ways to treat glaucoma. *Ophthalmology.* 2002;109(11):1955–1956.

8

Osmotic Drugs

PETER A. NETLAND AND ALLAN E. KOLKER

O smotically active ocular hypotensive agents were initially tried early in the twentieth century, when Andre Cantonnet described the oral use of sodium chloride and lactose for lowering intraocular pressure (IOP).[1] In 1914, Emil Hertel influenced IOP by intravenous injection of anisotonic solutions.[2] Many of these agents, such as concentrated saline, sodium carbonate, sugars, and gum acacia, while producing adequate ocular responses, did not stand the test of time because of their untoward side effects and the inadequate duration of their osmotic effect. After the ocular hypotensive effect of intravenous urea was described in 1958 and was further studied in glaucoma patients,[3,4] this drug became the first hyperosmotic agent to achieve widespread use in glaucoma therapy.

The use of urea has been superseded by other osmotic drugs in current ophthalmic clinical practice (figure 8.1). Orally administered mannitol is poorly absorbed from the gastrointestinal tract; however, in 1962, intravenous mannitol was shown to lower IOP.[5,6] Glycerol, introduced in 1963 by Virno et al.,[7] was the first practical oral osmotic drug for the reduction of IOP. In 1967, Becker, Kolker, and Krupin[8] described the use of oral isosorbide as preoperative medication and as therapy for patients with acute glaucomas.

Although osmotic agents for reduction of IOP are infrequently used, they may be more effective than other glaucoma medications in the short-term treatment of certain types of glaucomas. Osmotic drugs are useful in the preoperative preparation of select patients for intraocular surgery. These drugs are also effective in the initial treatment of acute and extreme elevation of IOP, including angle-closure glaucoma and certain secondary glaucomas.

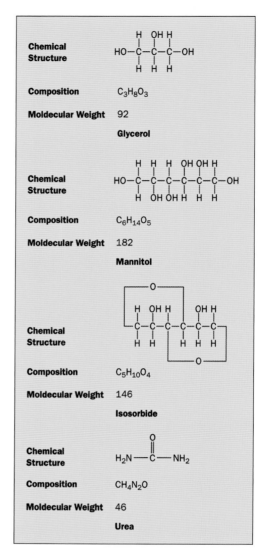

Figure 8.1. Osmotic drugs.

8.1 MECHANISM OF ACTION

Osmotic drugs lower IOP by increasing the osmotic gradient between the blood and the ocular fluids. Following administration of osmotic drugs, the blood osmolality is increased by up to 20 to 30 mOsm/L, which results in loss of water from the eye to the hyperosmotic plasma. This movement of water from the eye to the circulation is associated with a lowering of IOP.

The mechanism of reduction of IOP is likely due to reduction of vitreous volume, which probably results from the water transfer caused by the osmotic gradient

Table 8.1 Factors Affecting Osmotic Gradient

1. Ocular penetration
2. Distribution in body fluids
3. Molecular weight and concentration
4. Dosage
5. Rate and route of administration
6. Rate of systemic clearance
7. Type of diuresis

between the retina–choroid and the vitreous.[9,10] Water absorption by the iris appears to play an insignificant role in the hypotony induced by osmotic agents.[11] Although aqueous formation rates were not measured, conventional outflow facility does not change after administration of an osmotic agent.[12] A mechanism mediated by the central nervous system has been proposed,[13] perhaps via central osmoreceptors; however, this possibility has been disputed.[14]

The degree of IOP lowering is determined by the osmotic gradient caused by these drugs. The following factors influence degree and duration of the osmotic gradient (table 8.1)[15]:

1. *Ocular penetration.* Drugs that enter the eye rapidly produce less of an osmotic gradient compared with drugs that penetrate slowly or not at all. Ocular permeability to some drugs is greatly increased when the eye is inflamed and congested. This reduction of the osmotic gradient in inflamed eyes has been demonstrated after administration of urea, which is of relatively low molecular weight, and was less pronounced following treatment with glycerol and mannitol.[16,17] Although certain drugs (e.g., ethyl alcohol) enter the aqueous rapidly, part of their ocular hypotensive effect is due to relatively slow penetration in the avascular vitreous.

2. *Distribution in body fluids.* Drugs confined to the extracellular fluid space (e.g., mannitol) produce a greater effect on blood osmolality at the same dosage compared with drugs distributed in total body water (e.g., urea). For this reason, a larger dose in milliosmoles is required of urea compared with mannitol to produce the same osmotic gradient.

3. *Molecular weight and concentration.* Because the blood osmolality depends on the number of milliosmoles of substance administered, drugs with low molecular weight have potentially greater effect compared with compounds of high molecular weight at the same dosage in grams per kilogram. Thus, the lower molecular weight of urea compared with mannitol compensates for the greater distribution in body water of urea compared with mannitol. Also, osmotic drugs are administered as solutions, with osmolality directly proportional to the concentration. Drugs with low solubility require larger volumes of solution, with subsequently less effect on blood osmolality. Also, ingestion of fluids after osmotic drug use decreases blood osmolality, which decreases the osmotic gradient between the blood and the eye. This may occur following intake of fluids intended to make oral osmotic drugs more palatable.

4. *Dosage*. The change in blood osmolality depends on the total dose administered and the weight of the patient. With other factors being equal, a heavier patient has more body water and requires more drug compared with a lighter patient to achieve an equivalent osmotic gradient.

5. *Rate and route of administration*. Drugs administered intravenously bypass absorption from the gastrointestinal tract, generally producing a more rapid and greater osmotic gradient compared with orally administered drugs. When drugs are infused intravenously, a rate of 60 to 100 drops per minute is recommended.

6. *Rate of systemic clearance*. The rate of drug clearance from the systemic circulation influences the duration of action. Most osmotic drugs are excreted rapidly in the urine. Glycerol and ethyl alcohol, for example, are also metabolized.

7. *Type of diuresis*. Most osmotic drugs induce a diuresis, which may be hyper-, iso-, or hypoosmotic. After administration of ethyl alcohol, for example, the excreted urine is hypoosmotic, which can further increase the effect of the drug on blood osmolality.

8.2 INDICATIONS

Osmotic drugs are indicated for the short-term treatment of acute and marked elevation of IOP, including angle-closure glaucoma, aqueous misdirection (malignant glaucoma), and certain secondary glaucomas. These drugs are also indicated in the preoperative preparation of select patients for intraocular surgery. Long-term use is avoided because of the risk of dehydration, electrolyte imbalance, and other adverse effects.

8.3 CONTRAINDICATIONS

Osmotic drugs are contraindicated in patients with well-established anuria, severe dehydration, frank or impending acute pulmonary edema, severe cardiac decompensation, or hypersensitivity to any component of the preparations.

These drugs should be administered with caution to patients with cardiac, renal, or hepatic diseases. In patients with severe impairment of renal function, a test dose (0.2 g/kg of body weight, to produce urine flow of at least 30 to 50 mL/h) should be performed by the internist prior to use of intravenous mannitol. Caution should be exercised, in particular, in patients with congestive heart disease, hypervolemia, electrolyte abnormalities, confused mental states, and dehydration. Oral glycerol should be used with caution in diabetic patients because the blood glucose may rise after metabolism of the drug. When osmotic drugs are administered prior to surgery, the patient's bladder should be empty.

8.4 TREATMENT REGIMEN

Glycerol is also known as glycerin, which is available as a 99.5% anhydrous solution. Although a commercial product is unavailable, a 50% solution of glycerol can

Table 8.2 Dosage and Administration of Commonly Used
Osmotic Drugs

Drug	Solution	Route	Dose (g/kg)
Glycerol	50% (vol/vol)	Oral	1–1.5
Mannitol	20% (wt/vol)	Intravenous	0.5–2

be prepared by most pharmacies, which use glycerol to formulate other medications. Glycerol is prepared as a 50% vol/vol (0.628 g/mL) solution for oral administration and may be stored at room temperature. The usual dose is 1 to 1.5 g/kg, which is about 2 to 3 mL/kg body weight ($\sim$4 to 6 ounces per individual). Flavoring and pouring the glycerol solution over ice improve palatability.

Isosorbide for oral administration is no longer available as a commercial product. Isosorbide is prepared as a 45% wt/vol solution in a flavored vehicle and is chemically stable at room temperature. The usual dose is 1 to 2 g/kg of body weight, which is equivalent to 1.5 mL/lb body weight. Because the osmotic effect persists up to 5 or 6 hours, doses may be repeated two to four times per day during the short-term use of the drug.

The usual dose of mannitol for reduction of IOP is 0.5 to 2 g/kg of body weight, given as an intravenous infusion of a 20% solution over a period of 30 to 60 minutes. Doses as low as 0.25 g/kg may be effective. A single low dose of 12.5 g lowered IOP in normal subjects.[18] Alternative concentrations for ophthalmic use include 10%, 15%, and 25% mannitol. The dose may be lowered if the IOP is not too high or increased if there is pronounced intraocular inflammation. Less than the full dose may be administered by terminating the intravenous infusion when the desired effect on IOP is achieved. The solution is stored at room temperature, and higher concentrations may require slight warming for complete solution. Crystals may form at temperatures below room temperature. When mannitol concentrations of 20% or 25% are infused, the administration set should include a filter.

When an intravenous osmotic drug is required, mannitol is preferable to urea. Although urea is not commonly used, the dosage of intravenous urea is 2 to 7 mL/kg of a 30% solution. The solution of urea is unstable and must be prepared just prior to intravenous administration.

Osmotic drugs in common clinical use are shown in table 8.2.

8.5 SIDE EFFECTS

A potential ocular side effect of osmotic drugs is IOP "rebound." The creation of a blood–vitreous osmotic gradient causes transfer of water from the eye into the blood, thereby increasing the osmolality of the vitreous. During clearance of the drug from the circulation, the osmolality of the blood may decrease to a level below that in the vitreous. The hyperosmotic vitreous may then draw water into the eye, which may increase IOP. If the cause of glaucoma is not relieved after administration of the drug, IOP rebound may occur later. The osmotic drug itself may also enter the eye and then clear more slowly from the eye than from the systemic circulation. Thus, IOP rebound may be less common with glycerol and mannitol, which have poor ocular penetration compared with other osmotic drugs (e.g., urea).

A transient increased aqueous flare (aqueous protein concentration) has been observed after intravenous mannitol;[19] however, the clinical significance of this finding is unknown. Severe intraocular hemorrhage has been reported following administration of urea.[20]

Systemic side effects ranging from mild to life-threatening may develop following treatment with osmotic drugs.[15,21–23] The most frequent side effects are nausea, vomiting, and headache, which may exacerbate the symptoms of the patient with acute glaucoma. Also, these untoward side effects may be hazardous when the drugs are used perioperatively. Antiemetic drugs may reduce these symptoms when administered prior to the osmotic agent.

Hyperosmolality and electrolyte disturbances may cause various central nervous system side effects, including thirst, chills, fever, confusion, and disorientation. Subdural hematoma has been described after administration of urea.[24] This potentially fatal complication probably results from brain shrinkage and retraction, causing traction and tearing of the bridging veins between the sagittal sinus or the dura and the surface of the brain.

The diuresis that follows administration of osmotic drugs may lead to urinary retention requiring catheterization, especially in men with prostatic hypertrophy. Some patients who are treated with osmotic drugs perioperatively may require a catheter to avoid the need to void during surgery. Osmotic drugs may cause severe dehydration, and glycerol, in particular, may cause hyperglycemia.[25,26] Glycerol is metabolized to glucose (figure 8.2), and therefore, use of this drug should be avoided in diabetic patients, especially when multiple administrations are anticipated. Renal failure has been described in previously normal patients following infusion of mannitol.[27]

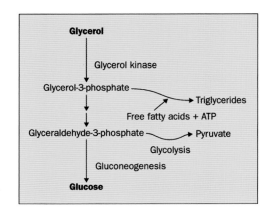

Figure 8.2. Biochemical pathway for glycerol metabolism.

Iatrogenic intoxication with osmotic drugs may occur, especially after treatment with mannitol.[28,29] Because it is confined to the extracellular fluid space, mannitol may greatly increase the blood volume. The ensuing dehydration of the brain may lead to central nervous system involvement, including lethargy and disorientation. Patients with mannitol intoxication may develop severe hyponatremia, a large osmolality gap (high measured minus calculated serum osmolality), and fluid overload. The treatment for this disorder is hemodialysis or peritoneal dialysis.

Increased blood volume after administration of osmotic drugs may overload the cardiac reserve, causing congestive heart failure or pulmonary edema. Elderly patients with borderline cardiac or renal function are especially at risk for these problems. Mannitol is retained in the extracellular fluid space, which causes expansion of blood volume, and intravenous administration may be more rapid than the gastrointestinal absorption of oral osmotic drugs. Thus, patients may be at higher risk for cardiovascular complications after treatment with mannitol compared with oral osmotic drugs.

Although hypersensitivity to osmotic drugs is uncommon, serious allergic reactions have been reported after the administration of intravenous mannitol.[30,31] Patients with a history of atopy and asthma may be at high risk for hypersensitivity reaction to mannitol. High-risk patients may be identified with skin testing, which can produce a positive reaction shortly after lightly scratching the skin where a drop of mannitol has been placed.[30] If a reaction occurs, mannitol infusion is discontinued and supportive therapy is instituted, including, as warranted, epinephrine, diphenhydramine, corticosteroids, or aminophylline.

Side effects of osmotic drugs are summarized in table 8.3.

Table 8.3 Side Effects of Osmotic Drugs

Ocular	Central Nervous System
IOP rebound	Headache
Intraocular hemorrhage	Backache
	Chills
	Fever
Gastrointestinal	Thirst
	Lethargy
Nausea	Confusion
Vomiting	Disorientation
Abdominal cramping	Subdural hematoma
Diarrhea	
	Cardiovascular
Genitourinary	Angina
	Pulmonary edema
Diuresis	Congestive heart failure
Electrolyte abnormalities	
Dehydration	Others
Hypervolemia	
Urinary retention	Hyperglycemia
Anuria	Hypersensitivity

8.6 DRUG INTERACTIONS

Drugs that may compromise renal or cardiovascular status should be used with caution in combination with osmotic drugs. Systemic absorption of topically administered beta blocker, for example, may further compromise patients at risk for congestive heart failure, predisposing them to untoward effects due to osmotic drugs. Osmotic diuretic drugs given to patients receiving angiotensin-converting enzyme inhibitors or other drugs for the treatment of high blood pressure may produce systemic hypotension.

A white flocculent precipitate may form from contact of mannitol with polyvinyl chloride surfaces. Mannitol, therefore, should not be placed in a polyvinyl chloride bag prior to intravenous administration.

8.7 CLINICAL USE

Although osmotic drugs are not useful in the long-term medical management of chronic glaucoma, they may be invaluable in the therapy of acutely elevated IOP and in the perioperative treatment of certain glaucoma patients.[15,21–23]

8.7.1 *Angle-Closure Glaucoma.* The therapy of acute angle-closure glaucoma is directed at lowering IOP and opening the anterior chamber angle. Osmotic drugs are one of the mainstays in the treatment of angle-closure glaucoma because they not only lower IOP but also facilitate opening of the angle. Vitreous dehydration caused by osmotic drugs allows the lens and iris to move posteriorly, thereby deepening the anterior chamber. In addition, the iris sphincter is often nonreactive due to relative ischemia when IOP is elevated. Rapid reduction of IOP by osmotic drugs may relieve this ischemia, permitting sphincter function and miosis and facilitating opening of the anterior chamber angle.

In many instances, therapy with osmotic drugs may be adequate to open the anterior chamber angle, thereby terminating the attack of acute glaucoma. Laser iridectomy may then be performed immediately or several days later, when the eye is less congested. If the angle remains closed after treatment with an osmotic drug, IOP will likely be lowered for a period of time, which may reduce corneal edema and facilitate iridectomy.

Oral isosorbide or glycerol is easier to administer in an office setting compared with intravenous mannitol. Isosorbide may cause less nausea and vomiting than does glycerol, and isosorbide is not metabolized to glucose, which is an advantage in diabetic patients. However, isosorbide is no longer commercially available. When nausea and vomiting or blood sugar considerations preclude the use of an oral osmotic drug, intravenous mannitol may be administered.

8.7.2 *Secondary Glaucomas.* In the secondary glaucomas, osmotic drugs are useful in the treatment of disorders characterized by transient but highly elevated IOP, glaucomas requiring control of IOP until the underlying problem is corrected, and disorders requiring glaucoma surgery that would benefit from preoperative reduction of IOP. Oral osmotic drugs have been given daily or even up to two or three times daily for up to several weeks without complications. In this situation, use of isosorbide avoids the large caloric load that would be ingested with glycerol therapy.

Patients with certain uveitic and posttraumatic glaucomas may be treated with osmotic drugs when they present with markedly elevated IOP that is expected to improve, as is the case in eyes with inflammation or blood in the anterior segment. The transiently and highly elevated IOP sometimes observed after cataract surgery or penetrating keratoplasty may be treated with osmotic drugs.[32]

These drugs are also helpful when reduction of IOP is beneficial prior to correction of the underlying cause, such as a tight scleral buckle or an intumescent lens. Surgery for lens-induced glaucoma is safer when performed at normal IOP following osmotic therapy. Dehydration and shrinkage of the vitreous may facilitate opening the angle and normalizing IOP prior to lens removal for phacomorphic glaucoma.

Osmotic drugs may be used preoperatively in eyes with extremely high IOP that require glaucoma surgery, such as neovascular glaucoma, to minimize the degree of intraoperative decompression. These drugs may delay the need for surgery, which can allow, for example, reduction of inflammation with corticosteroid therapy. In markedly inflamed eyes, glycerol or mannitol may be preferable because they penetrate the eye poorly.

8.7.3 *Aqueous Misdirection.* Although initial medical therapy for aqueous misdirection is with mydriatic-cycloplegic drugs and aqueous suppressants, the influence of osmotic drugs on the vitreous may be helpful in the therapy of this disorder.[33–35] These drugs at least temporarily dehydrate the vitreous and reduce its volume, which may facilitate correction of aqueous misdirection.

8.7.4 *Perioperative Use.* Some glaucoma patients may benefit from osmotic therapy during the perioperative period. In combined cataract and filtration surgery, for example, softening of the eye may be desirable, especially when IOP is even mildly elevated. Osmotic drugs may be used preoperatively or intraoperatively to reduce positive vitreous pressure, or postoperatively to treat transient elevation of IOP. This situation may be encountered, for example, in the open-angle glaucoma patient who undergoes cataract surgery without concomitant filtration surgery. Some glaucoma patients may be treated with osmotic drugs prior to surgical therapy for corneal, retinal, or other disorders.

8.8 ORAL OSMOTIC DRUGS

Orally administered osmotic drugs tend to be somewhat slower in their action but are safer compared with intravenous drugs (figure 8.3).

8.8.1 *Glycerol.* Glycerol has an onset of action from 10 to 30 minutes after ingestion, reaches a maximal effect in 45 to 120 minutes, and has a duration of action of 4 to 5

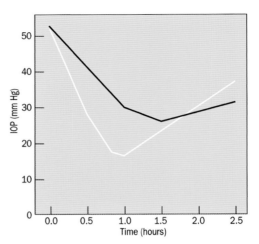

Figure 8.3. Representation of composite effects of mannitol (white line) and glycerol (black line) on IOP in glaucomatous patients with similar initial IOP. Oral glycerol is somewhat slower and less profound in its effect on IOP compared with intravenous mannitol. Data from Galin MA, Davidson R, Shachter N. Ophthalmological use of osmotic therapy. *Am J Ophthalmol.* 1966;62:629–634.

hours.[7,36,37] Glycerol is absorbed rapidly, is distributed in extracellular water, and has poor ocular penetration (table 8.4). These properties enhance the osmotic effect of the drug.

Approximately 80% of glycerol metabolism occurs in the liver, while 10% to 20% occurs in the kidney.[38] Because the majority of glycerol is metabolized by the liver, it has a greater margin of safety compared with mannitol in patients with decreased renal function. Glycerol is filtered and almost completely reabsorbed by the renal tubules until high serum levels are achieved; when serum carrying capacity is exceeded, glycerol appears in the urine and osmotic diuresis occurs. Both the metabolism and the reabsorption of glycerol attenuate the osmotic diuresis after ingestion of this drug. About 10% to 30% of glycerol is combined with free fatty acids to form triglyceride, while the majority is converted to glucose. Glycerol produces 4.34 cal/g when oxidized to carbon dioxide and water.[38] Diabetic patients, therefore, may develop hyperglycemia and ketosis if treated with glycerol.

In addition to hyperglycemia, patients frequently experience nausea and vomiting following ingestion of glycerol. This is a problem in the therapy of acute glaucoma and an even greater disadvantage for perioperative use.

8.8.2 *Other Oral Osmotic Drugs*

Isosorbide. is not commercially available at this time. After oral administration, isosorbide and glycerol are similar in their onset of action, time to maximal effect, and duration of effect.[8,39,40] Although isosorbide is rapidly absorbed, it is distributed in total body water and penetrates the eye slowly. These properties may lessen the osmotic effect of the drug, especially in inflamed eyes. From 1 to 3 hours after oral administration of isosorbide, anterior chamber aqueous levels averaged 55% of plasma levels.[8]

More than 95% of the administered dose of isosorbide is excreted unchanged in the urine. Isosorbide produces no caloric load after ingestion because it is not metabolized, which is a major advantage when compared with glycerol for use in diabetic patients. Isosorbide is less likely than glycerol to produce nausea and

Table 9.1 Systemic Beta-Adrenergic Blockers

Drug	Usual Dosage	
	Range[a] (total mg/day)	Frequency (times/day)
Nonselective Beta Blockers		
Nadolol[b] Corgard	40–120	1
Propranolol[b] Inderal	40–160	2
Propranolol long acting[b] Inderal LA	60–180	1
Timolol[b] Blocadren	20–40	2
Beta Blockers With Intrinsic Sympathomimetic Activity		
Acebutolol[b] Sectral	200–800	2
Penbutolol Levatol	10–40	1
Pindolol[b] Generic	10–40	2
Cardioselective (Beta-1–Selective) Beta Blockers		
Atenolol[b] Tenormin	25–100	1
Betaxolol[b] Kerlone	5–20	1
Bisoprolol[b] Zebeta	2.5–10	1
Metoprolol[b] Lopressor	50–100	1 or 2
Metoprolol extended release Toprol XL	50–100	1
Combined Alpha and Beta Blockers		
Carvedilol Coreg	12.5–50	2
Labetalol[b] Normodyne, Trandate	200–800	2

[a]The lower dose indicated is the preferred initial dose, and the higher dose is the maximum daily dose for treatment of systemic hypertension.

[b]Generic is available.

Source: Modified from Chobanian AV, Bakris GL, Black HR, et al. The seventh report of the Joint National Committee on Detection, Evaluation, and Treatment of High Blood Pressure. JAMA. 2003;289:2560–2572.

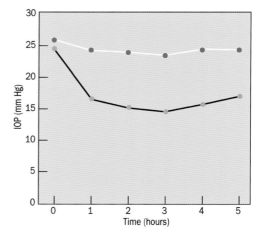

Figure 9.1. Significant reaction of mean IOP in six ocular hypertensive patients after oral administration of placebo (blue circles) or 80 mg propranolol (orange circles). Data from Wettrell K, Pandolfi M. Early dose response analysis of ocular hypotensive effects of propranolol in patients with ocular hypertension. *Br J Ophthalmol.* 1976;60:680–683.

of IOP to topical timolol treatment was influenced by the dose of the systemic beta blocker, with the expected effect at low doses, moderate response at intermediate doses, and little or no response at high doses of oral propranolol.[19] In patients using concurrent systemic beta blocker therapy, the ocular hypotensive efficacy of topical timolol was reduced, whereas the effect of brimonidine was not altered.[20] For this reason, topical beta blockers may not be the optimal therapy in patients treated with high-dose systemic beta blockers.

Initiation of topical treatment with beta blocker is unlikely to cause additional systemic side effects in patients already treated with oral beta blockers. Systemic absorption of timolol instilled into one eye of propranolol-treated patients had no effect on the pulse or the blood pressure.[19] In patients on long-term therapy with timolol eye drops, addition of systemic propranolol therapy may cause a significant reduction of IOP, presumably due to blockade of additional beta receptors by the systemic drug.[21]

9.1.2 *Central Sympatholytics.* The blood-pressure–lowering effect of central sympatholytics results from the passage of the drug through the blood–brain barrier and the stimulation of alpha-adrenergic receptors, resulting in decreased efferent sympathetic activity and increased vagal activity. After systemic administration, an initial direct stimulation of peripheral alpha-adrenergic receptors may cause a transient vasoconstriction, which is eventually inhibited by the central effect of the drug. Central sympatholytic drugs (table 9.2) are potent medications used for the treatment of systemic hypertension.

Clonidine was developed in 1962 as a potential decongestive drug and was unexpectedly found to cause decreased systemic blood pressure, which later proved therapeutically useful. This drug is a lipophilic alpha-2 agonist with some alpha-1–agonist activity. In 1966, Makabe[22] reported a reduction of normal and elevated IOP following intravenous administration of clonidine. In addition to oral and intravenous routes of administration, instillation of clonidine eye drops effectively lowered IOP.[23,24] However, topical use of the drug was limited because systemic

Table 9.2 Systemic Central Sympatholytics (Alpha-2 Agonists)

| Drug | Usual Dosage | |
	Range[a] (total mg/day)	Frequency
Clonidine[b] Catapres	0.1–0.8	2 per d
Clonidine patch Catapres-TTS	0.1–0.3	1 per wk
Guanfacine[b] Generic	0.5–2	1 per d
Methyldopa[b] Aldomet	250–1,000	2 per d
Reserpine[b] Generic	0.05–0.25	1[c]

[a]The lower dose indicated is the preferred initial dose, and the higher dose is the maximum daily dose for treatment of systemic hypertension.

[b]Generic is available.

[c]A 0.1 mg dose may be given every other day.

Source: Modified from Chobanian AV, Bakris GL, Black HR, et al. The seventh report of the Joint National Committee on Detection, Evaluation, and Treatment of High Blood Pressure. JAMA. 2003;289:2560–2572.

absorption and penetration of the blood–brain barrier caused significant systemic hypotension.[25]

The reduction of IOP after systemic administration of clonidine is primarily due to reduced aqueous formation, probably mediated by both central and peripheral adrenergic mechanisms.[25,26] This drug also causes a reduction of episcleral venous pressure.[25]

9.1.3 *Calcium Channel Blockers*. Calcium channel blockers were introduced for use in the management of patients with angina pectoris and have had a major impact in the therapy of patients with cardiac and vascular disease. These agents affect blood vessels by reducing their resistance and preventing vasospasm, which reduces systemic blood pressure. In addition, calcium channel blockers also have a moderate ocular hypotensive effect.[27,28]

Calcium channel blockers are a heterogeneous group of drugs that may have varying effects on different types of calcium channels. Several voltage-dependent types of calcium channels have been described, including L-, T-, N-, P-, Q-, and R-channels. There are at least four chemically distinct families of calcium antagonists: phenylalkylamines (e.g., verapamil), benzothiazepines (e.g., diltiazem), dihydropyridines (e.g., nifedipine), and piperazines (e.g., flunarizine, cinnarizine). Piperazine-type calcium channel blockers are not used for treatment of systemic hypertension.

Because of their varying effects on different calcium channels, dihydropyridine antagonists, such as nifedipine, are more selective for the vasculature compared with phenylalkylamines, such as verapamil. Certain drugs, such as nimodipine, cross the blood–brain barrier and can affect the cerebral vasculature.

Calcium channel blockers available for treatment of systemic hypertension in the United States and their usual systemic dosages are shown in Table 9.3. For

Table 9.3 Systemic Calcium Channel Blockers Available in the United States

Drug	Usual Dosage	
	Range[a] (total mg/day)	Frequency (times/day)
Non-Dihydropyridine-Based Antagonists		
Phenylalkylamine-Based Antagonists		
Verapamil immediate release[b] Calan, Isoptin	80–320	2
Verapamil long-acting[b] Calan SR, Isoptin SR	120–360	1 or 2
Verapamil controlled-onset extended release Covera HS, Verelan PM	120–360	1
Benzothiazepine-Based Antagonists		
Diltiazem extended release[b] Dilacor XR, Tiazac, Cardizem CD	180–420	1
Diltiazem long acting Cardizem LA	120–540	1
Dihydropyridine-Based Antagonists[c]		
Amlodipine Norvasc	2.5–10	1
Felodipine Plendil	2.5–20	1
Isradipine DynaCirc CR	2.5–10	2
Nicardipine sustained release Cardene SR	60–120	2
Nifedipine long-acting Procardia XL, Adalat CC	30–60	1
Nisoldipine Sular	10–40	1

[a]The lower dose indicated is the preferred initial dose, and the higher dose is the maximum daily dose for treatment of systemic hypertension.

[b]Generic is available.

[c]Another dihydropyridine-based calcium antagonist is nimodipine (Nimotop), which is used for subarachnoid hemorrhage in usual dosage of 60 mg (two 30-mg capsules) every 4 hours for 21 days.

Source: Modified from Chobanian AV, Bakris GL, Black HR, et al. The seventh report of the Joint National Committee on Detection, Evaluation, and Treatment of High Blood Pressure. JAMA. 2003;289:2560–2572.

simplification, antihypertensive calcium channel blockers have been grouped into dihydropyridine-based and non-dihydropyridine-based antagonists.[1] The "non-dihydropyridine" antagonists include both benzothiazepines and phenylalkyl-amines. The World Health Organization has divided calcium channel blockers into six types based on both their clinical and their pharmacologic effects.[29]

Systemic administration of these drugs has demonstrated variable effects on IOP, with a trend toward reduction of IOP. Topical administration of verapamil in humans has generally resulted in a mild-to-moderate reduction of IOP. The more consistent reduction of IOP following topical administration compared with systemic administration may be due to different local drug concentrations in the eye following these differing routes of administration. After topical administration of verapamil 0.125%, the peak concentration in the aqueous was in the 10^{-6} M range, which was 200-fold higher than the concentration observed following high-dose systemic administration.[30]

In rabbits, intravenous administration of verapamil or nifedipine caused a reduction of IOP.[31,32] Oral administration of verapamil in rabbits, however, had no effect on IOP.[33] This lack of effect may have been due to lower concentrations in the eye following oral administration compared with intravenous administration.

In patients with systemic hypertension, Monica et al.[34] found a significant reduction of IOP after oral nitrendipine. Similarly, Schnell[35] reported significant reduction of IOP up to 13% in open-angle glaucoma patients following a single sublingual administration of nifedipine. In contrast, oral verapamil,[30] oral or intravenous nifedipine,[36] and oral diltiazem[37] did not have significant effect on IOP in normal human subjects.

Topical administration of calcium channel blockers has been found to have a moderate ocular hypotensive effect, with a more consistent reduction of IOP than has been observed following systemic administration.[27] Topical calcium channel blockers are for investigational use only and are not available for therapeutic use in the United States.

Verapamil causes a dose-related increase in outflow facility in human eyes, which may explain the mechanism of the effect on IOP following topical administration of this calcium channel blocker.[38] In addition, episcleral venous pressure is significantly reduced in normal subjects following topical administration of verapamil.[39]

Topical beta blockers and systemic calcium channel blockers should be used concurrently with caution, especially in patients with impaired cardiovascular function. There have been two reports of severe bradycardia with concomitant use of timolol eye drops and oral verapamil.[40,41] Calcium channel blockers appear to have a favorable ocular safety profile. In patients treated with high doses of oral verapamil for hypertrophic cardiomyopathy, there were no adverse ocular effects compared with controls following 1 year of therapy.[42]

9.1.4 *Angiotensin-Converting Enzyme Inhibitors*. Angiotensinogen is converted by renin to angiotensin I, which is then converted to angiotensin II by the action of angiotensin-converting enzyme (ACE). Angiotensin II is the principal active component of the renin–angiotensin system, which has potent vasoconstricting and other effects. ACE inhibitors (table 9.4) are effective and well-tolerated medications

Table 9.4 Systemic Angiotensin-Converting Enzyme
Inhibitors

Drug	Usual Dosage	
	Range[a] (total mg/day)	Frequency (times/day)
Benazepril[b] Lotensin	10–40	1 or 2
Captopril[b] Capoten	25–100	2
Enalapril[b] Vasotec	2.5–40	1 or 2
Fosinopril Monopril	10–40	1
Lisinopril[b] Prinivil, Zestril	10–40	1
Moexipril Univasc	7.5–30	1
Perindopril Aceon	4–8	1 or 2
Quinapril Accupril	10–40	1
Ramipril Altace	2.5–20	1
Trandolapril Mavik	1–4	1

[a]The lower dose indicated is the preferred initial dose, and the higher
dose is the maximum daily dose for treatment of systemic hypertension.

[b]Generic is available.

Source: Modified from Chobanian AV, Bakris GL, Black HR, et al. The
seventh report of the Joint National Committee on Detection, Evaluation, and Treatment of High Blood Pressure. JAMA. 2003;289:2560–2572.

for the treatment of systemic hypertension. They are less effective, but are not necessarily ineffective, in blacks.

Several components of the renin–angiotensin system have been identified in the
eye. Oral administration of 25 mg of the ACE inhibitor captopril significantly
lowered IOP in patients with normal IOP and primary open-angle glaucoma.[43]
Topical ACE inhibitors have also been shown to lower IOP in humans.[44] Outflow
facility, measured by tonography, increased significantly after oral administration
of captopril,[43] although this drug has other effects on aqueous dynamics.

9.1.5 *Other Hypertensive Medications.* Dopamine agonists and antagonists, which can
affect blood pressure, can lower IOP in humans.[45]

Several hypertensive agents may *increase* IOP by causing lens swelling and angle-
closure glaucoma in patients with narrow anterior chamber angles. Diuretics that
may cause angle-closure glaucoma include thiazides and related drugs (chlorothi-
azide, chlorthalidone, hydrochlorothiazide, polythiazide, and trichlormethiazide)

and potassium-sparing diuretics (spironolactone).[46] The direct vasodilator hydralazine has also been found to cause idiopathic swelling of the lens and angle-closure glaucoma.[46]

9.2 ANTIEPILEPTIC DRUGS

The antiseizure drug topiramate (Topamax) has been associated with an ocular syndrome characterized by acute myopia and secondary angle-closure glaucoma.[47-53] This syndrome is associated with supraciliary effusion resulting in anterior displacement of the lens and iris, with secondary angle-closure glaucoma. Symptoms typically occur within a month of initiating therapy. Secondary angle-closure glaucoma associated with topiramate has been reported in pediatric patients as well as adults. Blurred vision is frequently the first presenting symptom. The primary treatment to reverse symptoms is discontinuation of topiramate.[53] Peripheral iridectomy is generally ineffective for this syndrome.

9.3 MARIJUANA

The *Cannabis sativa* plant and its close relatives are used to make hashish and marijuana, which are illicit and psychoactive substances with widespread consumption in society. The major active compound in these substances is tetrahydrocannabinol (THC), although marijuana is a heterogeneous mixture of chemicals. Many ophthalmologists who care for glaucoma patients have been asked by their patients about the ocular hypotensive effect of marijuana and its potential for therapy of glaucoma.

Ocular effects of marijuana include decrease in pupillary size with preservation of normal responsiveness to light, decrease in tear secretion, conjunctival hyperemia, and decrease in IOP.[54] In one study, IOP was reduced in 9 of 11 normal subjects, with a mean decrease of 25%, 1 hour after pipe smoking 2 g of marijuana containing approximately 18 mg THC.[55] When patients with ocular hypertension or glaucoma were tested, 7 of 11 showed a reduction in IOP averaging 30%.[56] In 31 glaucomatous eyes in 18 patients with different types of glaucoma, the maximum decrease in IOP was 6.6 mm Hg (~23% less than baseline) 90 minutes after inhalation of marijuana (figure 9.2).[57] In various human studies, the maximal reduction in IOP occurred at 60 to 90 minutes, and the duration of the decrease was approximately 4 to 5 hours, despite various routes of administration.[58]

On average, smoking marijuana reduces IOP in at least 60% to 65% of users; however, continued use leads to substantial systemic toxic effects.[59] In one study, initial decreases in IOP were not sustained over time, and all nine patients enrolled in the study elected to discontinue treatment within 1 to 9 months for various reasons.[60]

Clinical studies have not clearly defined the effects of marijuana on aqueous dynamics, which may involve a local effect on the eye and a central nervous system effect. However, preclinical testing on animals has shown that the reduction in IOP

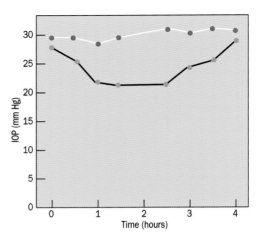

Figure 9.2. Effect of marijuana smoking on mean IOP in 31 eyes in 18 patients with different types of glaucoma (blue circles, placebo; orange circles, marijuana). After marijuana inhalation, IOP was significantly reduced, with maximal response at 90 minutes and duration of effect up to 4 hours. Data from Merritt JC, Crawford WJ, Alexander PC, et al. Effect of marihuana on intraocular and blood pressure in glaucoma. *Ophthalmology.* 1980;87:222–228.

is associated with increased outflow facility.[61] In addition to increased outflow facility, THC may cause reduced perfusion pressure to the ciliary body, decreased aqueous formation, a central nervous system effect, and both alpha- and beta-adrenergic effects in the eye.[58] In a single glaucoma patient studied in detail, the predominant effect observed was increased uveoscleral outflow, with a small effect on outflow facility.[62]

Marijuana has been designated a schedule I compound classified as having no medical benefit. Smoking cannabis or oral administration of THC does not seem a reasonable recommendation to make for patients with glaucoma, many of whom are elderly. There are many other alternatives to marijuana for reducing IOP with fewer attendant side effects. Although cannabinoid analogs have been tried, most have been limited by adverse effects or inconsistent clinical effects.[58–61] In general, attempts at topical application of cannabinoids have been unsatisfactory because of ocular irritation and other side effects or lack of effect on IOP,[58,63] although it may be possible to develop improved compounds and formulations in the future.[59]

9.4 ALCOHOL

Ethyl alcohol is widely used as a licit and socially acceptable albeit nonprescription drug. Alcohol has many ocular effects, including influences on eye movements, nystagmus, and amblyopia. At relatively high doses, alcohol also affects IOP. The mechanism of lowering IOP is an osmotic effect, which may be limited in degree and duration due to rapid penetration into the eye. However, alcohol also induces a hypotonic diuresis by inhibiting production of antidiuretic hormone, which may prolong and increase the osmotic gradient.

Lower doses of alcohol have little or no effect on IOP. Oral administration of 21 mL of 86- or 90-proof alcohol (43% or 45% alcohol, respectively) had no significant effect on IOP compared with controls.[64] Higher doses, however, may reduce IOP (see chapter 8). The oral dose of ethyl alcohol for lowering IOP is 0.8 to

1.5 g/kg, which is approximately 2 to 3 mL/kg of body weight of 40% to 50% solution (80 to 100 proof). Oral ingestion of 120 cc (4 oz, approximately equivalent to two cocktails) of whiskey or 1 L of beer (5% alcohol content) was equally effective in reducing IOP for at least 4 to 5 hours.[65]

Ethyl alcohol has many well-known short- and long-term side effects that limit the therapeutic use of this drug. At the higher doses required to lower IOP, alcohol has central nervous system side effects and may cause nausea and vomiting. The hypotonic diuresis may cause dehydration, and the metabolism of alcohol causes increased caloric load after ingestion, which may cause side effects in diabetic patients and even in nondiabetic individuals.

Because of its adverse effects, long-term treatment with alcohol is not recommended for treatment of elevated IOP. Short-term therapy with alcohol is rarely, if ever, necessary, such as in an emergency situation when no other osmotic IOP-lowering drug is available. However, IOP measurements may be temporarily lowered by alcohol and may deceive clinicians trying to monitor and interpret these measurements. Patients may not state that they have ingested alcohol, although the alert clinician is usually aware of this possibility.

9.5 ALTERNATIVE MEDICINE

Glaucoma patients may seek complementary and alternative medicine treatments to replace or supplement their traditional medicine management. In an urban referral glaucoma practice setting, approximately 5% of glaucoma patients reported use of complementary and alternative medicines specifically for glaucoma.[66] Numerous nontraditional treatments have been described, including ginkgo biloba, bilberry, taurine, magnesium, and vitamin B_{12}, most of which have putative benefits in glaucoma besides IOP reduction.[67] Vitamin C (ascorbate) may lower IOP, probably by an osmotic effect (see chapter 8). Topical application of forskolin may have a transient IOP-reducing effect.[67] Available evidence does not support the use of alternative medicines for glaucoma therapy.[68,69]

REFERENCES

1. Chobanian AV, Bakris GL, Black HR, et al. The seventh report of the Joint National Committee on Detection, Evaluation, and Treatment of High Blood Pressure. *JAMA*. 2003;289:2560–2572.
2. Langman MJ, Lancashire RJ, Cheng KK, Stewart PM. Systemic hypertension and glaucoma: mechanisms in common and co-occurrence. *Br J Ophthalmol*. 2005;89: 960–963.
3. Phillips CI, Howitt G, Rowlands DJ. Propranolol as ocular hypotensive agent. *Br J Ophthalmol*. 1967;51:222–226.
4. Coté G, Drance SM. The effect of propranolol on human intraocular pressure. *Can J Ophthalmol*. 1968;3:207–212.
5. Bucci MG, Missiroli A, Giraldi JP, Virno M. Local administration of propranolol in the treatment of glaucoma. *Boli Oculist*. 1968;47:51–80.

6. Musini A, Fabbri B, Bergamaschi M, et al. Comparison of the effect of propranolol, lignocaine, and other drugs on normal and raised intraocular pressure in man. *Am J Ophthalmol.* 1971;72:773–781.

7. Zimmerman TJ, Kaufman HE. Timolol: a beta-adrenergic blocking agent for the treatment of glaucoma. *Arch Ophthalmol.* 1977;95:601–604.

8. Wettrell K, Pandolfi M. Early dose response analysis of ocular hypotensive effects of propranolol in patients with ocular hypertension. *Br J Ophthalmol.* 1976;60:680–683.

9. Wettrell K, Pandolfi M. Propranolol vs acetazolamide: a long-term double-masked study of the effect on intraocular pressure and blood pressure. *Arch Ophthalmol.* 1979;97:280–283.

10. Öhrström A, Pandolfi M. Long-term treatment of glaucoma with systemic propranolol. *Am J Ophthalmol.* 1978;86:340–344.

11. Wettrell K, Pandolfi M. Effect of oral administration of various beta-blocking agents on the intraocular pressure in healthy volunteers. *Exp Eye Res.* 1975;21:451–456.

12. Rahi AH, Chapman CM, Garner A, Wright P. Pathology of practolol-induced ocular toxicity. *Br J Ophthalmol.* 1976;60:312–323.

13. Skegg DC, Doll R. Frequency of eye complaints and rashes among patients receiving practolol and propranolol. *Lancet.* 1977;2:475–478.

14. Elliot MJ, Cullen PM, Phillips CI. Ocular hypotensive effect of atenolol (Tenormin, I.C.I.): a new beta-adrenergic blocker. *Br J Ophthalmol.* 1975;59:296–300.

15. MacDonald MJ, Cullen PM, Phillips CI. Atenolol versus propranolol: a comparison of ocular hypotensive effect of an oral dose. *Br J Ophthalmol.* 1976;60:789–791.

16. Bonomi L, Steindler P. Effect of pindolol on intraocular pressure. *Br J Ophthalmol.* 1975;59:301–303.

17. el-Sharaf ED, Haroun EA, Ishaac Z, et al. The effect of some beta-adrenergic blockers on human intraocular pressure. *Exp Eye Res.* 1974;19:223–225.

18. Rennie IG, Smerdon DL. The effect of a once-daily oral dose of nadolol on intraocular pressure in normal volunteers. *Am J Ophthalmol.* 1985;100:445–447.

19. Blondeau P, Côté M, Tétrault L. Effect of timolol eye drops in subjects receiving systemic propranolol therapy. *Can J Ophthalmol.* 1983;18:18–21.

20. Schuman JS. Effects of systemic beta-blocker therapy on the efficacy and safety of topical brimonidine and timolol. Brimonidine Study Groups 1 and 2. *Ophthalmology.* 2000;107:1171–1177.

21. Öhrström A, Kättström Ö. A combination of oral and topical beta-blockers with additive effects on intraocular pressure. *Acta Ophthalmol.* 1983;61:1021–1028.

22. Makabe R. Ophthalmological studies with dichlorophenylamino-imidazoline. *Dtsch Med Wochenschr.* 1966;91:1686–1688.

23. Hasslinger C. Catapresan (2-(2,6-dichlorphenylamino)-2-imidazoline-hydrochloride): a new intaocular pressure lowering agent. *Klin Monatsbl Augenheilkd.* 1969;154:95–105.

24. Heilmann K. Examinations of the effect of Catapres in intraocular pressure. *Klin Monatsbl Augenheilkd.* 1970;157:182–192.

25. Hoskins HD Jr, Kass MA. Adrenergic agonists. In Hoskins HD Jr, Kass MA, eds. *Becker-Schaffer's Diagnosis and Therapy of the Glaucomas.* 6th ed. St Louis, MO: CV Mosby Co; 1989:435–452.

26. Liu JH, Neufeld AH. Study of central regulation of intraocular pressure using ventriculocisternal perfusion. *Invest Ophthalmol Vis Sci.* 1985;26:136–143.

27. Netland PA. Calcium channel blockers in glaucoma therapy. *Ophthalmol Clin North Am.* 1997;10:357–364.

28. Kanellopoulos AJ, Erickson KA, Netland PA. Systemic calcium channel blockers and glaucoma. *J Glaucoma.* 1996;5:357–362.

29. Vanhoutte PM, Paoletti R. The WHO classification of calcium antagonists. *Trends Pharmacol Sci.* 1987;8:4–5.

30. Siegner SW, Giovanoni RL, Erickson KA, Netland PA. Distribution of verapamil and norverapamil in the eye and systemic circulation after topical administration of verapamil in rabbits. *J Ocul Pharmacol Ther.* 1998;14:159–168.

31. Green K, Kim K. Papaverine and verapamil interaction with prostaglandin E_2 and $\triangle^9$-tetrahydrocannabinol in the eye. *Exp Eye Res.* 1977;24:207–212.

32. Payne LJ, Slagle TM, Cheeks LT, Green K. Effect of calcium channel blockers on intraocular pressure. *Ophthalmic Res.* 1990;22:337–341.

33. Beatty JF, Krupin T, Nichols PF, Becker B. Elevation of intraocular pressure by calcium channel blockers. *Arch Ophthalmol.* 1984;102:1072–1076.

34. Monica ML, Hesse RJ, Messerli FH. The effect of a calcium-channel blocking agent on intraocular pressure. *Am J Ophthalmol.* 1983;96:814.

35. Schnell D. Response of intraocular pressure in normal subjects and glaucoma patients to single and repeated doses of the coronary drug Adalat. In: Lochner W, Engel HJ, Lichtlen PR, eds. *Second International Adalat Symposium.* Berlin: Springer-Verlag; 1975:290–302.

36. Kelly SP, Walley TJ. Effect of the calcium antagonist nifedipine on intraocular pressure in normal subjects. *Br J Ophthalmol.* 1988;72:216–218.

37. Suzuki R, Hanada M, Fujii H, Kurimoto S. Effects of orally administered â-adrenergic blockers and calcium-channel blockers on the intraocular pressure of patients with treated hypertension. *Ann Ophthalmol.* 1992;24:220–223.

38. Erickson KA, Schroeder A, Netland PA. Verapamil increases outflow facility in the human eye. *Exp Eye Res.* 1995;61:565–567.

39. Abreu MM, Kim YY, Shin DH, Netland PA. Topical verapamil and episcleral venous pressure. *Ophthalmology.* 1998;105:2251–2255.

40. Pringle SD, MacEwen CJ. Severe bradycardia due to interaction of timolol eye drops and verapamil. *BMJ.* 1987;294:155–156.

41. Sinclair NI, Benzie JL. Timolol eye drops and verapamil: a dangerous combination. *Med J Aust.* 1983;1:548.

42. Hockwin O, Dragomirescu V, Laser H, et al. Evaluation of the ocular safety of verapamil: Scheimpflug photography with densitometric image analysis of lens transparency in patients with hypertrophic cardiomyopathy subjected to long-term therapy with high doses of verapamil. *Ophthalmic Res.* 1984;16:264–275.

43. Costagliola C, Di Benedetto R, De Caprio L, et al. Effect of oral captopril (SQ 14225) on intraocular pressure in man. *Eur J Ophthalmol.* 1995;5:19–25.

44. Constad WH, Fiore P, Samson C, Cinotti AA. Use of an angiotensin converting enzyme inhibitor in ocular hypertension and primary open-angle glaucoma. *Am J Ophthalmol.* 1988;105:674–677.

45. Wax MB, Burchfield JC, Lin C. Future directions for medical therapy of glaucoma. In: Ritch R, Shields MB, Krupin T, eds. *The Glaucomas.* 2nd ed. St Louis, MO: CV Mosby Co; 1996:1489–1503.

46. Mandelkorn RM. Nonsteroidal drugs and glaucoma. In: Ritch R, Shields MB, Krupin T, eds. *The Glaucomas.* 2nd ed. St Louis, MO: CV Mosby Co; 1996:1189–1204.

47. Banta JT, Hoffman K, Budenz DL, et al. Presumed topiramate-induced bilateral acute angle-closure glaucoma. *Am J Ophthalmol.* 2001;132:112–114.

48. Sankar PS, Pasquale LR, Grosskreutz CL. Uveal effusion and secondary angle-closure glaucoma associated with topiramate use. *Arch Ophthalmol.* 2001;119:1210–1211.

49. Rhee DJ, Goldberg MJ, Parrish RK. Bilateral angle-closure glaucoma and ciliary body swelling from topiramate. *Arch Ophthalmol.* 2001;119:1721–1723.

50. Medeiros FA, Zhang XY, Bernd AS, Weinreb RN. Angle-closure glaucoma associated with ciliary body detachment in patients using topiramate. *Arch Ophthalmol.* 2003;121:282–285.

51. Chen TC, Chao CW, Sorkin JA. Topiramate induced myopic shift and angle closure glaucoma. *Br J Ophthalmol.* 2003;87:648–649.

52. Craig JE, Ong TJ, Louis DL, Wells JM. Mechanism of topiramate-induced acute-onset myopia and angle closure glaucoma. *Am J Ophthalmol.* 2004;137:193–195.

53. Fraunfelder FW, Fraunfelder FT, Keates EU. Topiramate-associated acute, bilateral, secondary angle-closure glaucoma. *Ophthalmology.* 2004;111:109–111.

54. Hepler RS, Frank IM, Ungerleider JT. Pupillary constriction after marijuana smoking. *Am J Ophthalmol.* 1972;74:1185–1190.

55. Hepler RS, Frank IM. Marihuana smoking and intraocular pressure. *JAMA.* 1971;217:1392.

56. Hepler RS, Frank IM, Petrus R. Ocular effects of marihuana smoking. In: Braude MC, Szara S, eds. *The Pharmacology of Marihuana.* New York: Raven Press; 1976:815–828.

57. Merritt JC, Crawford WJ, Alexander PC, et al. Effect of marihuana on intraocular and blood pressure in glaucoma. *Ophthalmology.* 1980;87:222–228.

58. Green K, Roth M. Marijuana in the medical management of glaucoma. *Perspect Ophthalmol.* 1980;4:101–105.

59. Green K. Marijuana smoking vs cannabinoids for glaucoma therapy. *Arch Ophthalmol.* 1998;116:1433–1437.

60. Flach AJ. Delta-9-tetrahydrocannabinol (THC) in the treatment of end-stage open-angle glaucoma. *Trans Am Ophthalmol Soc.* 2002;100:215–222.

61. Tiedeman JS, Shields MB, Weber PA, et al. Effect of synthetic cannabinoids on elevated intraocular pressure. *Ophthalmology.* 1981;88:270–277.

62. Zhan GL, Camras CB, Palmberg PF, Toris CB. Effects of marijuana on aqueous humor dynamics in a glaucoma patient. *J Glaucoma.* 2005;14:175–177.

63. Jay WM, Green K. Multiple-drop study of topically applied 1% $\triangle^9$-tetrahydrocannabinol in human eyes. *Arch Ophthalmol.* 1983;101:591–593.

64. Obstbaum SA, Podos SM, Kolker AE. Low-dose oral alcohol and intraocular pressure. *Am J Ophthalmol.* 1973;76:926–928.

65. Peczon JD, Grant WM. Glaucoma, alcohol, and intraocular pressure. *Arch Ophthalmol.* 1965;73:495–501.

66. Rhee DJ, Spaeth GL, Myers JS, et al. Prevalence of the use of complementary and alternative medicine for glaucoma. *Ophthalmology.* 2002;109:438–443.

67. Ritch R. Complementary therapy for the treatment of glaucoma: a perspective. *Ophthalmol Clin North Am.* 2005;18:597–609.

68. Rhee DJ, Katz LJ, Spaeth GL, Myers JS. Complementary and alternative medicine for glaucoma. *Surv Ophthalmol.* 2001;46:43–55.

69. West AL, Oren GA, Moroi SE. Evidence for the use of nutritional supplements and herbal medicines in common eye diseases. *Am J Ophthalmol.* 2006;141:157–166.

10

Initial Medical Treatment

NAUMAN R. IMAMI AND R. RAND ALLINGHAM

lthough options for the initial management of most forms of open-angle glaucoma include laser and incisional surgery, medical therapy is typically initiated first. There are currently many medications from which to choose. Fortunately, results from several recent, randomized clinical trials are now available to provide evidence-based guidance to ophthalmologists.

Glaucoma is the leading cause of irreversible blindness worldwide.[1] In the past, glaucoma was primarily defined by elevated intraocular pressure (IOP). Although elevated IOP is recognized as a significant risk factor for glaucoma, it is not the only one. Of patients with open-angle glaucoma, 17% never exhibit IOP greater than normal.[2] In some populations, including Hispanics of Mexican descent and the Japanese, fewer than 20% of those with glaucoma initially have elevated IOP.[3,4]

Primary open-angle glaucoma (POAG) is now defined by the American Academy of Ophthalmology (AAO) as a progressive, chronic optic neuropathy where IOP and other currently unknown factors contribute to damage of the optic nerve, resulting in acquired atrophy with loss of retinal ganglion cells and their axons.[5] POAG also requires adult onset, an open anterior-chamber angle, and the absence of known secondary causes of glaucoma. IOP elevation is considered a risk factor but is not a necessary criterion for diagnosing POAG.

POAG is a chronic, slowly progressive disease for which there is no cure. To maximize treatment efficacy, physicians must partner with patients. This is best achieved when physicians clearly discuss diagnoses, current treatment options, and potential future outcomes. After understanding their illness, patients are in a better position to make informed decisions regarding treatment options and are more likely to be compliant with their treatment regimen.

179

10.1 PATIENT HISTORY AND RISK FACTORS

Prior to the initiation of treatment, a comprehensive ocular examination is required. This includes a complete ophthalmic history, with an emphasis on previous glaucoma diagnosis and therapy. The time of initial diagnosis, maximum IOP, recent IOP measurements, and corneal thickness should be noted. All previous glaucoma medications used, as well as their efficacy and side effects, must be recorded. Secondary causes of glaucoma (e.g., pigmentary, exfoliation, corticosteroid use, trauma, uveitis, or previous ocular surgery) should also be noted. Where available, copies of prior visual fields, optic nerve photographs, and nerve fiber layer measurements should be obtained. Systemic medical conditions and drug allergies must be noted. A family history of ocular diseases, including glaucoma and visual impairment, is important.

Several risk factors have been closely associated with the development and progression of POAG. These include IOP, age, race, family history, thinner central corneal thickness, and increased cup-to-disk ratio.[6–9] Of these risk factors, IOP is the only one that is amenable to treatment.

Experimental studies have shown that raising IOP in animals produces typical glaucomatous optic nerve cupping.[10,11] Clinical examples of patients with asymmetric glaucoma, with worse damage occurring in the eye with higher IOP, have been documented.[12,13] The Collaborative Glaucoma Study found that the relative risk for developing glaucoma was 10.5 times greater in persons who had baseline IOPs of 24 mm Hg or greater compared with those who had IOPs less than 16 mm Hg.[6] The study also found that the relative risk of developing glaucoma rises in a dose–response fashion with baseline IOP. Several randomized, prospective clinical trials have shown that lowering IOP can delay the development and progression of glaucoma.[14–16] Improvement in optic nerve cupping with significant lowering of IOP has also been reported.[17]

However, even though recent clinical trials have shown the benefits of lowering IOP in managing glaucoma, some patients continue to lose visual function from glaucoma despite what may appear to be adequately controlled IOP. Of course, IOP-related factors such as nonadherence with medical therapy and IOP fluctuation may contribute to this phenomenon. Other factors, however, may play a role. Research continues to look for IOP independent treatment modalities.[18,19] Current areas of research include ocular blood flow, calcium metabolism, blockage of glutamate excitotoxicity, inhibition of nitric oxide production, prevention of tumor necrosis factor activation, modulation of heat-shock protein expression, free radicals, neurotrophins, alpha-2–adrenergic receptor agonists, and other approaches to inhibit apoptosis. The results from a large randomized clinical trial investigating the use of memantine, an *N*-methyl-D-aspartate receptor antagonist, as a potential neuroprotectant are expected in the near future. Until more definitive data are available, IOP reduction remains the only proven glaucoma treatment.

10.2 GLAUCOMA TREATMENT TRIALS

Treatment of POAG and other forms of open-angle glaucoma has been addressed by several large clinical trials comparing medical, laser, and surgical intervention. Two of these trials assessed early surgical intervention. In the Scottish Glaucoma Trial,[20] 99 patients with newly diagnosed glaucoma were randomly assigned to initial trabeculectomy (46 patients) or conventional medical therapy followed by trabeculectomy if medical therapy failed (53 patients). After a 3- to 5-year follow-up, a greater decrease in IOP was noted in those treated with surgery. More than half of those treated with medical therapy required surgical intervention. There was no difference in final visual acuity between the two groups, but there was greater visual field loss in the medically treated group.

The Moorfields Primary Treatment Trial[21] randomized 168 newly diagnosed glaucoma patients into three groups: initial medical therapy, initial laser trabeculoplasty, or initial trabeculectomy. With a minimum follow-up of 5 years, the study found that the greatest decrease in IOP occurred in the trabeculectomy group. In the medical arm and the laser arm, there was equal IOP lowering. There was no difference in visual acuity among the three groups. There was a greater loss of visual field, as measured by the number of absolute defects on Friedmann visual fields, in the medically treated group and the laser-treated group compared to the trabeculectomy group.

These two trials have influenced some aspects of glaucoma management. Prior to these studies, glaucoma therapy followed a well-defined course. First, medical treatment was instituted and increased until maximum tolerated levels were reached. Laser trabeculoplasty was the second-line treatment. After the failure of both medical therapy and laser trabeculoplasty, trabeculectomy was undertaken. However, some have proposed that filtering surgery may be more successful prior to chronic IOP-lowering therapy.[22] It is important to note that these trials preceded the introduction of prostaglandin analogs, which are the most potent currently available medical treatment and are administered once daily, which could improve adherence. The outcomes may have been different if these agents were available for the medical treatment arm of these studies. By highlighting the potential benefits of early surgical intervention, these studies questioned our traditional therapeutic sequence and were an important impetus for the Collaborative Initial Glaucoma Treatment Study (discussed further below).

The Glaucoma Laser Trial[23] and the Glaucoma Laser Trial Follow-up Study[23] compared initial treatment with laser trabeculoplasty and a stepwise medical regimen in the treatment of newly diagnosed POAG. In the Glaucoma Laser Trial, 271 patients with similar IOP elevation, optic nerve damage, and visual field loss bilaterally had one eye randomized to initial laser trabeculoplasty and the fellow eye randomized to a stepwise medical regimen. Argon laser trabeculoplasty (ALT) was performed in two 180° sessions approximately 4 weeks apart. The medically treated eye was started on timolol 0.5% twice daily (step 1). If an appropriate IOP was not maintained, timolol was replaced with dipivefrin (step 2). This was followed by replacement with low-dose pilocarpine (step 3) and then high-dose pilocarpine (step 4). Combination timolol and high-dose pilocarpine (step 5) and combination dipivefrin and high-dose pilocarpine (step 6) followed. After this regimen, treatment options were opened to the best judgment of the treating physician. With 2.5 to 5.5 years of follow-up, this study concluded that initial treatment with laser trabeculoplasty was at least as effective as initial treatment with timolol.

The Glaucoma Laser Trial Follow-up Study continued to observe 203 patients from the Glaucoma Laser Trial. Median follow-up was 7 years, with a range from 6 to 9 years. This study showed that eyes initially treated with laser trabeculoplasty had a greater reduction in IOP of 1.2 mm Hg and a greater improvement in visual field of 0.6 dB. Because the difference in end points was small, the study group maintained its earlier conclusion that initial treatment with ALT was at least as effective as initial treatment with timolol.

These two studies highlight the benefits of laser trabeculoplasty as a safe and effective initial treatment for glaucoma. However, a significant number of patients initially treated with laser trabeculoplasty subsequently required medical therapy. At 2-year follow-up, 56% of laser-treated patients were using one or more glaucoma medications. These studies were also performed prior to the advent of newer glaucoma medications.

There is a resurgence of interest in laser trabeculoplasty with the advent of the frequency-doubled Q-switched 532-nm Nd:YAG (neodymium-doped yttrium aluminum garnet) selective laser. Selective laser trabeculoplasty (SLT) lowers IOP without coagulative damage to the trabecular meshwork. Several studies have shown efficacy similar to ALT in controlling IOP.[24,25] Since there is less structural damage to the trabecular meshwork, SLT may allow for more retreatment than ALT.[26] SLT has been shown to reduce the number of medications needed to control IOP over a 1-year period.[27] However, one recent study showed a 68% to 75% SLT failure rate at 6-month follow-up.[28]

The Fluorouracil Filtering Surgery Study[29] examined the role of postoperative subconjunctival 5-fluorouracil (5-FU) in patients who were at high risk for filtration surgery failure. A total of 213 patients who had undergone either filtration surgery and failed or previous cataract surgery were randomized to traditional trabeculectomy or trabeculectomy augmented with postoperative 5-FU. The 5-FU was administered twice daily for 1 week and then once daily for the second week. After 5 years of follow-up, 51% of eyes treated with 5-FU and 74% of eyes not treated with 5-FU were considered surgical failures. Risk factors for surgical failure included high preoperative IOP, short time interval since last surgery involving conjunctival manipulation, number of previous surgeries with conjunctival manipulation, and Hispanic ancestry. Patients in the 5-FU group had a higher incidence of late bleb leaks (9% vs. 2%). The study members recommended the use of 5-FU after trabeculectomy in eyes that had previous cataract surgery or unsuccessful filtering surgery.

The Fluorouracil Filtering Surgery Study clearly showed the benefits of pharmacologic manipulation of wound healing in filtering surgery. Currently, 5-FU is also used intraoperatively as a one-time application.[30] Postoperative 5-FU is generally titrated to bleb appearance. With the advent of mitomycin C, a stronger antimetabolite that can be applied intraoperatively, the surgical options continue to broaden. However, there is an increased risk of bleb leak, hypotony, and late-onset endophthalmitis with antimetabolite use.[31,32]

The Advanced Glaucoma Intervention Study (AGIS)[33] is a long-term study evaluating the outcome of glaucoma uncontrolled with medical therapy. A total of 789 eyes of 591 subjects were randomized between (1) ALT followed by trabeculectomy followed by a second trabeculectomy and (2) trabeculectomy followed by ALT followed by a second trabeculectomy. With 10 years of follow-up, this study highlighted a racial difference in outcomes. Although the IOP lowering was greater in the trabeculectomy-first group for both Caucasians and African Americans, visual function (as measured by visual field, visual acuity, and vision parameters) was better preserved in African Americans in the ALT-first group and in Caucasians in the trabeculectomy-first group.

Initial trabeculectomy increased the risk of cataract formation by 78% and a second trabeculectomy increased risk by almost 300% compared to the first trabeculectomy.[34] It is important to remember that when this study began in 1992, antimetabolites were primarily used in higher risk eyes; therefore, fewer than 1% of initial trabeculectomies utilized antimetabolites. Also, prostaglandin agents, topical carbonic anhydrase inhibitors (CAIs), and topical selective alpha-2–adrenergic agonists were not available early in the study.

AGIS data highlight the importance of IOP control in reducing the risk of glaucoma progression. Retrospective analysis showed that the group of patients who maintained IOP less than 18 mm Hg (mean IOP, 12.3 mm Hg) at all visits over a 6-year period showed no change in their mean AGIS visual field score.[35] AGIS also highlights the importance of IOP fluctuation as a risk factor for visual field progression. Patients with IOP fluctuations as measured by standard deviation of office-measured IOPs of 3 mm Hg or more had a statistically greater risk of progression compared to patients with IOP standard deviations less than 3 mm Hg. Each 1 mm Hg increase in IOP fluctuation increased the risk of visual field progression by 30%.[36]

The Collaborative Normal-Tension Glaucoma Study (CNTGS)[14,37] enrolled 230 patients with unilateral or bilateral normal tension glaucoma (NTG). The diagnosis of NTG was based upon characteristic optic disk and visual field findings in the absence of any documented IOP greater than 24 mm Hg. Study patients had a median IOP of 20 mm Hg or less from 10 baseline measurements. One eye of each patient was randomized to either observation or aggressive treatment to lower IOP by 30%. Randomization occurred immediately if there was evidence of recent visual field progression or if fixation was threatened. Eyes not meeting these criteria were observed without treatment until visual field change, optic nerve head change, or a disk hemorrhage was documented, at which time they were randomized. Sixty-two percent of eyes were randomized. Study end points were optic disk progression or visual field loss. When visual field progression was evaluated, baseline data in the control group were obtained at the time of randomization, whereas in the treatment group, a new baseline was established when the 30% IOP reduction was realized. Stabilization occurred an average of 219 days after randomization. End points were significantly more common in the control group (35% vs. 12%) when the effect of cataract was removed. The rate of cataract formation was significantly less in the control group (14% vs. 38%). There was no statistically significant difference in the rate of cataract formation between the control group and the medically treated subgroup.

If visual fields at the time of randomization were used as the initial baseline, the rate of progression of visual fields between the treatment group and the control group were statistically indistinguishable.[37] A significant decline in the mean deviation values occurred in the treatment group from the time of randomization to the time of IOP stabilization. The decline in mean deviation disappeared after adjustment for reduction in foveal threshold. Because glaucomatous progression usually does not affect only the foveal threshold, the study authors postulated that the progression of visual field loss in the treated group between randomization and stabilization of IOP reduction might be related to cataract formation. When the effects of cataract were addressed in the analysis, visual field progression was greater in the control group at both 3-year and 5-year follow-up.

The CNTGS confirmed the role of IOP in the progression of visual field loss in this patient population. It also showed the potential complications induced by treatments aimed at reducing IOP. Since this study was done prior to the introduction of topical CAIs and prostaglandin analogs, and since beta blockers and alpha-adrenergic agents were not allowed by the study protocol, in actual clinical practice, surgical intervention to reach the 30% IOP reduction may be needed less often. The CNTGS identified variable rates of visual field progression with some patients showing progression within several months; however, 50% of patients who received no treatment showed no visual field progression in 5 years.[38] Individual factors that increased the risk of progression included migraine, female sex, and disk hemorrhage at the time of diagnosis. Asian patients had a longer mean time to progression than did Caucasian patients. Therefore, it may be prudent to follow lower risk patients without treatment to obtain adequate baseline studies to identify individual stability.

The Ocular Hypertension Treatment Study (OHTS)[9,15] was designed to determine whether medical treatment of elevated IOP in the absence of optic nerve or visual field abnormalities is beneficial. Sixteen hundred thirty-six subjects whose IOP was between 24 and 32 mm Hg in one eye and at least 21 mm Hg in the fellow eye, with normal optic nerves and visual fields, were randomized to observation or medical treatment designed to lower IOP by at least 20%. With 5 years of follow-up, the risk of progressing to glaucoma was 4.4% in the treated group and 9.5% in the untreated group. Of these end points, slightly more than 50% were only optic disk changes, thus highlighting the importance of careful, continued optic disk examination.[15] Individual risk factors for progression included older age, higher IOP, larger cup-to-disk ratio, greater pattern standard deviation, and thinner central corneal thickness. Interestingly, the presence of diabetes was found to be protective. However, the diagnosis of diabetes was based only upon patient self-reporting, and no independent testing or confirmation was obtained. Also, the presence of any diabetic retinopathy was an exclusion criterion at baseline. The reliability of these predictive factors in creating a risk calculator has been recently supported.[39]

The OHTS data clearly shows the benefits of reducing IOP in ocular hypertensive patients. However, it is important to consider that 90.5% of untreated patients showed no evidence of progression over 5 years. Therefore, not all ocular hypertensive patients require treatment, and individual patient risk assessment is needed prior to initiating therapy.

The Early Manifest Glaucoma Trial (EMGT)[16] randomized 255 patients with POAG, NTG, or exfoliation glaucoma to topical beta blocker therapy followed by laser trabeculoplasty as needed or observation with the option of delayed treatment if there was sustained IOP elevation greater than 34 mm Hg. Outcome parameters were progression of visual field and optic nerve changes, as documented by stereoscopic disk photography. The median entry IOP was 20 mm Hg. The treated group achieved an average IOP reduction of 25%, while the observation group had no significant IOP reduction. The risk of glaucoma progression was 45% in the treated group and 62% in the control group after average follow-up of 6 years. Individual risk factors that increased the risk of glaucoma progression included increased baseline IOP, exfoliation syndrome, bilateral disease, worse mean deviation on automated visual fields, older age, and frequent disk hemorrhage. Each 1 mm Hg reduction in IOP was associated with approximately a 10% reduction in risk of glaucoma progression.[40]

The EMGT prospectively shows the benefits of IOP reduction in lowering the risk of glaucoma progression in patients with preexisting glaucoma. Since there remained a 45% risk of glaucoma progression in those patients who achieved on average a 25% IOP reduction, this study tends to indicate that a lower initial target pressure may be needed when managing this patient population.

The Collaborative Initial Glaucoma Treatment Study (CIGTS)[41,42] compared filtering surgery with medical treatment in newly diagnosed POAG, pigmentary glaucoma, and exfoliation glaucoma in 607 patients. Each arm is followed by laser trabeculoplasty if there is treatment failure. The surgically treated group had a mean IOP at follow-up of 14 to 15 mm Hg (48% reduction), and the medically treated group had a mean IOP at follow-up of 17 to 18 mm Hg (35% reduction). After 5 years of follow-up, the mean visual field scores of each group were similar. The risk of significant loss of visual field as defined by an increase of at least 3 units of the visual field score was 10.7% in the medically treated arm and 13.5% in the surgically treated arm. The likelihood of cataract surgery was about three times greater in the surgically treated group (17.3% vs. 6.2%). Quality of life analyses were generally similar between the two groups, with the exception of local eye symptoms, which were statistically greater in the surgically treated group.

The CIGTS data are relevant to current ophthalmic practice. It shows that despite obtaining lower IOPs in this group of early glaucoma patients, initial trabeculectomy (with the use of antimetabolites—primarily 5-FU—at the surgeon's discretion) has similar glaucoma stabilization rates over 5 years compared to initial medical treatment. Given that 45% of treated patients in EMGT progressed despite achieving a 25% target IOP reduction, the relative stability in the visual field scores with medically obtained IOP reductions of 35% in the CIGTS study tend to indicate that a lower initial target pressure may be more efficacious.

The European Glaucoma Prevention Study (EGPS)[43] is a randomized double-masked controlled clinical trial evaluating the effect of dorzolamide versus placebo on the development of glaucoma in 1,081 patients. Interestingly, IOP reduction at

5 years was 22% in the treated group and 19% in the placebo group. End points were defined as visual field worsening, optic disk change, or an IOP of 35 mm Hg or greater in the same eye on two visits within 1 week. The rates of end point occurrences (13.7% dorzolamide vs. 16.4% placebo) were not statistically different.

The EGPS results must be considered in context with evidence from OHTS, CNTGS, and EMGT and the retrospective but consistent evidence obtained from AGIS that strongly support the benefit of IOP reduction. Several issues are concerning when evaluating the EGPS data.[44] The "placebo effect" was much higher than one would normally anticipate. A significant number of patients were lost to follow-up studying EGPS, which could skew the results. Finally, in the absence of a clinically significant IOP reduction between the two arms, the study will not be able to identify the benefit of lowering IOP in reducing the risk of glaucoma development. It will be interesting to see follow-up results from this study and the outcomes of an expected combined evaluation with the OHTS data set.

These clinical trials provide an excellent framework of rigorous evidence-based medicine to direct our management of glaucoma (table 10.1). IOP appears to have a dose–response relationship with glaucoma development and progression. Lowering IOP with medications, trabeculoplasty, and surgery are all effective in reducing the risk of glaucoma progression.

10.3 TO TREAT OR NOT TO TREAT

Data from these clinical trials are very helpful in broadly guiding our treatment plans; however, glaucoma treatment must be individualized. After evaluating all available information for a given patient, a decision must first be made whether treatment is necessary. In certain rare circumstances, patients' life expectancies may be limited, and their visual loss from glaucoma may not be very advanced. In this situation, a determination must be made regarding the likelihood that these patients will become visually handicapped from glaucoma without treatment. If they are considered to be at low risk, treatment may not be required. Clinicians must be very careful in pursuing this course, because it is notoriously difficult to predict the life expectancy of individual patients. Also, with the relatively low side effect profile of newer glaucoma medications and SLT, a conservative, safe, and effective treatment protocol can be instituted in most cases.

10.4 TARGET INTRAOCULAR PRESSURE

After the decision to treat has been made, a treatment goal must be set. Glaucoma medications lower IOP, but how low should the IOP be? Target IOP is defined as the IOP that is expected to confer optic nerve stability in a patient with glaucoma. Once the target IOP is reached, ideally the rate of ganglion cell loss is lowered to that of age-matched controls or it will be lowered to a rate at which patients will not become visually handicapped during their lifetime.

Table 10.1 Overview of Glaucoma Trials

Name	Study Design	Results
Scottish Glaucoma Trial[20]	116 newly diagnosed POAG patients randomized to medical therapy vs. trabeculectomy	Trabeculectomy lowered IOP more and had less visual field loss *Caveat*: limited medication options
Moorfields Primary Treatment Trial[21]	168 newly diagnosed POAG patients randomized to medical therapy, trabeculoplasty, and trabeculectomy	Trabeculectomy lowered IOP more and had less visual field loss *Caveat*: limited medications and 98% surgical success at 5 years
Glaucoma Laser Trial[23]	271 newly diagnosed POAG patients randomized to medical therapy vs. laser trabeculoplasty	Initial trabeculoplasty at least as effective as initial timolol *Caveat*: limited medication options
Glaucoma Laser Trial Follow-up Study[23]	203 patients from Glaucoma Laser Trial followed for 6 to 9 years	Confirmed Glaucoma Laser Trial findings with extended follow-up *Caveat*: limited medication options
Fluorouracil Filtering Surgery Study[29]	213 high-risk patients undergoing trabeculectomy randomized between postoperative 5-FU or no antimetabolite	5-FU reduced 5 year *failure* rate from 74% to 51% *Caveat*: increased risk of bleb leak
Advanced Glaucoma Intervention Study (AGIS)[32–34]	591 patients with medically uncontrolled glaucoma randomized to trabeculectomy or trabeculoplasty	African Americans had better results with trabeculoplasty as initial treatment, while Caucasians had better results with trabeculectomy Mean IOP of 12.3 mm Hg limits glaucoma progression *Caveat*: retrospective analysis
Collaborative Normal-Tension Glaucoma Study (CNTGS)[14,37,38]	230 NTG patients observed until increased risk of progression, and randomized to observation or 30% IOP lowering	Lowering IOP in NTG by 30% reduced the risk of progression from 35% to 12% *Caveat*: only after effect of cataract is removed; 50% of patients with no treatment did not progress over 5 years

(continued)

Table 10.1 (*Continued*)

Name	Study Design	Results
Ocular Hypertension Treatment Study (OHTS)[9,15]	1,637 ocular hypertensive patients randomized to medical treatment to lower IOP by 20% or observation	Lowering IOP by 20% reduced risk of glaucoma development in ocular hypertensive patients from 9.5% to 4.4% over 5 years Thinner central corneal thickness is a risk factor for glaucoma development
Early Manifest Glaucoma Trial (EMGT)[16,40]	255 glaucoma patients randomized to observation or treatment with betaxolol and trabeculoplasty	Lowering IOP 25% reduced risk of glaucoma progression from 62% to 45% over 6 years *Caveat*: 45% of treated patients still progressed; may need lower IOP target
Collaborative Initial Glaucoma Treatment Study (CIGTS)[41,42]	607 newly diagnosed glaucoma patients randomized to medical treatment vs. trabeculectomy	Lowering IOP with medication was as effective as lowering IOP with trabeculectomy in limiting glaucoma progression *Caveat*: IOP was lowered more in surgical group 48% vs. 35%
European Glaucoma Prevention Study (EGPS)[43]	1,077 ocular hypertensive patients randomized to medical therapy with dorzolamide or placebo (dorzolamide vehicle)	Medical therapy lowered IOP by 22% and placebo lowered IOP by 19% No difference in rates of glaucoma development *Caveat*: data do not match with other trials, and placebo effect is unexpectedly high

There is no well-defined method of choosing a target IOP. Several theories are inherent in setting a target IOP. It is generally believed that damaged optic nerves require greater IOP reduction. Dr. Morton Grant summarized this concept as follows: "[T]he worse the initial condition of the eye, the lower the tension needs to be to prevent further vision loss or blindness."[45] Visual field loss and optic nerve cupping are the best indicators of such damage. Future glaucomatous visual field loss can be correlated with the current degree of field loss and with the current IOP compared with the IOP at which visual field loss is believed to have occurred.[46]

Finally, because IOP is the only currently addressable risk factor for the progression of glaucoma, individuals with additional risk factors may benefit from greater IOP reduction.[47]

In its 2005 *Primary Open-Angle Glaucoma Preferred Practice Pattern*,[5] the AAO recommends that the initial target IOP be at least 20% below that of pretreatment levels, assuming that damage occurred at those pressure levels. The AAO further recommends an adjustment downward of target IOP based on responses to the following questions:

1. How severe is the existing optic nerve damage?
2. How high is the IOP?
3. How rapidly has the optic nerve damage occurred?
4. How many additional risk factors are present?

One method of grading the severity of damage recommended by the AAO is as follows:

1. *Mild:* Characteristic optic nerve abnormalities are consistent with glaucoma, but the visual field is normal.
2. *Moderate:* Visual field abnormalities exist in one hemifield and are not within 5° of fixation.
3. *Severe:* Visual field abnormalities exist in both hemifields or visual field loss is within 5° of fixation.

This grading system assists in quantifying the degree of preexisting glaucomatous damage while selecting a target IOP. With mild damage, an initial goal of 20% reduction in IOP is reasonable. A 30% reduction with moderate damage and 35% to 40% reduction with severe damage may be more appropriate. With the potential of "preperimetric" glaucoma being identified with newer nerve fiber layer analyzers we may begin to identify patients with more *mild* glaucoma. Currently, most glaucoma diagnoses are made in conjunction with visual field loss and would, by definition, be at least *moderate* requiring an initial target IOP reduction of at least 30%. This fits nicely with EMGT and CIGTS data, which indicate that lower target pressures may be more appropriate. With very advanced disease and near-total optic nerve cupping, most glaucoma specialists believe the IOP should be maintained below 15 mm Hg. Some glaucoma specialists are recommending an upper limit in the single digits to low teens for these advanced cases. AGIS data showing average visual field stability in patients with IOPs consistently below 18 mm Hg, with a mean IOP of 12.3 mm Hg, support this position.[35]

Once a target IOP has been selected, it is important to remember that it is not a fixed target, but the target can be adjusted according to the patient's clinical course. If the patient continues to show optic nerve or visual field deterioration despite consistent maintenance at the target IOP and adherence to the medical regimen, it would be reasonable to further reduce the target IOP. Similarly, if visual fields and optic nerves have remained stable at the target IOP for a long time, the clinician could consider reducing medications and temporarily raising the target IOP.

Lower target pressures are associated with increased financial costs and treatment-related side effects. Without the potential downside to treatment, a very low target IOP would be selected for all glaucoma patients. The target IOP can also be adjusted depending on the ease with which it can be reached. Some patients may easily reach their target IOP on one medication used only once a day. If further IOP lowering can be achieved by adding another drop, which the patients tolerate well and are willing to take, it may be reasonable to aim for an IOP lower than the target IOP. On the other hand, if patients are having difficulty reaching the target IOP despite multiple medications and laser treatment, the next step may be surgery. If patients cannot increase their medical regimen and if they are hesitant to undergo surgery, the importance of reaching the IOP goal must be reassessed. If the potential benefit of reaching the target IOP is outweighed by the potential risks of further treatment, IOP greater than the target IOP may be acceptable. However, these patients must be observed closely to detect evidence of progression.

10.5 INITIAL TREATMENT MODALITY

After setting a target IOP, the ophthalmologist must decide how to reach it. As discussed above, there is support for initial medical, laser, and surgical intervention.[20,21,23,41] Therefore, before selecting one of these treatment protocols, it is imperative to have a frank discussion with patients about the status of their disease and all treatment options. Only after all the options have been reviewed and patients' questions answered can patients properly give informed consent to the treatment regimen. If more invasive treatments are not chosen initially, patients will be aware of possible future options. The negative effect of prior long-term medical therapy on the success of filtration surgery is important to consider. With newer medications, maximum medical therapy may be achieved with as few as three medications.

The most common approach is to begin with medical treatment. Glaucoma is a slowly progressive disease. Therefore, obtaining a baseline set of data prior to performing an irreversible procedure is useful. Although studies highlight the benefits of early trabeculectomy and laser trabeculoplasty, these trials did not include the newest generation of medications, which are potent and generally well tolerated. In contrast, CIGTS showed equivalent visual field stability between the medically treated and surgically treated patients over 5 years.[41]

The failure to adhere to medical therapy is a major problem. Nonadherence has been estimated to cause approximately 10% of all visual loss from glaucoma and is a leading cause of blindness.[48] Patients may improperly use medications or use medications only prior to visiting their physician. Side effects discourage patients from using medicines. Complicated dosage regimens can be difficult to follow. Medications containing a combination of drugs may be preferable to separate agents. To help improve patient adherence, pharmaceutical companies are creating medication reminder aids for patients. Theoretically, such devices may be helpful in reminding patients to use their medications; however, actual efficacy remains to be studied. Cost is another important issue. Patients may not be able to afford the high prices of glaucoma medications, especially since the treatment program may be life-long. Patients must also maintain follow-up with their physicians to monitor the efficacy of medical management. If there are serious concerns regarding adherence, laser trabeculoplasty is a reasonable first-line therapy. Trabeculoplasty has generally been found to be effective for about 5 years in 50% of patients.[49]

Primary filtering surgery is an appropriate alternative for patients who have advanced initial damage or significantly elevated IOP and whose target IOP is considered not achievable through any other treatment modality. Even in these patients, a trial of medical treatment is warranted if for no other reason than to control IOP prior to surgery. This trial may reduce progressive optic nerve damage and visual field loss in the eye scheduled for initial surgery. In a subset of such patients, an unexpectedly good response to medical therapy may obviate the need for initial surgery.

Regardless of which therapy is initially selected, treatment effect must be followed closely. If, after an adequate trial, one line of therapy does not achieve the target IOP, the clinician should not hesitate to advance to an alternate treatment modality. A common mistake in glaucoma management is not being aggressive enough in achieving the target IOP.

10.6 INITIAL MEDICAL MANAGEMENT

Once a decision has been made to pursue medical therapy, the ophthalmologist must choose among the many medical options available. Prior to selecting a medication, the physician should review the patient's medical history, allergies, and experience with previous glaucoma medications. Documenting efficacy and side effects of medications previously used in a dedicated location in the medical record will reduce the likelihood of repeating unsuccessful therapeutic trials in the future.

Beta blockers are contraindicated in patients with asthma, chronic obstructive pulmonary disease (COPD) or bradycardia. Systemic CAIs should be avoided in patients with a history of calcific kidney stones or potential problems with metabolic acidosis. Systemic CAIs may be used with caution in patients with a sulfa allergy.[50]

Ocular conditions can also affect the choice of medications. Uveitis and cystoid macular edema (CME) are infrequently associated with prostaglandin analogs.[51-55] Although rarely used, dipivefrin and epinephrine are associated with CME in aphakic patients. Echothiophate iodide is not used in phakic patients because of its cataractogenic properties, but it is a very effective treatment in pseudophakic and aphakic individuals. Miosis from any cholinergic agent can decrease visual function in patients with cataracts, especially central posterior subcapsular cataracts, and in patients with advanced glaucoma.

If there are no contraindications, one of the three available prostaglandin analogs (bimatoprost, latanoprost, and travoprost) is an excellent initial treatment choice. These medications are more efficacious than timolol in lowering IOP[56-58] and require only once-daily dosing. Some studies have noted slight efficacy differences among these medications; however, these differences are of questionable practical clinical relevance from an initial treatment perspective.[57,59,60] Additionally, there is increasing attention to IOP fluctuation as an independent, major risk factor for glaucoma progression.[36,61] Since prostaglandin analogs appear to provide better diurnal pressure control than do other IOP-lowering medication classes,[62,63] there is additional support for using prostaglandin analogs as first-line glaucoma therapy. In many cases, increasing medication cost and insurance-mandated formulary coverage will become the primary driver of which prostaglandin agent is initially chosen.

It is very important to review medication side effects with patients prior to beginning therapy. Iris color change, periorbital hyperpigmentation, and hypertrichosis are unique to the prostaglandin class of drugs.[64–66] Periorbital hyperpigmentation and hypertrichosis may improve with medication stoppage. There is a tendency for less conjunctival hyperemia with latanoprost.[60] Some patients who do not respond to latanoprost have shown an IOP lowering when switched to bimatoprost;[67] therefore, if there is not an initial response to one prostaglandin agent, changing medication within this class may be a reasonable next step.

If there are no contraindications, a nonselective beta blocker may also be considered as initial therapy. Beta blockers function by reducing aqueous production. They have a long history of efficacy in lowering IOP in normal, ocular hypertensive, and glaucomatous patients.[68] Patients have been maintained on these drugs for many years, and the side effect profile is well documented. These drugs are generally well tolerated. For patient adherence, timolol and levobunolol allow reliable once-daily dosing. In patients with abnormal lipid profiles, carteolol is a good choice because it has a less negative effect on serum lipids.[69] Due to the availability of generic options, beta blockers may be an ideal choice when medication cost is a priority.

In a patient with a history of mild asthma or COPD, betaxolol provides a safer alternative. However, most studies have shown its efficacy in lowering IOP to be less than that of nonselective beta blockers.[70] Furthermore, betaxolol has been associated with adverse pulmonary side effects in at-risk populations.[71] Given the availability of alternate medications, the use of *any* beta blocker should be carefully considered in the presence of a relative contraindication.

Brimonidine, an alpha-2–selective agonist, can also be considered as initial treatment in select cases. Brimonidine reduces aqueous production and increases uveoscleral outflow. The Brimonidine Study Group compared the IOP-lowering effect of brimonidine 0.2% with timolol 0.5%, each administered twice daily for 1 year.[72] Both medications maintained a significant reduction in IOP from baseline throughout the study. At peak times, the IOP-lowering effect of brimonidine was greater than or equal to that of timolol. The IOP-lowering effect of timolol was greater than that of brimonidine for all follow-up visits at trough times. Additionally, timolol is used once or twice daily compared with brimonidine, which requires three-times-daily administration for complete coverage despite the fact that it is used twice daily in most cases. Brimonidine has been associated with dry mouth, ocular hyperemia, and ocular burning. From a cardiopulmonary perspective, brimonidine may be safer than beta blockers. Patients with cardiopulmonary disease may benefit from brimonidine as initial treatment.

Topical CAIs, such as dorzolamide and brinzolamide, are useful because they lower IOP without the systemic problems of acetazolamide or methazolamide. Several studies highlight the IOP-lowering efficacy of both dorzolamide and brinzola-mide.[73,74] These medications can also be considered as first-line treatment for glau-coma. However, when compared to beta blockers and latanoprost, which can often be used once daily, topical CAIs require twice-daily or three-times-daily dosing.

Cholinergic agonists, dipivefrin, epinephrine, apraclonidine, and systemic CAIs have become less popular early in the course of glaucoma management because of their side effect profiles and dosing intervals. Combination agents are not usually considered for initial therapy unless urgent, significant IOP reduction in needed.

10.7 PATIENT FOLLOW-UP

The physician–patient relationship cannot be overemphasized. Good communica-tion can greatly improve patient adherence with medications and follow-up. The side effect profiles of proposed treatments must be reviewed. Patients need to be clearly informed about the dosage regimen. Written instructions with charts are invaluable, especially when multiple medications are used. Appropriate techniques for administering eye drops need to be taught. Observing patients using eye drops in the office can be very informative. Techniques to reduce systemic absorption and toxicity, such as nasolacrimal occlusion and eyelid closure, should be discussed.[75]

Once a therapeutic course has been initiated, its efficacy must be documented. A monocular trial in patients with bilateral elevated IOP can be a helpful approach to assess treatment effect. In this manner, the fellow eye is used as an internal control. A lower IOP in the treated eye helps document a positive treatment effect, whereas a lower IOP in both eyes probably indicates baseline IOP fluctuations. Some recent studies have raised questions regarding the potential benefits of monocular trials due to independent IOP variability between eyes and varying efficacy of the same medication between eyes.[76,77] Beta blockers can have a contralateral IOP-lowering effect through systemic absorption.[78] This effect is usually small and generally does not interfere with a monocular trial.

Because of the chronic nature of glaucoma, appropriate follow-up is mandatory. The AAO has developed guidelines for glaucoma management (table 10.2).[5] Every follow-up patient visit should include interval ocular history, general medical his-tory, local or systemic problems with medications, general assessment of impact of

Table 10.2 AAO-Recommended Guidelines for Follow-up

Target IOP Achieved	Progression of Damage	Duration of Control	Follow-up Interval
Yes	No	<6 months	1 to 6 months
Yes	No	>6 months	3 to 12 months
Yes	Yes	—	1 week to 4 months
No	—	—	1 day to 4 months

Source: *Primary Open-Angle Glaucoma Preferred Practice Pattern*. San Francisco, CA: American Academy of Ophthalmology; 2005.

Table 10.3 AAO-Recommended Guidelines for Optic Disk Examination

Target IOP Achieved	Progression of Damage	Duration of Control	Follow-up Interval
Yes	No	<6 months	6 to 12 months
Yes	No	>6 months	6 to 18 months
Yes	Yes	—	2 to 12 months
No	Yes/no	—	2 to 12 months

Source: *Primary Open-Angle Glaucoma Preferred Practice Pattern*. San Francisco, CA: American Academy of Ophthalmology; 2005.

visual function on daily living, and the frequency and time of last glaucoma medications. Visual acuity, IOP check, and slit-lamp examination should be performed in each eye, as well as detailed examination of the optic disk (table 10.3).

Having an appropriate baseline visual field is a prerequisite to accurately identify visual field changes. Obtaining a baseline may require two or more visual field tests for adequate reliability and to eliminate learning effect. In most cases, two visual field tests are satisfactory. If visual field change is identified, it is wise to confirm this with another test to rule out long-term fluctuation as a cause (table 10.4). Newer visual field machines have sophisticated statistical packages to assist in the determination of progression.

If visual function continues to deteriorate, the therapeutic goal and methods must be reevaluated. Signs of nonadherence with prescribed therapy should be sought. The possibility of an alternate diagnosis or the development of a new disease process should also be considered.

10.8 GLAUCOMA SUSPECTS

Many people who are at high risk of developing POAG currently do not manifest optic nerve or visual field damage. These people, generally referred to as *POAG suspects*, should be identified early and observed at regular intervals for possible progression to POAG. With the development of sophisticated nerve fiber layer

Table 10.4 AAO-Recommended Guidelines for Visual Field Testing

Target IOP Achieved	Progression of Damage	Duration of Control	Follow-up Interval
Yes	No	<6 months	6 to 18 months
Yes	No	>6 months	6 to 24 months
Yes	Yes	—	1 to 6 months
No	Yes/no	—	1 to 6 months

Source: *Primary Open-Angle Glaucoma Preferred Practice Pattern*. San Francisco, CA: American Academy of Ophthalmology; 2005.

analyzers, eventually, it may be possible to detect glaucomatous damage prior to optic nerve or visual field changes.

The AAO uses several criteria to identify glaucoma suspects.[79] These people can have an abnormal-appearing optic nerve suggestive of glaucoma as indicated by a large cup-to-disk ratio, narrowed neuroretinal rim tissue, asymmetric cupping, focal abnormalities of the neuroretinal rim (e.g., notching or hemorrhage), and abnormalities of the nerve fiber layer. Borderline visual fields and elevated IOP also identify glaucoma suspects. These people have normal open angles and no secondary cause for elevated IOP. Their risk for developing POAG can be further stratified by assessing the number of additional risk factors present and the degree of IOP elevation if present. People with definite evidence of optic nerve, nerve fiber layer, or visual field changes should be considered as having POAG.

As with diagnosed POAG patients, an adequate baseline evaluation of POAG suspects is essential. Individuals considered at high risk are those with elevated IOP, thin corneas, age greater than 50 years, African American or Hispanic ancestry, family history of glaucoma, and optic nerve findings consistent with early glaucomatous damage.

The OHTS[9,15] is an excellent resource for managing glaucoma suspects with elevated IOP. In multivariate analysis, risk factors for development of glaucoma are increasing age, larger vertical or horizontal cup-to-disk ratio, higher IOP, greater pattern standard deviation, and thinner central corneal measurement. Clearly, extrapolating individual patient outcomes from data obtained from clinical trials can be difficult. Patients should be stratified according to their individual risk profiles. For example, a patient with an IOP less than 24 mm Hg and a corneal thickness greater than 588 μm has a 2% risk of glaucoma development over 6 years, whereas a patient with an IOP greater than 26 mm Hg and a corneal thickness less than 555 μm has a 36% risk of glaucoma development. A recently introduced risk calculator has been created using the OHTS data. This may prove helpful as a guide to determine the need for treatment in patients at risk of progression to glaucoma.[39]

The risk of glaucoma development combined with the potential benefits of early intervention versus the cost and risk of early treatment in a normally slowly progressive disease process should be carefully discussed with the patient. If the clinician feels the risk of glaucoma damage outweighs the downsides of early treatment, therapeutic intervention should be recommended.

If a high-risk glaucoma suspect is to be treated, the same protocol used in treating POAG should be followed. A target IOP should be set, although it is generally not as low as that in POAG because preexisting damage, if present, is not detectable. A 20% reduction in IOP is a reasonable initial target. Generally, only medical therapy is instituted in the absence of optic nerve damage unless IOP is extremely high; however, in select cases, trabeculoplasty may also be appropriate. As with POAG, follow-up is very important. AAO guidelines state that untreated low-risk glaucoma suspects with stable optic nerves and IOP should be observed every 6 to 24 months, with a complete eye examination and visual fields. Untreated high-risk glaucoma suspects with stable optic nerves and IOP should be observed every 3 to 12 months. Treated high-risk patients with controlled IOP should be seen every 3 to 12 months, after which visits can be slowly extended if optic nerve and visual field stability has been clearly documented. Treated high-risk patients with uncontrolled IOP should be seen at least every 4 months until the target IOP has been achieved.

REFERENCES

1. Quigley HA. Number of people with glaucoma worldwide. *Br J Ophthalmol.* 1996; 80:389–393.
2. Sommer A, Tielsch JM, Katz J, et al. Relationship between intraocular pressure and primary open angle glaucoma among white and black Americans: the Baltimore Eye Survey. *Arch Ophthalmol.* 1991;109:1090–1095.
3. Quigley HA, West SK, Rodriguez J, et al. The prevalence of glaucoma in a population-based study of Hispanic subjects: Proyecto VER. *Arch Ophthalmol.* 2001;119:1819–1826.
4. Iwase A, Suzuki Y, Araie M, et al. The prevalence of open angle glaucoma in Japanese: the Tajimi Study. *Ophthalmology* 2004;111:1641–1648.
5. *Primary Open-Angle Glaucoma Preferred Practice Pattern.* San Francisco, CA: American Academy of Ophthalmology; 2005. www.aao.org/education/guidelines/ppp/poag_new.cfm.
6. Armaly MF, Krueger DE, Maunder L, et al. Biostatistical analysis of the Collaborative Glaucoma Study, I: summary report of the risk factors for glaucomatous visual-field defects. *Arch Ophthalmol.* 1980;98:2163–2171.
7. Tielsch JM, Sommer A, Katz J, et al. Racial variations in the prevalence of primary open-angle glaucoma: the Baltimore Eye Survey. *JAMA.* 1991;266:369–374.
8. Tielsch JM, Katz J, Sommer A, et al. Family history and the risk of primary open-angle glaucoma: the Baltimore Eye Survey. *Arch Ophthalmol.* 1994;112:69–73.
9. Gordon MA, Heuer DK, Higginbotham EJ, et al. The Ocular Hypertension Treatment Study: Baseline factors that predict the onset of primary open angle glaucoma. *Arch Ophthalmol.* 2002; 120:714–20.
10. Gaasterland D, Tanishima T, Kuwabara T. Axoplasmic flow during chronic experimental glaucoma, I: light and electron microscopic studies of the monkey optic nervehead during development of glaucomatous cupping. *Invest Ophthalmol Vis Sci.* 1978;17:838–846.
11. Quigley HA, Addicks EM. Chronic experimental glaucoma in primates, II: effect of extended intraocular pressure elevation on optic nerve head and axonal transport. *Invest Ophthalmol Vis Sci.* 1980;19:137–152.
12. Cartwright MJ, Anderson DR. Correlation of asymmetric damage with asymmetric intraocular pressure in normal-tension glaucoma (low-tension glaucoma). *Arch Ophthalmol.* 1988;106:898–900.
13. Crichton A, Drance SM, Douglas GR, Schulzer M. Unequal intraocular pressure and its relation to asymmetric visual field defects in low-tension glaucoma. *Ophthalmology.* 1989;96:1312–1314.
14. Collaborative Normal-Tension Glaucoma Study Group. The effectiveness of intraocular pressure reduction in the treatment of normal-tension glaucoma. *Am J Ophthalmol.* 1998;126:498–505.
15. Kass MA, Heuer DK, Higginbotham EJ, et al. The Ocular Hypertension Treatment Study. A randomized trial determines that topical ocular hypertensive medication delays or prevents the onset of primary open-angle glaucoma. *Arch Ophthalmol.* 2002; 120:701–713.

16. Heijl A, Leske MC, Bengtsson B, et al. Reduction of intraocular pressure and glaucoma progression. Results from the Early Manifest Glaucoma Trial. *Arch Ophthalmol.* 2002; 120:1268–1279.

17. Shin DH, Bielik M, Hong YJ, et al. Reversal of glaucomatous optic disc cupping in adult patients. *Arch Ophthalmol.* 1989;107:1599–1603.

18. Marcic TS, Belyes DA, Katz B. Neuroprotection in glaucoma: a model for neuroprotection in optic neuropathies. *Curr Opin Ophthalmol.* 2003;14:353–356.

19. Levin LA. Neuroprotection and regeneration in glaucoma. *Ophthalmol Clin North Am.* 2005;18:585–596.

20. Jay JL, Allan D. The benefit of early trabeculectomy versus conventional management in primary open angle glaucoma relative to severity of disease. *Eye.* 1989;3: 528–535.

21. Migdal C, Gregory W, Hitchings R. Long-term functional outcome after early surgery compared with laser and medicine in open-angle glaucoma. *Ophthalmology.* 1994; 101:1651–1657.

22. Lavin MJ, Wormald RP, Migdal CS, Hitchings RA. The influence of prior therapy on the success of trabeculectomy. *Arch Ophthalmol.* 1990;108:1543–1548.

23. Glaucoma Laser Trial Research Group. The Glaucoma Laser Trial (GLT) and Glaucoma Laser Trial Follow-up Study, 7: results. *Am J Ophthalmol.* 1995;120:718–731.

24. Damji KF, Shah KC, Rock WJ et al. Selective laser trabeculoplasty V argon laser trabeculoplasty: a prospective randomized clinical trial. *Br J Ophthalmol.* 1999;83: 718–722.

25. Juzych MS, Chopra V, Banitt MR, et al. Comparison of long-term outcomes of argon laser trabeculoplasty in open-angle glaucoma. *Ophthalmology.* 2004; 111:1853–1859.

26. Latina MA, Sibayan SA, Shin DH et al. Q-switched 532-nm ND:YAG laser trabeculoplasty (selective laser trabeculoplasty): a multicenter, pilot clinical study. *Ophthalmology.* 1998;105:2082–2088.

27. Francis BA, Ianchulev T, Schofield JK, Minckler DS. Selective laser trabeculoplasty as a replacement for medical therapy in open-angle glaucoma. *Am J Ophthalmol* 2005; 140:524–525.

28. Song J, Lee PP, Epstein DL et al. High failure rate associated with 180 degrees selective laser trabeculoplasty. *J Glaucoma.* 2005;14:400–408.

29. Fluorouracil Filtering Surgery Study Group. Five-year follow-up of the Fluorouracil Filtering Surgery Study. *Am J Ophthalmol.* 1996;121:349–366.

30. Singh K, Egbert PR, Byrd S, et al. Trabeculectomy with intraoperative 5-fluorouracil vs mitomycin C. *Am J Ophthalmol.* 1997;123:48–53.

31. Greenfield DS, Suner IJ, Miller MP, et al. Endophthalmitis after filtering surgery with mitomycin. *Arch Ophthalmol.* 1996;114:943–949.

32. Greenfield DS, Liebmann JM, Jee J, Ritch R. Late-onset bleb leaks after glaucoma filtering surgery. *Arch Ophthalmol.* 1998;116:443–447.

33. Ederer F, Gaasterland DA, Dally LG et al. The Advanced Glaucoma Intervention Study (AGIS): 13. Comparison of treatment outcomes within race: 10-year results. *Ophthalmology.* 2004;111:651–664.

34. AGIS Investigators. The Advanced Glaucoma Intervention Study: 8. Risk of cataract formation after trabeculectomy. *Arch Ophthalmol.* 2001;119:1771–1779.

35. AGIS Investigators. The Advanced Glaucoma Intervention Study (AGIS): 7. The relationship between control of intraocular pressure and visual field deterioration. *Am J Ophthalmol.* 2000;130:429–440.

36. Nouri-Mahdavi K, Hoffman D, Coleman AL, et al. Predictive factors for glaucoma-tous visual field progression in the Advanced Glaucoma Intervention Study. *Ophthalmology*. 2004;111:1627–1635.

37. Collaborative Normal-Tension Glaucoma Study Group. Comparison of glaucomatous progression between untreated patients with normal-tension glaucoma and patients with therapeutically reduced intraocular pressures. *Am J Ophthalmol*. 1998;126: 487–497.

38. Drance S, Anderson DR, Schulzer M, et al. Risk factors for progression of visual field abnormalities in normal-tension glaucoma. *Am J Ophthalmol*. 2001;131:6997–6708.

39. Medeiros FA, Weinreb RN, Sample PA, et al. Validation of a predictive model to estimate the risk of conversion from ocular hypertension to glaucoma. *Arch Ophthalmol*. 2005;123:1351–1360.

40. Leske MC, Heijl A, Hussien M, et al. Factors for glaucoma progression and the effect of treatment. *Arch Ophthalmol*. 2003;121:48–56.

41. Lichter PR, Musch DC, Gillespie BW, et al. Interim clinical outcomes in the Collaborative Initial Glaucoma Treatment Study comparing initial treatment randomized to medications or surgery. *Ophthalmology*. 2001;108:1943–1953.

42. Janz NK, Wren PA, Lichter PA, et al. Quality of life in newly diagnosed glaucoma patients. Collaborative Initial Glaucoma Treatment Study. *Ophthalmology*. 2001;108: 887–897.

43. European Glaucoma Prevention Study (EGPS) Group. Results of the European Glaucoma Prevention Study. *Ophthalmology*. 2005;112:366–375.

44. Quigley HA. Letters to the Editor. European Glaucoma Prevention Study. *Ophthalmology*. 2005;112:1642–1643.

45. Grant WM, Burke JF Jr. Why do some people go blind from glaucoma? *Ophthalmology*. 1982;89:991–998.

46. Anderson DR. Glaucoma: the damage caused by pressure [XLVI Edward Jackson Memorial Lecture]. *Am J Ophthalmol*. 1989;108:485–495.

47. Jampel HD. Target pressure in glaucoma therapy. *J Glaucoma*. 1997;6:133–138.

48. Ashburn FS Jr, Goldberg I, Kass MA. Compliance with ocular therapy. *Surv Ophthalmol*. 1980;24:237–248.

49. Chung PY, Schuman TS, Netland PA, et al. Five-year results of a randomized, prospective clinical trial of diode vs argon laser trabeculoplasty for open-angle glaucoma. *Am J Ophthalmol*. 1998;126:185–190.

50. Lee AG, Anderson R, Kardon RH, et al. Presumed "sulfa allergy" in patients with intracranial hypertension treated with acetazolamide or furosemide: cross-reactivity, myth or reality? *Am J Ophthalmol*. 2004;138:114–118.

51. Warwar RE, Bullock JD, Ballal D. Cystoid macular edema and anterior uveitis associated with latanoprost use: experience and incidence in a retrospective review of 94 patients. *Ophthalmology*. 1998;105:263–268.

52. Packer M, Fine IH, Hoffmann RS. Bilateral nongranulomatous anterior uveitis associated with bimatoprost. *J Cataract Refract Surg*. 2003;11:2242–2243.

53. Kumarasamy M, Desai S. Anterior uveitis associated with travoprost. *BMJ*. 2004; 329(7459):205.

54. Faulkner WJ, Burk SE. Acute anterior uveitis and corneal edema associated with travoprost. *Arch Ophthalmol*. 2003;121:1054–1055.

55. Wand M, Gaudio AR. Cystoid macular edema associated with ocular hypotensive lipids. *Am J Ophthalmol*. 2002;133:393–397.

56. Hedman K, Larsson LI. The effect of latanoprost compared with timolol in African-American, Asian, Caucasian and Mexican open-angle glaucoma or ocular hypertensive patients. *Surv Ophthalmol.* 2002;47(suppl 1):S77–S89.

57. Netland PA, Landry T, Sullivan EK, et al. Travoprost compared with latanoprost and timolol in patients with open-angle glaucoma or ocular hypertension. *Am J Ophthalmol.* 2001;132:472–484.

58. Brandt JD, VanDenburgh AM, Chen K, et al. Comparison of once or twice daily bimatoprost with twice-daily timolol in patients with elevated IOP: a 3-month clinical trial. *Ophthalmology.* 2001;108:1023–1031.

59. Noecker RS, Dirks MS, Choplin N, et al. Comparison of latanoprost, bimatoprost, and travoprost in patients with elevated intraocular pressure: a 12-week, randomized, masked-evaluator multicenter study. *Am J Ophthalmol.* 2003;135:688–703.

60. Parrish RK, Palmberg P, Sheu WP, et al. A comparison of latanoprost, bimatoprost, and travoprost in patients with elevated intraocular pressure. a 12-week, randomized, masked-evaluator multicenter study. *Am J Ophthalmol.* 2003;135:688–703.

61. Asrani S, Zeimer R, Wilensky J, et al. Large diurnal fluctuations in intraocular pressure are an independent risk factor in patients with glaucoma. *J Glaucoma.* 2000;9:134–142.

62. Larsson LI, Mishima HK, Takamatsu M, et al. The effect of latanoprost on circadian intraocular pressure. *Surv Ophthalmol.* 2002;47(suppl 1):S90–S96.

63. Orzalesi N, Rossetti L, Bottoli A, et al. Comparison of the effects of latanoprost, travoprost and bimatoprost on circadian intraocular pressure in patients with glaucoma or ocular hypertension. *Ophthalmology.* 2006;113:239–246.

64. Schumer RA, Camras CB, Mandahl AK. Putative side effects of prostaglandin analogs. *Surv Ophthalmol.* 2002;47(suppl 1):S219–s230.

65. Wand M, Ritch R, Isbey EK Jr, et al. Latanoprost and periocular skin color changes. *Arch Ophthalmol.* 2001;119:614–615.

66. Johnstone MA, Albert DM. Prostaglandin-induced hair growth. *Surv Ophthalmol.* 2002;47(suppl 1):S185–S202.

67. Gandolfi SA, Cimino L. Effect of bimatoprost on patients with primary open-angle glaucoma or ocular hypertension who are nonresponders to latanoprost. *Ophthalmology.* 2003;110:609–614.

68. Zimmerman TJ, Kaufman HE. Timolol: a beta-adrenergic blocking agent for the treatment of glaucoma. *Arch Ophthalmol.* 1977;95:601–604.

69. Freedman SF, Freedman NJ, Shields MB, et al. Effects of ocular carteolol and timolol on plasma high-density lipoprotein cholesterol level. *Am J Ophthalmol.* 1993;116: 600–611.

70. Allen RC, Epstein DL. Additive effect of betaxolol and epinephrine in primary open angle glaucoma. *Arch Ophthalmol.* 1986;104:1178–1184.

71. Harris LS, Greenstein SH, Bloom AF. Respiratory difficulties with betaxolol. *Am J Ophthalmol.* 1986;102:274–275.

72. Katz LJ. Brimonidine tartrate 0.2% twice daily vs timolol 0.5% twice daily: 1-year results in glaucoma patients. Brimonidine Study Group. *Am J Ophthalmol.* 1999; 127:20–26.

73. Adamsons IA, Polis A, Ostrov CS, Boyle JE. Two-year safety study of dorzolamide as monotherapy and with timolol and pilocarpine. Dorzolamide Safety Study Group. *J Glaucoma.* 1998;7:395–401.

74. Silver LH. Clinical efficacy and safety of brinzolamide (Azopt), a new topical carbonic anhydrase inhibitor for primary open-angle glaucoma and ocular hypertension. Brinzolamide Primary Therapy Study Group. *Am J Ophthalmol.* 1998;126:400–408.

75. Zimmerman TJ, Kooner KS, Kandarakis AS, Ziegler LP. Improving the therapeutic index of topically applied ocular drugs. *Arch Ophthalmol.* 1984;102:551–553.

76. Realini T, Fechtner R, Atreides SP, Gollance S. The uniocular drug trial and second-eye response to glaucoma medications. *Ophthalmology.* 2004;111:421–426.

77. Sit AJ, Liu JHK, Weinreb RN. Asymmetry of right versus left intraocular pressures over 24 hours in glaucoma patients. *Ophthalmology.* 2006;113:425–430.

78. Zimmerman TJ, Kass MA, Yablonski ME, Becker B. Timolol maleate: efficacy and safety. *Arch Ophthalmol.* 1979;97:656–658.

79. *Primary Open-Angle Glaucoma Suspect Preferred Practice Pattern.* San Francisco, CA: American Academy of Ophthalmology; 2005. www.aao.org/education/guidelines/ppp/poags_new.cfm

11

Adjunctive Medical Therapy

MALIK Y. KAHOOK, LISA S. GAMELL, AND JOEL S. SCHUMAN

A fter diagnosing a patient with glaucoma, in the United States the clinician usually prescribes topical medication as the initial treatment regimen. Ophthalmologists are fortunate to have many drugs in their arsenal today that are effective at lowering intraocular pressure (IOP) while requiring less frequent dosing and causing fewer systemic and ocular side effects than previous generations of glaucoma medications. While this provides the clinician with more options, it can also cause confusion. The ophthalmologist must choose one from among more than a handful of drops as initial single therapy. This decision is more clear-cut when patients have relative contraindications to particular drugs, such as avoiding beta blockers in patients with asthma or heart block or trying alternatives to carbonic anhydrase inhibitors (CAIs) in patients who are sulfa allergic. Otherwise, decisions may often be based upon experience or the clinician's comfort level with a particular medication.

More difficult decisions arise when disease progresses and a change in therapy is indicated. Options include adding additional medications, substituting one medication for another, or performing a surgical procedure, such as laser or filtration surgery. Which path the ophthalmologist follows depends not only upon clinical parameters such as disease severity but also upon patient parameters, including age, compliance, and quality-of-life issues. Preceding chapters provide pharmacologic information on the various classes of drugs: adrenergic agents, beta blockers, CAIs, cholinergics, osmotics, and prostaglandin analogs (PAs). The goal of this chapter is to guide the clinician in using these drugs to the patient's maximal benefit.

11.1 ADJUNCTIVE THERAPY: FIRST-LINE DRUGS

Which drug to use as initial single therapy depends on many factors, including the patient's health, allergies, and the amount of pressure reduction needed to reach target pressure. In the past (1980s, 1990s, and very early twenty-first century), beta blockers were the preferred first-line glaucoma drug because they were effective for lowering IOP and were relatively well tolerated when compared to other available medications. In addition, until the introduction in the United States of apraclonidine in 1989 and PAs in 1996, beta blockers and direct- and indirect-acting cholinergics were the most potent topical agents available. The current list of medications for glaucoma, including alpha agonists, CAIs, and PAs, provides multiple alternatives for initial therapy. Most ophthalmologists would agree that PAs, with once-daily dosing, excellent IOP-lowering effect, and few side effects, have replaced beta blockers as the most commonly used agent for first-line therapy.

Regardless of which drug is chosen as the first-line agent, the clinician should have a clear goal for IOP reduction in mind. The term *target pressure* is not the most accurate, since there is no magic number that will guarantee disease stability. A reasonable goal is approximately a 20–30% reduction in IOP;[1] it is often useful to perform a monocular drug trial, where the drop is given in one eye alone to see if an adequate IOP-lowering effect is achieved.[2] If an acceptable IOP reduction results, the drug may be added to the other eye. If the drug does not appear to be efficacious, an alternative drug may be tried. Bear in mind that a monocular trial provides the most information when the IOP is similar in both eyes. In addition, caution should be used if the IOP is very high in a patient with notable retinal nerve fiber layer or visual field damage. In such a patient, a monocular trial is not appropriate, and the clinician should attempt to quickly and effectively lower IOP in both eyes.

11.2 COMBINATION THERAPY

The need to add more medications to the patient's regimen becomes evident when there is progression of disease or when a single drug does not sustain a reduced pressure. In the case of advancing disease, optic nerve or visual field changes may occur despite a seemingly adequate initial pressure reduction. This should prompt the addition of medications to further reduce the IOP. For patients with early glaucoma and little optic nerve damage and visual field loss, an IOP in the high teens or low 20s may suffice, while for a patient with visual field loss on one side of the horizontal meridian or the other, an IOP in the mid to high teens may be required. For a patient with advanced disease, an IOP of 12 or less might be targeted as the goal to halt disease progression.[3] On the other hand, usually a clinician will recalibrate the goal IOP through a process of trial and error for any given patient. In general, if target IOP is not adequate to control the disease, the aim should be approximately 20–30% reduction in IOP when there is evidence of progressive disease.

When the IOP rises to levels previously associated with disease progression, more aggressive treatment is needed. The reason for IOP elevation may be a loss of drug efficacy or refractory disease. A loss of drug efficacy can be assessed by performing a reverse monocular drug trial, where a drug is discontinued in one eye. If the IOP rises considerably, then the drug most likely is helping and advancing disease is the culprit.[4] In the case of dramatic elevations of IOP, however, it is more prudent to add or change to another drug unilaterally or bilaterally than to take one away and risk a potentially damaging IOP spike.

11.3 ADDITION OR SUBSTITUTION?

Many practitioners tend to add medications, assuming that more is better. Remember, however, that it is the patient who must take all of the medications. Each time patients add a new drop to their regimen, they add new potential side effects, drug or preservative allergies, and inconveniences to their daily schedule. As a general rule of thumb, additional medications are needed when disease progresses despite an already reduced IOP. Substitution is more appropriate in patients with less advanced disease who display tolerance or a loss of drug efficacy over time.

In both addition and substitution, the new medication should belong to a different drug class. For example, adding or substituting a nonselective beta blocker for a selective beta blocker will not produce a dramatic change in IOP and is usually not an appropriate choice (unless such a change is, e.g., from betaxolol to timolol for dose scheduling purposes).

11.4 ADDITIVITY OF MEDICATIONS

How well two or more medications achieve IOP reduction also depends upon drug class, or their mechanisms of action. Two beta blockers used together will have little added IOP-lowering effect, since they both decrease aqueous humor formation by the same mechanism. Likewise, two PAs used simultaneously will add little to IOP lowering and, in fact, may be less effective than either medication alone.[5] On the other hand, a beta blocker and a CAI both decrease aqueous humor production, but by different mechanisms, the beta blocker by occupying adrenergic receptors and the CAI by reducing the activity of the enzyme carbonic anhydrase, which is responsible for catalyzing the reaction converting bicarbonate to carbon dioxide and water. In fact, IOP may drop an additional 13–21% when dorzolamide 2% (Trusopt) is added to timolol 0.5%.[6] Alpha-adrenergic agonists can also effectively reduce IOP in patients on maximal medical therapy.[7]

The PAs contribute positively to the IOP-lowering effect of beta blockers, alpha agonists, and CAIs, which all act by decreasing aqueous production. Studies investigating the addition of a beta blocker to a PA showed an IOP reduction of 15–35%.[8,9] The mechanism of action for all PAs contributes to this additivity by increasing pressure-independent (uveoscleral) outflow, and to some extent, pressure-dependent

Table 11.1 General Guidelines for Combination Therapy for Glaucoma

If medication is not working or significant side effects occur, stop the drug!
If a medication is working, but is not adequate, switch to or add another drug.
A monocular therapeutic trial can determine if a drug is effective.
Use the lowest dose and frequency possible, and increase as needed.
If medications are not adequate, move on to laser trabeculoplasty or filtration surgery.

outflow (facility), as well. As a result, however, this class of agents is less effective when used in conjunction with cholinergic agents. Drugs such as pilocarpine decrease uveoscleral outflow and therefore are antagonistic to PAs, as indicated by several clinical studies.[10,11]

Multiple studies have verified the IOP-lowering effect of adding a CAI to a PA.[12–14] This result appears to be similar to combining a beta blocker with a PA but greater than that of combined alpha-agonist–PA therapy. These differences are yet to be unequivocally proven, and future prospective randomized studies are needed to determine the differences in additive therapy with the various PA agents.

In view of the apparent additive IOP-lowering effect of beta blockers to the PA class of glaucoma medications, newer drop formulations containing both medications in one bottle are currently being studied.[15–17] Published data indicate that fixed combinations of a PA and a beta blocker appear to provide near-equal IOP-lowering effects compared to concomitant use of the two drugs while providing the benefit of decreasing dosing frequency, reducing preservative exposure, and possibly improving compliance. These medications may prove advantageous in treating patients while offering the added benefit of saving on cost of medications (depending on drug pricing).

A monocular therapeutic trial of 3 or 4 weeks can determine if a drug is effective; however, beta blockers and brimonidine can have significant crossover activity (you may see IOP lowering in the eye *not* being treated). An in-office monocular therapeutic trial can be used for all glaucoma medications except PAs. The drop is given in one eye, and IOP is checked 2 hours after dosing. Other general guidelines for combination medical therapy are given in table 11.1.

While there is no hard-and-fast rule determining which drugs should be used as first-line agents and in which order new drugs should be added or substituted, figure 11.1 provides some general guidelines. It is important to remember that this is only a general strategy for combination therapy, which may vary dramatically from patient to patient depending upon individual response, systemic considerations, side effects, and patient lifestyle.

11.5 PROGRESSING TO MAXIMAL MEDICAL THERAPY: INDIVIDUALIZING TREATMENT

In an attempt to control IOP and prevent progression of glaucomatous optic nerve damage, clinicians often place patients on multiple medications. Using every avail-

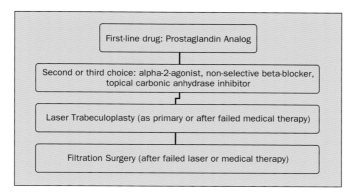

Figure 11.1. General strategy for combination therapy for glaucoma.

able glaucoma medication that the patient can topically or systemically tolerate is considered *maximal medical therapy*. The word "tolerate" is key, since the number of medications a patient may simultaneously use is often limited by surface irritation, allergy, systemic side effects, or inconvenience. Some patients simply do not want to take five different eye drops a day, and there is often very little the clinician can do to change their minds.

An important implication of the term "maximal medical therapy" is that it is the last resort before surgical interventions, such as laser trabeculoplasty (LTP) or trabeculectomy. If patients are cognizant of this, they are often prompted to be more compliant with their medications. On the other hand, some would rather have laser surgery, in the hopes that it will obviate the need for multiple medications, even if the effect is not permanent.

Just as no two cases of glaucoma are the same, no two patients are the same with regard to their response to medications. Each patient's eye drop regimen, therefore, should be constructed and then modified to meet the individual patient's needs. When it was widely used, pilocarpine might not have been a good choice for a healthy, young professional, due to not only accommodative effects but also frequent dosing. Now, for such an individual, a PA at bedtime may be best tolerated until additional medications are needed. Particularly for noncompliant patients, a fixed-dose combination drug may be appropriate early in treatment. Communication with the patient and the patient's primary care physician is instrumental in assuring a safe and acceptable drug regimen.

11.6 IMPROVEMENT OF COMPLIANCE

The relatively recent introduction of topical CAIs, PAs, and alpha agonists has made life easier for our glaucoma patients compared to those treated just 10 to 15 years ago. Maximal medical therapy is now a combination of the nonselective beta blocker timolol and topical CAI dorzolamide morning and night, a PA at night, and an alpha agonist twice a day, for a total of five drops in each eye over the course of the day. The number of drops has been almost halved compared to the previous use of twice-daily beta blockers, twice-daily epinephrine, and miotic agents four times per day. It is still not easy to be on this medical regimen!

Even the most conscientious patient can forget when to take particular drops. In addition, most pharmacies print prescription instructions in small type that is often difficult for some glaucoma patients to read clearly. This has improved recently, with many pharmacies providing larger type when requested, but this is by no means universal. We have found that the use of a medication card along with specific verbal instruction enhances compliance. A recent study by Kharod et al.[18] verified that written instructions improved patients' knowledge of their prescribed regimens. If the patient has a family member, friend, or health aide who will assist with drop instillation, make sure this party is present when the card is reviewed with the patient. The card includes the medication name and cap color, drop dosage and laterality, and specific times to take the medication. Patients may get anxious and worry that they are not spacing their medications properly during the day. By talking to the patient about daily waking, sleeping, and work activities, a reasonable schedule can be devised, and revised in the future if needed (figure 11.2).

Clinicians should ensure that patients know how to instill their eye drops. When prescribing a medication for the first time, or when faced with patients whose IOP does not improve despite seemingly adequate therapy, the clinician should have them demonstrate in the office how they administer the eye drops. This provides important information for the clinician and allows immediate feedback for the patient.

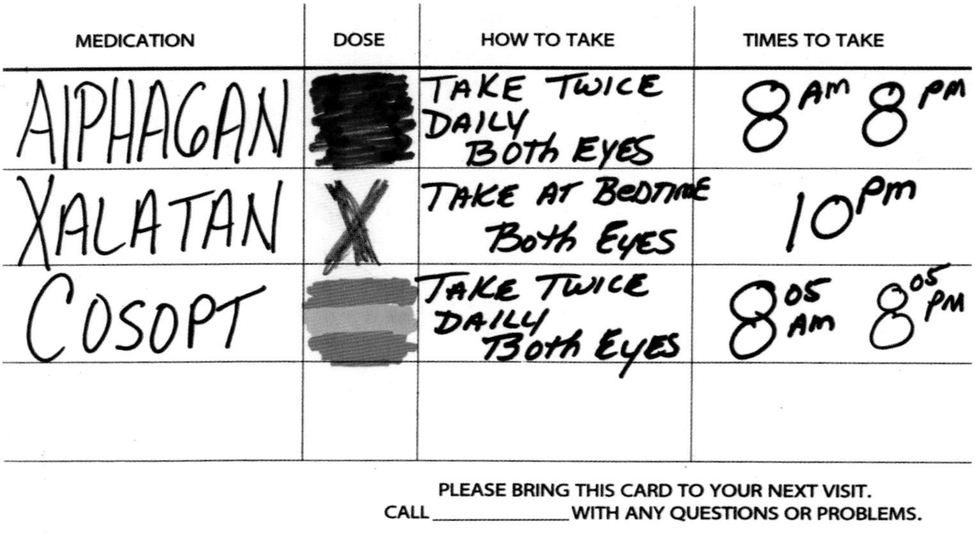

MEDICATION	DOSE	HOW TO TAKE	TIMES TO TAKE
ALPHAGAN	■	TAKE TWICE DAILY BOTH EYES	8 AM 8 PM
XALATAN	X	TAKE AT BEDTIME BOTH EYES	10 PM
COSOPT	▬	TAKE TWICE DAILY BOTH EYES	8 05 AM 8 05 PM

PLEASE BRING THIS CARD TO YOUR NEXT VISIT.
CALL_____WITH ANY QUESTIONS OR PROBLEMS.

Figure 11.2. Medication card listing medications, frequency of dosing, eye that receives medication, and exact times of day for dosing. This card shows color of bottle top, label, or pill to assist patient in recognizing correct drug.

Clinicians should also inform patients about their disease. Patients will have little incentive to take three or more medications a day if they do not know why they are taking them. Patients need to be given information about their disease, why treatment is required, and what the potential side effects of treatment or treatment failure may be. This can be accomplished verbally by the physician or nurse or technician, and then reinforced with video or written materials, if appropriate for the patient's level of sight or intellect.

Additionally, new dosing and compliance aids have been introduced to assist patients in taking their drops. These aids vary, offering support for patients who lack the dexterity to use drops, providing audible and visible reminders to take drops, and in one case, making a digital record of patients' dosing history for the physician to review. These new devices could allow physicians to better identify patients who are nonadherent to therapeutic regimens and may alternatively benefit from reeducation, laser treatment, or more invasive surgical intervention.[19,20]

11.7 ENHANCEMENT OF SURVEILLANCE

Once patients are receiving maximal tolerated medical therapy for their glaucoma, they should be seen more frequently. A patient with a stable optic nerve head, IOP, and visual fields may be seen every 4 to 6 months. Patients are usually placed on maximal medical therapy, however, due to evidence of more progressive or unstable disease. As a result, examinations ranging from every 2 to 4 months may be in order. These exams should document not only IOP but also the optic nerve head for any changes, even if through an undilated pupil. If progressive changes in the cup or nerve fiber layer are evident, as revealed by physical examination and perhaps structural imaging, then repeat visual field testing is appropriate. In today's environment of managed care, it is important to remember that insurance companies should not determine when a patient with progressive glaucomatous changes should have functional testing; however, the financial consequence of unreimbursible diagnostic evaluation should be considered by the patient and physician.

Increased frequency of visits helps the clinician not only to monitor more closely possible disease progression but also to detect potential medication side effects or allergies that may affect treatment. If patients suspect that a medication is making their eyes irritated or uncomfortable, they will often stop taking the medication without consulting their physician. This will make it difficult to determine which drug is the true culprit. Patients should be encouraged to call the office in the event of adverse drug effects or schedule an earlier follow-up visit to avoid these situations. In the case of the noncompliant patient who is reluctant to undergo surgical procedures, visits as frequently as every 1 to 3 months may be helpful. Such enhanced surveillance will ensure that the patient gets adequate prescription refills and will document the history of noncompliance and uncontrolled disease. This information coupled with the inconvenience of office visits can convince a previously unwilling patient to have a necessary surgical intervention, especially if it means taking fewer eye drops and seeing the doctor less often.

11.8 HIGH IOP ON INITIAL PRESENTATION

Patients presenting with extremely elevated IOP (e.g., >50 mm Hg) usually have symptoms. Unlike the chronically elevated IOP found with primary open-angle glaucoma or some forms of secondary glaucoma, acutely elevated IOP can cause blurry vision, pain, haloes around lights, nausea, vomiting, red eye, and corneal swelling.[21] On the other hand, optic nerve or visual field damage is less frequently found with acutely elevated IOP, because the symptoms bring attention to the disorder early on. With chronic IOP elevation, however, disease progression is indolent and may present with severe optic nerve damage despite a lack of symptoms. Table 11.2 lists the most common causes of acutely elevated IOP.

When patients with extremely elevated IOP are evaluated, it is important to perform a complete ophthalmic examination, including gonioscopy. Zeiss gonioscopy is adequate, but in situations where symptoms are uniocular, Koeppe gonioscopy or even ultrasound biomicroscopy or anterior segment optical coherence tomography may be helpful to evaluate possible angle recession or questionably narrow angles. In addition, a thorough history will also provide useful information to help identify the cause of the elevated IOP. A history of diabetes may suggest neovascular glaucoma. A history of sudden visual loss may suggest central retinal vein occlusion with subsequent neovascular glaucoma. Previous surgery may be a clue to angle closure, inflammatory glaucoma, or a steroid response. Intermittent pain and blurred vision may suggest chronic angle-closure glaucoma, while sudden pain and visual loss may suggest acute angle-closure glaucoma. The medical history is also important to elicit any conditions that may be relative contraindications to glaucoma therapy. For example, a history of chronic obstructive pulmonary disease, heart block, or congestive heart failure may make one wary of using beta blockers. CAIs are a poor option in patients with poorly controlled diabetes mellitus, sickle cell anemia, or sulfa allergy.

Once the etiology of the elevated IOP is known, the goal is to lower the pressure as rapidly as possible. In general, the goal IOP is one that is considered safe for the optic nerve. In a young, otherwise healthy patient, an acceptable IOP might be

Table 11.2 Causes of Acute IOP Elevation

Angle-Closure Glaucomas	Open-Angle Glaucomas
Primary Angle Closure	Juvenile open-angle glaucoma
Acute angle closure	Secondary open-angle glaucoma
Chronic angle closure	Postoperative changes
Secondary angle closure	Pseudoexfoliation syndrome
Neovascular glaucoma	Pigment dispersion syndrome
Uveitic glaucoma with synechiae	Angle recession
Iris bombe	Uveitic glaucoma
Malignant glaucoma	Steroid response
Intraocular tumors	Carotid-cavernous fistula

Table 11.3 Medical Treatment of Extremely Elevated IOP[a]

Medication	Marked IOP and Symptoms	High IOP With Mild Symptoms
Beta blockers	Q 10min × 2, then Q 12 hours	Q 10min × 2, then Q 12 hours
Alpha agonists	Q 10min × 2, then Q 12 hours	Q 10min × 2, then Q 12 hours
Carbonic anhydrase inhibitors	CAI Q 10min × 2, then Q 8 hours or acetazolamide 500 mg iv	CAI Q 10min × 2, then Q 8 hours or acetazolamide 500 orally
Osmotics	Mannitol 1–2 g/kg iv (20% solution)	Oral glycerine 1–1.5 g/kg po (50% solution)

[a]Pilocarpine is often used in angle-closure glaucoma.

slightly higher than in an elderly patient with other underlying systemic illnesses, such as diabetes mellitus. The mainstay of therapy for extremely elevated IOP includes aqueous suppressants and osmotics. Miotics are generally used in cases of angle-closure glaucoma or open-angle glaucoma without inflammation. Table 11.3 lists general guidelines for managing acutely elevated IOP.

After receiving medication in the office for severely elevated IOP, patients should have their IOP rechecked after 45 minutes to 1 hour. If the IOP level is acceptable, patients may be sent home with detailed medication cards, with the understanding that they must be seen the next day to ensure that the IOP remains controlled with medications. If compliance issues or a lack of an adequate support system makes return visits seem unlikely, then the decision to admit the patient to the hospital for eye drop administration and closer observation may be appropriate. In addition, if the IOP is not adequately reduced after initial treatment, the patient may also be admitted for overnight observation and repeat IOP checks during the course of the day or night. If IOP cannot be adequately controlled with appropriate medical and/ or laser treatment—in the case of angle-closure glaucoma—then incisional surgery, such as a trabeculectomy, should be considered.

11.9 WHEN MEDICAL THERAPY FAILS

A surgical procedure is indicated when medical therapy no longer adequately controls IOP. While some feel surgery should be the initial treatment for glaucoma, most clinicians in the United States use LTP, either with an argon laser (argon LTP [ALT]) or a frequency-doubled Q-switched Nd:YAG (neodymium-doped yttrium aluminum garnet) laser (selective LTP [SLT]), and trabeculectomy when medical therapy fails. Although the Glaucoma Laser Trial has shown at least equal efficacy for initial medical therapy and for initial ALT, ALT causes a permanent anatomic alteration of the body and has potential significant adverse effects.[22] Although the likelihood of such serious ALT side effects is small, most clinicians in the United States favor reserving ALT until after medical therapy has failed. An even stronger statement can be made for withholding filtering surgery until after the failure of medical therapy and ALT. Filtration surgery is at least as effective at IOP reduction as medical therapy, perhaps even more so.[23] However, the potential adverse side effects of filtration surgery make topical therapy a favored first-line option.

Which procedure to choose when disease can no longer be controlled with medications will depend upon the type of glaucoma, the severity of disease, and the patient. LTP is a less invasive procedure than filtration surgery and is often the initial surgical intervention performed. It is an effective IOP-lowering procedure in patients with primary open-angle glaucoma, pigmentary glaucoma, and pseudoexfoliation glaucoma.[24] LTP is less effective in patients with congenital or juvenile open-angle glaucoma, angle recession, and uveitic glaucoma.[25] ALT reduces the IOP in approximately 85% of all patients 1 year after treatment and has an efficacy of 50% at 5 years[26,27] Initially, IOP reductions range from 20% to 30% or a mean of 9 mm Hg.[28]

In patients who have difficulty complying with complicated medication regimens, LTP may be helpful in reducing the number of glaucoma medications needed to achieve IOP control. LTP in combination with medical therapy has been shown to control IOP in a slightly higher percentage of patients than medical therapy alone.[28] However, LTP does not reveal its maximal pressure-lowering effect until 4 to 6 weeks after treatment. In patients with rapidly progressing disease and severe field loss, this latency period may allow further damage to occur. In such patients, filtration surgery is a better option. It has also been shown that patients with higher IOP—greater than 35 mm Hg—have a higher failure rate with LTP, mainly because the absolute pressure reduction is not adequate even though a 40% to 50% change may be evident after the procedure.[29,30]

Complications of LTP include corneal irritation or abrasions, mild postoperative iritis, peripheral anterior synechiae, or worsening of glaucoma. In addition, a steroid response can occur, since topical steroids are usually used to suppress postoperative inflammation. The most common adverse effect of LTP is a rise in IOP usually seen in the immediate postoperative period in approximately 20% of patients.[31] This transient rise in IOP has been associated with loss of visual field.[32] Apraclonidine and brimonidine are the most effective at preventing postoperative IOP spikes after LTP.[33,34] In patients with severe disk damage and field loss from glaucoma, LTP is still a viable treatment option as long as postoperative IOP is monitored closely during the first 24 hours.

LTP has traditionally been done using an argon laser. Recently, SLT has found a role in treating glaucoma patients. SLT uses a Q-switched, 3-nanosecond, frequency-doubled Nd:YAG laser that delivers a fraction of the laser energy (<1%) to tissue compared to ALT. The short pulse of energy delivered to the target is shorter than the thermal relaxation time of tissue, resulting in selective photothermolysis, minimizing generalized destruction and collateral damage.[35]

Latina et al.[35] were first to describe SLT for use in decreasing IOP in a group of glaucoma patients, including those with previous ALT or history of maximal medical therapy. Since its introduction, multiple studies have been done to support the clinical efficacy of SLT compared to ALT and medical therapy. Prospective studies have indicated that SLT can decrease IOP by 30% to 35% when used as primary therapy. Melamed et al.[36] showed that SLT is safe and effective as primary treatment for open-angle glaucoma in eyes not previously treated with medicines. IOP dropped an average of 7.7 ± 3.5 mm Hg after SLT. In addition, when comparing SLT to ALT, a similar IOP-lowering effect is demonstrated with long-term follow-up.[37,38]

In histological evaluation done by Kramer and Noecker,[39] less structural damage to the trabecular meshwork was witnessed after SLT in comparison with ALT. Scanning electron microscopy of human cadaver eyes following ALT and SLT revealed coagulated tissue and crater formation with the former and no significant physical alteration to the meshwork in the latter. This makes SLT a potentially repeatable treatment, although this hypothesis requires further study and long-term follow-up.

When LTP (argon or selective) fails to control IOP or if a patient is a poor candidate for laser surgery in the setting of failed maximal medical therapy, the procedure of choice is usually trabeculectomy.

11.10 CONCLUSIONS

When prescribing multiple medications in the treatment of glaucoma, the clinician considers the mechanism of action of various drugs, the patient's general health, and the patient's lifestyle and ability to comply with medical therapy. In general, when a patient does not have adequate glaucoma control or suffers disease progression while on maximal medical therapy, a surgical procedure should be performed. LTP (argon or selective) is generally an appropriate first choice after failing medical treatment. If adequate IOP reduction does not occur, then trabeculectomy or shunt placement should be considered. It is the clinician's responsibility to make sure that the patient with glaucoma understands the disease, treatment options, and potential for visual loss both with and without adequate therapy.

REFERENCES

1. Epstein DL. In: Epstein DL, Allingham R, Schuman JS, eds. *Chandler and Grant's Glaucoma.* 4th ed. Philadelphia: Williams & Wilkins; 1997.
2. Smith J, Wandel T. Rationale for the one-eye therapeutic trial. *Ann Ophthalmol.* 1986;18:8.
3. Grant WM, Burke JF Jr. Why do some people go blind from glaucoma? *Ophthalmology.* 1982;89:991–998.
4. Ritch R, Shields MB, Krupin T. Chronic open-angle glaucoma: treatment overview. In: Ritch R, Shields MB, Krupin T, eds. *The Glaucomas: Glaucoma Therapy.* Boston: Mosby; 1996:1513.
5. Doi LM, Melo LA Jr, Prata JA Jr. Effects of the combination of bimatoprost and latanoprost on intraocular pressure in primary open angle glaucoma: a randomised clinical trial. *Br J Ophthalmol.* 2005;89(5):547–549.
6. Nardin G, et al. Activity of the topical CAI MK-507 bid when added to timolol bid. *Invest Ophthalmol Vis Sci.* 1991;32(suppl):989.
7. Serle JB, Podos SM, Abundo GP, et al. The effect of brimonidine tartrate in glaucoma patients on maximal medical therapy. *Invest Ophthalmol Vis Sci.* 1993;34(suppl): 1137.

8. Racz P, Ruzsonyi MR, Nagy ZT, Gaygi Z, Bito LZ. Around-the-clock intraocular pressure reduction with once-daily application of latanoprost by itself or in combination with timolol. *Arch Ophthalmol.* 1996;114(3):268–273.

9. Alm A, Widengard I, Kjellgren D, Soderstrom M, Fristrom B, Heijl A, Stjerschantz J. Latanoprost administered once daily caused a maintained reduction of intraocular pressure in glaucoma patients treated concomitantly with timolol. *Br J Ophthalmol.* 1995;79(1):12–16.

10. Villumsen J, Alm A. Effect of the prostaglandin F_{2alpha} analogue PhXA41 in eyes treated with pilocarpine and timolol. *Invest Ophthalmol Vis Sci.* 1992;33(suppl): 1248.

11. Fristrom B, Nilsson SE. Interaction of PhXA41, a new prostaglandin analogue, with pilocarpine. A study on patients with elevated intraocular pressure. *Arch Ophthalmol.* 1993;111(5):662–665.

12. Shoji N, Ogata H, Suyama H, et al. Intraocular pressure lowering effect of brinzolamide 1.0% as adjunctive therapy to latanoprost 0.005% in patients with open angle glaucoma or ocular hypertension: an uncontrolled, open-label study. *Curr Med Res Opin.* 2005;21(4):503–508.

13. Reis R, Queiroz CF, Santos LC, Avila MP, Magacho L. A randomized, investigator-masked, 4-week study comparing timolol maleate 0.5%, brinzolamide 1%, and brimonidine tartrate 0.2% as adjunctive therapies to travoprost 0.004% in adults with primary open-angle glaucoma or ocular hypertension. *Clin Ther.* 2006;28(4):552–559.

14. O'Connor DJ, Martone if, Mead A. Additive intraocular pressure lowering effect of various medications with latanoprost. *Am J Ophthalmol.* 2002;133:836–837.

15. Magacho L, Reis R, Shetty RK, Santos LC, Avila MP. Efficacy of latanoprost or fixed-combination latanoprost-timolol in patients switched from a combination of timolol and a nonprostaglandin medication. *Ophthalmology.* 2006;113(3):442–445.

16. Hughes BA, Bacharach J, Craven ER, et al. A three-month, multicenter, double-masked study of the safety and efficacy of travoprost 0.004%/timolol 0.5% ophthalmic solution compared to travoprost 0.004% ophthalmic solution and timolol 0.5% dosed concomitantly in subjects with open angle glaucoma or ocular hypertension. *J Glaucoma.* 2005;14(5):392–399.

17. Schuman JS, Katz GJ, Lewis RA, et al. Efficacy and safety of a fixed combination of travoprost 0.004%/timolol 0.5% ophthalmic solution once daily for open-angle glaucoma or ocular hypertension. *Am J Ophthalmol.* 2005;140(2):242–250.

18. Kharod BV, Johnson PB, Nesti HA, Rhee DJ. Effect of written instructions on accuracy of self-reporting medication regimen in glaucoma patients. *J Glaucoma.* 2006; 15(3):244–247.

19. Rivers PH. Compliance aids—do they work? *Drugs Aging.* 1992;2(2):103–111.

20. Boden C, Sit A, Weinreb RN. Accuracy of an electronic monitoring and reminder device for use with travoprost eye drops. *J Glaucoma.* 2006;15(1):30–34.

21. Allingham RR. Management of highly elevated intraocular pressure. In: Epstein DL, Allingham RR, Schuman JS, eds. *Chandler and Grant's Glaucoma.* 4th ed. Baltimore, Md: Williams & Wilkins; 1997:177–180.

22. Glaucoma Laser Trial Research Group. The Glaucoma Laser Trial (GLT) and glaucoma laser trial follow-up study: 7. Results. *Am J Ophthalmol.* 1995;120(6):718–731.

23. Stewart WC, Sine CS, LoPresto C. Surgical vs. medical management of chronic open-angle glaucoma. *Am J Ophthalmol.* 1996;122:767–774.

24. Committee on Ophthalmic Procedure Assessment. Laser trabeculoplasty for primary open-angle glaucoma. *Ophthalmology.* 1996;103:1706–1712.

25. Weinreb RN, Tsai CS. Laser trabeculoplasty. In: Ritch R, Shields MB, Krupin T, eds. *The Glaucomas: Glaucoma Therapy*. 2nd ed. Boston: Mosby; 1996:1575–1590.

26. Shingleton BJ, Richter CU, Bellows AR, et al. Long-term efficacy of argon laser trabeculoplasty. *Ophthalmology*. 1987; 94:1513–1518.

27. Schwartz AL, Whitten ME, Bleiman B, Martin D. Argon laser trabecular surgery in uncontrolled phakic open angle glaucoma. *Ophthalmology*. 1981;88:203–212.

28. Glaucoma Laser Trial Research Group. The Glaucoma Laser Trial (GLT): 2. Results of argon laser trabeculoplasty versus topical medications. *Ophthalmology*. 1990;97:1403–1413.

29. Thomas JV, Simmons RJ, Belcher CD. Argon laser trabeculoplasty in the pre-surgical glaucoma patient. *Ophthalmology*. 1982;89:187–197.

30. Schwartz AL, Love DC, Schwartz MA. Long-term follow-up of argon laser trabeculoplasty for uncontrolled open angle glaucoma. *Arch Ophthalmol*. 1985;103:1482–1484.

31. Reiss GR, Wilensky JT, Higginbotham EJ. Laser trabeculoplasty. *Surv Ophthalmol*. 1991;35:407–428.

32. Thomas JV, Simmons RJ, Belcher CD. Complications of argon laser trabeculoplasty. *Glaucoma*. 1982;4:50.

33. Krupin T, Stank T, Feitl ME. Apraclonidine pretreatment decreases the acute intraocular pressure rise after laser trabeculoplasty or iridotomy. *J Glaucoma*. 1992;1:79–86.

34. The Brimonidine-ALT Study Group. Effect of brimonidine 0.5% on intraocular pressure spikes following 360 argon laser trabeculoplasty. *Ophthalmol Surg Lasers*. 1995;26:404–409.

35. Latina MA, Sibayan SA, Shin DH, et al. Q-switched 532-nm Nd:YAG laser trabeculoplasty (selective laser trabeculoplasty): a multicenter, pilot, clinical study. *Ophthalmology*. 1998;105:2082–2088.

36. Melamed S, Ben Simon GJ, Levkovitch-Verbin H. Selective laser trabeculoplasty as primary treatment of open-angle glaucoma. *Arch Ophthalmol*. 2003;121:957–960.

37. Juzych MS, Chopra V, Banitt MR, et al. Comparison of long-term outcomes of selective laser trabeculoplasty versus argon laser trabeculoplasty in open-angle glaucoma. *Ophthalmology*. 2004;111:1853–1859.

38. Damji KF, Shah KC, Rock WJ, et al. Selective laser trabeculoplasty v argon laser trabeculoplasty: a prospective randomised clinical trial. *Br J Ophthalmol*. 1999;83:18–722.

39. Kramer TR, Noecker RJ. Comparison of the morphologic changes after selective laser trabeculoplasty and argon laser trabeculoplasty in human eye bank eyes. *Ophthalmology*. 2001;108:773–779.

Special Therapeutic Situations

ROBERT RITCH, YANIV BARKANA, AND JEFFREY M. LIEBMANN

Certain discrete glaucomas and difficult clinical problems require the use of multiple medications or require medications to be used in conjunction with laser treatment or filtration surgery. The specific medications used may differ from those used in primary open-angle glaucoma. Directed therapy, when applicable, should be a strong consideration in treatment.

Directed therapy is conceptually simple. It merely means devising specific treatments for specific diseases. This fundamental tenet of medicine has been applied infrequently in the treatment of glaucoma.

The simplification of glaucoma into congenital, open-angle, and angle-closure glaucoma has led us to focus on glaucoma as the disease and intraocular pressure (IOP) as its treatable aspect. Specific glaucomas, however, lead to trabecular dysfunction by specific series of events. In theory, intervention could be applied at each of these steps. Little emphasis has been placed on preventive treatment or disease-specific therapy, and more could be done even with our present knowledge. Other potentially damaging abnormalities bypass the meshwork and affect the optic nerve head directly. These include disorders affecting ocular perfusion, the extracellular matrix of the optic nerve head and lamina cribrosa, and perhaps factors within the central nervous system. These other risk factors are also potentially treatable, now or in the future.

12.1 ANGLE-CLOSURE GLAUCOMA

Angle closure is an anatomic disorder comprising a final common pathway of iris apposition to the trabecular meshwork. By recent convention, the term "glaucoma" is applied to eyes with visual field and/or optic nerve damage, analogous to the differentiation between ocular hypertension and glaucoma in eyes with open angles. Angle closure results from various abnormal relationships of anterior segment structures. These, in turn, result from one or more abnormalities in the relative or absolute sizes or positions of anterior segment structures or posterior segment forces that alter anterior segment anatomy.[1] Angle closure results from blockage of the meshwork by the iris, but the forces causing this blockage may be viewed as originating at four successive anatomic levels (figure 12.1):

1. Iris (pupillary block)
2. Ciliary body (plateau iris)
3. Lens (phacomorphic glaucoma)
4. Posterior to lens (aqueous misdirection, or malignant glaucoma)

The more posterior the level at which the angle closure originates, the more complex the diagnosis and treatment, because the operative mechanism specific to each level may also be accompanied by a component of the mechanism(s) peculiar to each of the levels preceding it and may require a combination of treatments appropriate to each of the mechanisms involved.

Indentation gonioscopy, or dynamic gonioscopy, is mandatory for accurate assessment and appropriate treatment of angle closure. Pressure applied to the cornea by the goniolens forces aqueous into the angle, widening it. The presence and extent of closure by peripheral anterior synechiae (PAS), the contour and insertion site of the iris, and the depth of the angle can be determined. Gonioscopy in a completely darkened room is of the utmost importance when assessing a narrow angle for occludability (figure 12.2), because any light shining through the pupil may suffice to eliminate iris apposition to the trabecular meshwork. The slit beam should consist of the smallest square of light available to avoid stimulating the pupillary light reflex. The quadrant of angle to be assessed is examined with the four-mirror lens without pressure on the cornea and with the patient looking sufficiently far in the direction of the mirror so that the examiner can see as deeply into the angle as possible. The angle is observed while the pupil dilates in the dark. The narrowest quadrant is usually the superior angle (inferior mirror).

12.1.1 *Acute Angle Closure.* Therapy in acute angle closure (AAC) is directed at decreasing IOP rapidly and opening the angle. Both medical and laser treatments play a role in opening the angle and eliminating pupillary block.

Hyperosmotic agents lower IOP by causing a rapid but transient increase in serum osmolality of between 20 and 30 mOsm/L.[2] The resulting blood–ocular osmotic gradient draws water from the eye via the retinal and uveal vasculature, primarily from the vitreous cavity. The decrease in vitreous volume lowers IOP and allows the lens to move posteriorly. Although the vitreous volume is decreased by only about 3%, this amounts to a volume of 0.12 mL, which is half the volume of the normal anterior chamber and twice the volume of the normal posterior chamber. IOP decreases within 30 to 60 minutes after administration, and the effect lasts about 5 to 6 hours. For maximal benefit, patients should limit fluid intake.

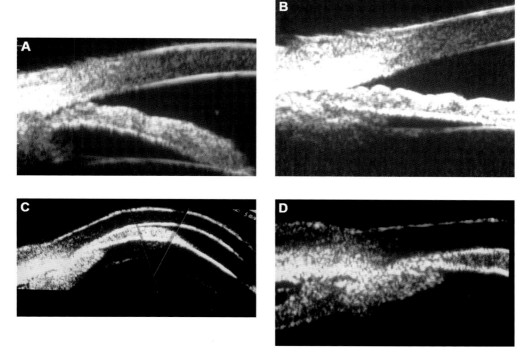

Figure 12.1. (A) Pupillary block (level 1). Force-producing iris apposition to the trabecular meshwork originates from the posterior chamber. Iridotomy provides definitive treatment. (B) Plateau iris (level 2). Force-producing iris apposition to the trabecular meshwork in this eye, which has already undergone laser iridotomy, originates from anteriorly positioned ciliary processes, holding the iris forward. Argon laser peripheral iridoplasty (ALPI) provides definitive treatment. (C) Phacomorphic glaucoma (level 3). Force-producing iris apposition to trabecular meshwork originates from an intumescent lens, pushing ciliary processes and the iris forward. ALPI can break an attack of acute angle-closure, and iridotomy can be performed to eliminate any component of pupillary block to give the eye time to quiet and the media time to clear so that lens extraction, the definitive procedure, can be safely performed. (D) Aqueous misdirection (level 4). Force-producing iris apposition to trabecular meshwork originates from behind the lens, pushing the lens, ciliary processes, and iris forward. Shallow supraciliary detachment is present, causing the lens–iris diaphragm to rotate anteriorly. The abnormal vitreociliary relationship that results causes posterior diversion of aqueous into the vitreous. Resultant increased posterior segment pressure pushes the lens farther forward, allowing more aqueous to be secreted into the vitreous and setting up a vicious cycle. Restoration of normal anatomic relationships is the definitive treatment, but achieving this can be difficult and entail complex combinations of medical, laser, and surgical treatment. Reprinted with permission from Ritch R, Lowe RF. Angle-closure glaucoma: mechanisms and epidemiology. In: Ritch R, Shields MB, Krupin T, eds. *The Glaucomas.* 2nd ed. St Louis, MO: CV Mosby Co; 1996:801–819.

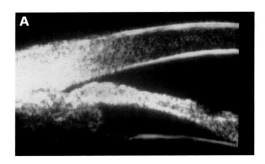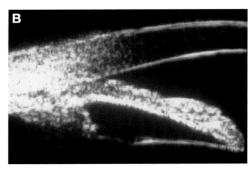

Figure 12.2. (A) Ultrasound biomicrograph of anterior chamber angle in bright illumination. The iris is slightly convex, consistent with relative pupillary block. Aqueous has access to the trabecular meshwork, which is between Schwalbe's line and the scleral spur. (B) In the dark, the pupil dilates and the peripheral iris moves against the trabecular meshwork, closing the angle. Reprinted with permission from Ritch R, Lowe RF. Angle-closure glaucoma: mechanisms and epidemiology. In: Ritch R, Shields MB, Krupin T, eds. *The Glaucomas*. 2nd ed. St Louis, MO: CV Mosby Co; 1996:801–819.

Glycerol is administered as a liquid in dosages of 1 to 1.5 g/kg of body weight,[3] either as a 100% solution mixed with an equal volume of iced juice or as a commercial preparation (Osmoglyn, 50% solution). Oral glycerol is rapidly absorbed, is distributed throughout the extracellular water, and penetrates the eye poorly. The drug is metabolized by the liver rather than excreted by the kidneys, producing less diuresis than do other hyperosmotic agents. Glycerol has an unpleasantly sweet taste and may cause vomiting. The caloric content is 4.32 cal/g, which, combined with the osmotic diuretic effect and resultant dehydration, mandates special caution when used in diabetic patients, who may develop hyperglycemia and ketosis.[4]

Isosorbide (Ismotic) is more palatable, causes less nausea and vomiting, and is not metabolized—a particular advantage in diabetic patients. Although isosorbide had advantages over other osmotic drugs (see chapter 8), this drug is not commercially available at this time. A solution of 20% mannitol (Osmitrol), 0.5 to 2 g/kg, given intravenously over 45 minutes, has a greater hypotensive effect and may be given when severe nausea and vomiting are present.

Administration of hyperosmotic agents is commonly accompanied by thirst and headache. Hyperosmolar coma can be a serious complication caused by severe dehydration of the central nervous system. Patients with renal or cardiovascular disease or those already dehydrated by vomiting are at risk. These agents should be used cautiously in patients with reduced cardiac function, because the sudden intravascular volume overload may lead to congestive heart failure and pulmonary edema.[5]

Acetazolamide (Ak-Zol, Dazamide, Diamox), a carbonic anhydrase inhibitor (CAI), is highly effective in AAC, even in the presence of ischemic iris atrophy and paralysis of the pupil. Rapid IOP reduction is most reliably achieved by giving 500 mg intravenously. Adverse reactions are uncommon. Acetazolamide tablets may be given orally as an alternative, but the onset of action is not as rapid. Following oral therapy, the maximum effect occurs at 2 hours, and high plasma levels persist for 4 to 6 hours but then drop rapidly because of excretion in the urine. Topical aqueous suppressants are additive with acetazolamide but take longer to act, and their absorption through the cornea is slowed by corneal edema and markedly elevated IOP. They should be used in conjunction with, but not as an alternative to, systemic medications. These topical agents are more useful in later stages of treatment and in maintaining reduced IOP prior to laser iridotomy.

The liberal use of miotics to constrict the pupil and pull the peripheral iris away from the angle wall was long the main approach to AAC. A typical recommended regimen was pilocarpine 4% every 5 minutes for four doses, every 15 minutes for four doses, then every hour for four doses or until the attack was broken. However, when IOP is extremely high, the pupil is unresponsive to miotics because of ischemia and paralysis of the iris sphincter. Pilocarpine not only may be ineffective but, in some eyes, may paradoxically worsen the situation, triggering aqueous misdirection.[6] Although the miotic effect of pilocarpine is blocked, ciliary muscle contraction causes thickening of the lens and forward lens movement, which results in further shallowing of the anterior chamber. For this reason, some clinicians use lower concentrations of pilocarpine (1% or 2%) with less frequent dosing. In eyes with level 3 block (phacomorphic glaucoma) or level 4 block (aqueous misdirection), pilocarpine treatment should be considered contraindicated. Unequal anterior chamber depths, progressive increase in myopia, and progressive shallowing of the anterior chamber are clues to the correct diagnosis.

High doses of pilocarpine may produce cholinergic toxicity, which may not be noticed because of the nausea and vomiting associated with the AAC glaucoma attack. Strong miotics, such as echothiophate (Phospholine Iodide), can increase both the pupillary block and the vascular congestion. Immediate treatment with intravenous acetazolamide and repeated instillation of pilocarpine 2% was not more successful in breaking attacks of AAC glaucoma than was treatment with acetazolamide and a single drop of pilocarpine given 3 hours later.[7] Similar results were obtained with topically administered timolol (Blocadren) in place of acetazolamide.[8]

Our preferred approach to the treatment of AAC is designed to prioritize reopening of the anterior chamber angle and to minimize the possibility of adverse responses to pilocarpine.[9] Examination of the affected eye and fellow eye, with attention to central and peripheral anterior chamber depth as well as the shape of the peripheral iris, is performed in an attempt to determine the underlying mechanisms of the angle closure (pupillary block, plateau iris, phacomorphic glaucoma, or aqueous misdirection). A detailed analysis of these mechanisms has been published elsewhere.[1]

In the absence of oral isosorbide, we use glycerol as our preferred hyperosmotic agent, along with one or more topical aqueous suppressants. Intravenous acetazolamide can be given according to the physician's preference. The patient is then placed supine to permit the lens to fall posteriorly with vitreous dehydration. The eye is reassessed after 1 hour. IOP is usually decreased, but the angle may remains appositionally closed. One drop of pilocarpine 4% is given and the patient is reexamined 30 minutes later. If IOP is reduced and the angle is open, the patient may be treated medically with topical low-dose pilocarpine, aqueous suppressants, and corticosteroids, until the eye quiets and laser iridotomy may be performed. However, if IOP is unchanged or elevated and the angle remains closed, lens-related angle closure should be suspected, further pilocarpine is withheld, and the attack is broken by argon laser peripheral iridoplasty (ALPI).[10,11]

AAC is associated with a marked inflammatory reaction. The instillation of prednisolone 1% or dexamethasone 0.1% is desirable from the start to reduce inflammation. Severe pain may be treated with analgesics, and vomiting with antiemetics.

Laser iridotomy is the procedure of choice for all cases of AAC with a component of pupillary block. Success requires gonioscopic confirmation of angle opening, because transient lowering of IOP may occur with medical therapy. Ideally, iridotomy should be performed after the acute attack has been terminated and the eye is no longer inflamed. Attacks of AAC that are unresponsive to medical treatment are almost always successfully broken with ALPI. Alternatively, ALPI with or without systemic medications may be used as immediate initial treatment, especially in eyes at risk for developing chronic angle-closure glaucoma, or eyes in which a dominant mechanism exists that is not pupillary block. It is highly effective in breaking the initial attack.[12–15] In the absence of oral isosorbide and our current disinclination to use intravenous acetazolamide, we have moved to performing ALPI as an initial procedure.

ALPI does not eliminate pupillary block and is not a substitute for laser iridotomy, which must be performed as soon as the eye is quiet. However, even in eyes with extensive PAS, IOP is lowered sufficiently for a few days for the inflammation to resolve. ALPI is much safer than attempting surgical iridectomy on an inflamed eye with elevated IOP. The risks of intraoperative surgery are avoided and, even if aqueous misdirection is present, the angle remains open long enough for inflammation to clear. The alternative of waiting and prolonging medical therapy for several days seriously increases the possibility of irreversible damage to the iris, lens, drainage pathways, and optic nerve head.

12.1.2 *Chronic Angle Closure.* Chronic angle-closure (CAC) refers to an eye in which portions of the anterior chamber angle are permanently closed by PAS. In the era of surgical iridectomy, an attack of AAC could arise in an eye that had developed PAS because of gradual angle closure prior to the development of the attack. Conversely, a prolonged acute attack or a series of subacute attacks could lead to progressive PAS formation. The presence of PAS defined "chronic." At present, we prefer the term "combined-mechanism glaucoma" for those eyes that have had angle closure eliminated by laser treatment and have residual elevated IOP, reserving the term "chronic angle-closure glaucoma" for those eyes that develop gradual sealing of the angle with PAS and gradual elevation of IOP in the absence of an acute attack.

It is important to recognize early stages of appositional angle closure in the absence of PAS and to recognize circumferential (creeping) angle closure. Laser iridotomy is indicated for all stages of CAC, opening areas of the angle not involved by PAS and preventing further synechial closure.

Prolonged miotic treatment in eyes with open-angle glaucoma and narrow angles may lead to pupillary block and angle-closure glaucoma. Zonular relaxation leads to anterior lens movement and increased lens thickness in combination with increased pupillary block produced by pilocarpine. When miotic-induced angle closure occurs, the approach to treatment should be determined by assessing the medications necessary to control the glaucoma. If the patient has been treated with miotics alone, substitution of aqueous suppressants may suffice. If the patient requires miotics for IOP control, then laser iridotomy is warranted.

If the angle remains appositionally closed or spontaneously occludable after laser iridotomy, mechanisms other than pupillary block are likely responsible and ALPI is indicated to prevent progressive damage to, or further appositional and/or synechial closure of, the angle. The need for continued medical treatment after iridotomy with or without ALPI is determined by the level of IOP and the extent of glaucomatous damage. Treatment is similar to that of open-angle glaucoma. In two trials, latanoprost lowered IOP more effectively than did timolol in patients with CAC glaucoma.[16–18] Latanoprost was also effective in eyes with circumferential PAS to the level of the trabecular meshwork.[19] Periodic gonioscopy is obviously warranted. Argon laser trabeculoplasty has been reported to be both successful[20] and unsuccessful[21] after iridotomy in combined-mechanism glaucoma. It remains to be evaluated whether selective laser trabeculoplasty is effective in this situation. If IOP remains uncontrolled and glaucomatous damage develops, filtration surgery is indicated. Patients who already present with glaucomatous optic neuropathy are unlikely to be adequately treated with iridotomy only and have a moderate chance to require filtration surgery. There is an increased chance of developing aqueous misdirection following filtration surgery in patients who have had angle-closure glaucoma.[22]

12.2 DISCRETE OPEN-ANGLE GLAUCOMAS

The term "primary open-angle glaucoma" refers to a condition characterized by elevated IOP and characteristic optic disk and/or visual field damage with no other identifiable cause at slit-lamp examination. However, the use of the word "primary" is suggestive of a single, discrete entity with a specific mechanism of disease causation. More likely, this category represents an assortment of disorders, as we are now seeing with the discovery of multiple genetic loci. Similarly, the term "normal-tension glaucoma" (or "low-tension glaucoma") has been used to define a group of patients with glaucomatous damage but IOP less than some arbitrarily defined number. This is an artificial distinction based on population statistics. Interpretation of this term as previously used in the literature is further complicated by the recent realization that Goldmann tonometry is influenced by corneal thickness, a factor not routinely measured previously. The term "idiopathic open-angle glaucoma," which reflects the present state of ignorance about the cause of the disease, would be more appropriate. As specific causes are discovered and named, the pool of idiopathic glaucoma patients will gradually decrease in size.

The concept of primary and secondary glaucomas is more a reflection of incomplete understanding regarding the pathophysiologic events that ultimately lead to glaucomatous optic atrophy and visual field loss than of any true division of the glaucomas into primary and secondary forms.[23] The term "discrete glaucomas" is used here to refer to well-defined entities for which there is a better understanding of causation and associated ocular findings. In the past, treatment of these glaucomas has been virtually identical to that of idiopathic (primary) open-angle glaucoma. This singularity of treatment was unfortunate, because it reduced the emphasis on accurate diagnosis and delayed the development of disease-specific treatment modalities. The sections that follow emphasize the differences in treatment of discrete glaucomas from that of idiopathic open-angle glaucoma. Some of these differences are inferential, based on logic and empirical findings, and have yet to be proven in clinical trials.

12.2.1 *Pigmentary Glaucoma.* Pigment dispersion syndrome (PDS) and pigmentary glaucoma (PG) are characterized by disruption of the iris pigment epithelium (IPE) and deposition of the dispersed pigment granules throughout the anterior segment. The classic diagnostic triad consists of

1. Corneal pigmentation (Krukenberg spindle)
2. Slitlike, radial, midperipheral iris transillumination defects
3. Dense trabecular pigmentation

The iris insertion is typically posterior, and the peripheral iris tends to have a concave configuration. The extent of iridolenticular contact is greater than normal, inhibiting aqueous equilibration between the posterior and the anterior chamber by preventing retrograde aqueous flow. Inhibition of blinking allows buildup of the aqueous in the posterior chamber. The act of blinking provides a mechanical pump to push aqueous from the posterior chamber to the anterior chamber.[24] Once in the anterior chamber, the increased aqueous volume or pressure pushes the iris backward, accentuating the concavity—a phenomenon termed *reverse pupillary block*.[25] Accommodation also increases the iris concavity (figure 12.3A).[26–28] Iris pigment is released by mechanical damage to the IPE due to friction between the posteriorly bowed iris and the anterior zonular bundles.

Treatment may be directed at lowering IOP or stopping the basic disease process. We do not generally treat normotensive patients. If IOP is elevated and pigment is noted in the anterior chamber either spontaneously or after dilation, then treatment is initiated. A case may be made for treating younger patients with high-normal IOP, but no prospective clinical trial of medical therapy or laser iridotomy has yet been performed.

Miotic therapy reverses the iris concavity and produces a convex configuration, completely eliminating iridozonular contact (figure 12.3B). By so doing, miotics may prevent further pigment liberation and the development or progression of trabecular damage and glaucoma by immobilizing the pupil and may allow existing damage to reverse more readily. Most patients requiring therapy for PG are between the ages of 20 and 45 years and tolerate miotic drops or gel poorly because of intolerable accommodative spasm, induced myopia, and blurred vision. Pilocarpine Ocuserts, which provided low-dose pilocarpine release at a constant rate and were well tolerated, are no longer manufactured.

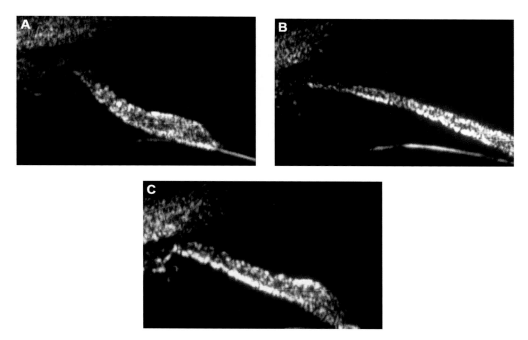

Figure 12.3. (A) Iris concavity in pigment dispersion syndrome. (B) Pilocarpine produces convex configuration. (C) Laser iridotomy produces planar configuration.

There is approximately a 7% incidence of retinal detachment in patients with PDS, irrespective of the presence or absence of glaucoma and of miotic treatment.[29] Approximately 80% of patients with PDS are myopic. The incidence of lattice degeneration and full-thickness retinal breaks appears to be more common in eyes with PDS or PG than in the unaffected population, when the degree of myopia is compared.[30] Before a miotic is prescribed for these patients, a thorough peripheral retinal examination should be performed and any retinal breaks or vitreous traction should be treated prophylactically.

In the absence of pilocarpine Ocuserts, we advocate treating patients with PDS and elevated IOP with prostaglandin analogs, to which this disease responds extremely well. Aqueous suppressants may lead to greater iridozonular contact by decreasing the volume of the posterior chamber, while decreased aqueous flow through the trabecular meshwork may allow greater blockage and dysfunction of the meshwork over the long term.[31] In one short-term study, latanoprost was shown to lower IOP more effectively than timolol in patients with PG.[32] It has also been noted that PDS seems to respond to epinephrine or dipivefrin with a greater mean drop in IOP than does any other glaucoma.[29,33,34]

Elimination of iridozonular contact and improvement of aqueous outflow rather than inhibition of its production are more desirable in preventing glaucomatous damage by reversing the pathophysiology of the disease. Laser iridotomy relieves reverse pupillary block by allowing aqueous to flow from the anterior to the posterior chamber and produces a planar iris configuration (figure 12.3C). Whereas pilocarpine completely inhibits exercise-induced pigment release and IOP elevation, iridotomy does so incompletely.[35,36]

If patients with PDS could be identified before they develop irreversible outflow obstruction, IOP elevation might be prevented with a prophylactic iridotomy. Before this treatment strategy can be recommended, however, diagnostic measures are needed to predict which patients with PDS have a sufficient risk of developing IOP elevation to justify the prophylactic iridotomy, and large, long-term trials are needed to prove that the iridotomy will prevent the eventual elevation of IOP. In a retrospective multicenter case series of 60 patients observed for a mean of 70.3 ± 26.0 months after iridotomy in one eye, no long-term benefit was observed.[37] Because the purpose of iridotomy is to prevent further pigment liberation from the iris, patients should still be in the pigment liberation stage (younger than ~ 45 years of age). If pigment is liberated into the anterior chamber with pupillary dilation, it is suggestive that the patient is still in this stage. Patients with uncontrolled glaucoma who are facing surgery are also poor candidates, because years may be necessary to achieve functional reconstitution of the meshwork. At present, we restrict iridotomy to patients who have elevated IOP with no damage or with early glaucomatous damage.

12.2.2 Exfoliation Syndrome.

Glaucoma associated with exfoliation syndrome tends to respond less well to medical therapy than does idiopathic open-angle glaucoma, is more difficult to treat, is more likely to require surgical intervention, and has a worse prognosis. Patients with exfoliative glaucoma have higher IOP and more severe damage at the time of detection, and their glaucomatous damage progresses more rapidly, compared with patients with primary open-angle glaucoma.[38] Patients with ocular hypertension who have exfoliation syndrome are twice as likely to develop glaucoma compared with patients without exfoliation.[39]

Treatment of exfoliative glaucoma is usually initiated with a prostaglandin analog or aqueous suppressants, similar to treatment of primary open-angle glaucoma. Latanoprost was more effective than 0.5% timolol[40] and as effective as timolol–dorzolamide fixed combination[41] in reducing IOP in patients with exfoliative glaucoma. On the other hand, as in PG, miotics may be a good choice of initial agent because they not only lower IOP and increase aqueous outflow but also, by inhibiting pupillary movement, decrease the amount of exfoliation material and pigment dispersed by iridolenticular contact. Miotics should enable the trabecular meshwork to clear and should slow the progression of the disease. However, many patients have nuclear sclerosis, and miotics may reduce visual acuity or dim vision sufficiently to create difficulty. Also, long-term use of miotics may lead to the development of posterior synechiae. We have found, however, that 2% pilocarpine taken at bedtime provides a nonreactive 3 mm pupil throughout the day without causing blurred vision for most patients.

Pupillary dilation in eyes with exfoliation syndrome may result in acute IOP rises accompanied by diffuse pigment dispersion in the anterior chamber.[42,43]

12.2.3 Corticosteroid-Induced Glaucoma.

Glaucoma is most commonly associated with topical application of corticosteroids, but may also result from systemic administration. Topical corticosteroid creams, lotions, or ointments placed on the eyelids, face, or even remote sites may also be associated with IOP elevation,[44,45] as may inhaled corticosteroids.[46] Elevated IOP may also be produced by an increase in endogenous corticosteroids, as seen in adrenal hyperplasia or Cushing's disease.[47] Because corticosteroids may be prescribed by general physicians and because some preparations are now available over the counter, physicians and patients alike should be educated regarding their potential risks.

Patients receiving corticosteroids may develop elevated IOP from days to years after initiating treatment.[48] With topical corticosteroids, IOP elevation typically occurs within 2 to 6 weeks. However, the period required and the magnitude of the IOP rise appear to depend on many factors, including the potency and dosage of the preparation, the frequency of application, the route of administration, the presence of other ocular or systemic diseases, and the individual responsiveness of the patient. In rare cases, an abrupt rise in IOP has been reported after corticosteroid administration in eyes with open angles.[49]

The clinical features depend on the age at presentation. In infants and very young children, corticosteroid-induced glaucoma may resemble typical findings of congenital glaucoma, with enlarged, edematous corneas.[50] In older children and adults, it is clinically similar to juvenile- or adult-onset idiopathic open-angle glaucoma. In patients with normal-tension glaucoma, the clinician should consider the possibility of damage from previously elevated IOP as a result of past corticosteroid use.

When corticosteroid-induced glaucoma is suspected, the agent of concern should be discontinued or used in a lower concentration. Alternatively, a weaker corticosteroid or a nonsteroidal anti-inflammatory agent (e.g., diclofenac) should be substituted. If IOP remains elevated despite discontinuation, the therapeutic approach is identical to that used for idiopathic open-angle glaucoma. If elevated IOP results from a periocular depot corticosteroid injection, excision of the depot may be necessary. IOP elevation associated with intravitreal steroid injection can be controlled with medical therapy in the large majority of cases.[51] Infrequently, surgical intervention is required, in the form of vitrectomy-assisted removal of the steroid, filtration surgery, or both. Steroid-releasing implants, however, often cause marked and intractable elevation of IOP, often requiring surgical treatment. Although laser trabeculoplasty may be less effective than in eyes with other forms of glaucoma, laser treatment may be attempted prior to surgical intervention in patients more than 40 years of age.

12.2.4 *Neovascular Glaucoma*. Medical treatment of neovascular glaucoma can be frustrating and is often ineffective. Panretinal photocoagulation (PRP) for proliferative retinopathy should be performed. When adequate PRP is performed early, there is extensive evidence for the regression of anterior segment neovascularization in eyes with central retinal vein occlusion and proliferative diabetic retinopathy. Adjunctive medical therapy with angiogenesis-inhibiting drugs may be useful and is under evaluation at this time. Control of blood sugar is also important because near-normal glycemia is associated with later development and lesser severity of diabetic retinopathy.[52]

When the angle is open, medical treatment for neovascular glaucoma includes aqueous suppressants, topical corticosteroids, and a cycloplegic. Pilocarpine has been considered relatively contraindicated because of its effect on the blood–aqueous barrier, but may be tried. Similarly, prostaglandin analogs may be tried cautiously in view of their reported association with disruption of blood–aqueous barrier and increased intraocular inflammation.

With extensive synechial angle closure, miotics are ineffective and should be considered contraindicated because of the inflammation and hyperemia they produce. Prostaglandin analogs and aqueous suppressants are beneficial but often do not lower IOP to a normal range. Hyperosmotic agents can be used intermittently. The most important medications remain topical cycloplegics and corticosteroids to decrease congestion and inflammation and prepare the eye for definitive surgery.

12.2.5 *Iridocorneal Endothelial Syndrome.* Patients with iridocorneal endothelial syndrome may require treatment for corneal edema, glaucoma, or both. The glaucoma can often be controlled medically in the early stages, especially with aqueous suppressants. Lowering IOP may also control the corneal edema, although the additional use of hypertonic saline solutions and soft contact lenses is often required. When medical control becomes ineffective as the disease progresses, surgical intervention is required. Argon laser trabeculoplasty is contraindicated.

12.3 TRAUMA AND GLAUCOMA

12.3.1 *Hyphema.* Elevated IOP associated with hyphema usually responds favorably to aqueous suppressants. CAIs may also be added to the treatment regimen. However, caution is warranted with systemic acetazolamide in patients with sickle cell hemoglobinopathy (or sickle trait), because the drug increases the concentration of ascorbic acid in the aqueous, which leads to more sickling in the anterior chamber.[53] Systemic acetazolamide also causes systemic acidosis, which may exacerbate erythrocyte sickling. Methazolamide may be safer because it causes less systemic acidosis than does acetazolamide.

Surgical intervention is warranted when IOP cannot be controlled medically and threatens to cause glaucomatous damage or if corneal blood staining develops. Unfortunately, the optic disk usually cannot be visually assessed, and many patients will manifest afferent pupillary defects caused by the presence of the blood itself, rather than by the optic nerve injury. Consequently, intervention may need to be undertaken based on somewhat arbitrary criteria. Although a healthy optic nerve may be able to tolerate IOP of 40 to 50 mm Hg for 1 week or longer, a glaucomatous disk may suffer further damage with substantially lower IOP within a shorter time period. Evaluation of the fellow eye for evidence of preexisting glaucomatous optic neuropathy may thus be helpful with regard to guiding therapy.

12.3.2 *Angle-Recession Glaucoma.* Angle-recession glaucoma usually develops years or even decades after blunt trauma with hyphema. In one series, the mean duration between injury and diagnosis of elevated IOP was 16 years.[54] In another, the time between injury and the diagnosis of glaucoma averaged 7.6 ± 9.5 years.[55] Late glaucoma is more common if the recession involves 180° or more of the angle. Patients with angle recession who develop glaucoma probably have a predisposition to it. The fellow eyes of patients with unilateral angle-recession glaucoma are more likely to have abnormalities of aqueous dynamics or open-angle glaucoma.

Medical therapy for angle-recession glaucoma is identical to that for idiopathic open-angle glaucoma. Pilocarpine may have little effect or a paradoxical effect on IOP. The response to medical treatment is worse, as is the response to argon laser trabeculoplasty.

12.3.3 Inflammation. Ocular inflammation is a common complication of blunt injury. In one series of 496 consecutive uveitis patients, the inflammation in 24 (4.8%) of the patients was attributed to nonpenetrating trauma.[56] Trauma-induced inflammation may compromise outflow and elevate IOP by several mechanisms, including the following:

1. Obstruction of outflow pathways with inflammatory cells, debris, protein, or other serum components that are liberated because of vascular incompetence
2. Inflammation-induced swelling of the trabecular meshwork that impairs outflow
3. Inflammatory damage to trabecular endothelial cells
4. Sclerosis of the trabecular meshwork as a result of chronic inflammation
5. Obstruction of the trabecular meshwork by a hyaline membrane

Treatment with topical corticosteroids and glaucoma medications frequently affords resolution of the intraocular inflammation and IOP reduction.

Inflammation is a common complication of penetrating injury and may be associated with posterior synechiae formation, pupillary block, iris bombe, and angle-closure glaucoma. Glaucoma may result from trabecular obstruction, with inflammatory cells and debris. If there is chronic inflammation in the fellow eye, sympathetic ophthalmia should be suspected.

12.3.4 Foreign Bodies. Whenever possible, foreign bodies should be removed to prevent the complications described above. Once glaucoma is present, a foreign body may be so encapsulated that standard extraction techniques may be problematic. Furthermore, the visual prognosis may already be limited by extensive retinal damage. Corticosteroids to avoid cyclitic membranes and scarring of the meshwork are also of primary importance during the early postinjury period. Antibiotics are required for endophthalmitis prophylaxis. Elevated IOP may be treated with aqueous suppressants. When medical therapy is insufficient, filtering surgery may be appropriate.

12.3.5 Chemical Burns. Management of elevated IOP in the early phase of a chemical burn is limited to aqueous suppressants. However, because re-epithelialization of the ocular surface may be impaired by topical medications, systemic medications may be preferred. Miotics are relatively contraindicated, because they may aggravate anterior segment inflammation, as well as contribute to the formation of posterior synechiae that may eventuate in pupillary block. Corticosteroids may be helpful with respect to minimizing anterior segment inflammation, but concern regarding the increased risk of corneal stromal melting may favor systemic administration.

12.4 OTHER SPECIAL SITUATIONS

12.4.1 *Infants and Children.* Initial surgical treatment should not be delayed in an attempt to achieve medical control of IOP in infants with congenital glaucoma. Medications are primarily used preoperatively to allow corneal edema to clear, improving visualization at the time of examination under anesthesia and surgery, and to help control any damage that might occur in the interim preoperatively (see also Chapter 13). If trabeculotomies and/or goniotomies fail and trabeculectomy is believed to be required, some surgeons would attempt medical control at this point.

Long-term medical therapy in infants and children can be difficult because of side effects and compliance problems. Serious adverse effects have been reported from ophthalmic drugs in infants, and parents should be instructed about side effects and taught to perform careful nasolacrimal occlusion. The introduction of new classes of topical agents in the past few years offers greater possibilities for achieving control of IOP.

Prior to the introduction of topical CAIs, acetazolamide suspension, 5 to 10 mg/kg body weight divided to three times daily, was considered the safest medication for infants. Topical CAIs should be considered as a first-line agent. Systemic CAIs have been noted to cause rapid and severe acidosis in infants.

Although studies of beta-adrenergic blocking agents in children have shown a minimum of side effects in short-term use, apnea has been reported in neonates. Parents should be cautioned to discontinue the medication if any side effects, such as asthmatic symptoms, develop. The selective beta-1 blockers, such as betaxolol, should have even fewer pulmonary side effects.

Latanoprost is well tolerated in children, with infrequent and mild local side effects. However, the iris color change associated with it could have serious psychological effects, and unilateral therapy should be approached cautiously. Also, while clinical trials have shown a benefit in some children, the responder rates have been lower than those observed in adults.

Brimonidine has been reported to cause serious side effects in infants, including systemic hypotension, severe fatigue, transient unarousability, unresponsiveness, and episodes of fainting.[57] Therefore, it should be used with extreme caution and restricted to older children.

Miotics can induce visually disabling myopia in the young patient and are not recommended for infants.

Older children are better able to tolerate topical medications. Again, parents should be carefully apprised of potential side effects of any glaucoma agents being used. If psychological or behavioral difficulties arise, a trial of discontinuing successive potentially causative medications should be undertaken.

12.4.2 Prepresbyopic Adults. Adults younger than about 45 years of age have two particular problems with glaucoma medications. As mentioned above, miotic drops or gels cause visually disabling side effects. When used, these should be initiated at the lowest commercially available concentration, with gradual increase as necessary according to therapeutic effect.

The second problem with glaucoma medications in younger patients is a greater frequency of, or sensitivity to, psychological and sexual side effects. These can include depression, anxiety, confusion, sleep disturbances, drowsiness, weakness, fatigue, memory loss, disorientation, emotional lability, loss of libido, and impotence. Central nervous system side effects of CAIs have been primarily associated with their systemic use and can be described as a complex consisting of general malaise, fatigue, weight loss, depression, anorexia, and loss of libido. Once again, careful instruction on nasolacrimal occlusion can result in reduced dosages of medications and decreased systemic absorption. This is especially important when topical medications are prescribed for pregnant or lactating women.

12.4.3 Patients With Cataracts. A major problem faced by patients with cataracts is dimming of vision and/or decreased visual acuity with miotic treatment. This visual effect can interfere with driving and other daily activities. Patients should be questioned about these effects. Some patients volunteer this information readily and express a desire to eliminate miotic treatment, whereas others exhibit an attitude of forbearance. Not all patients with cataracts have these side effects. Many patients with nuclear sclerosis find their vision improved, instead of worsened, with miotics or are able to read without glasses because of the pinhole effect, and are hesitant to discontinue the miotics once started.

A second problem associated with miotic therapy, noted above, is the increased tendency to posterior synechiae formation in patients with exfoliation syndrome, which increases in prevalence with age.

12.4.4 Panallergic Patients. The word "panallergic" can be used to describe patients who simply cannot tolerate virtually any medication for one reason or another. Allergic reactions to every topical glaucoma agent have been reported. Contact dermatitis is not uncommon with alpha-2 agonists, miotics, CAIs, and beta blockers. Also included in this category are patients who have multiple side effects to medications or who just cannot tolerate the baseline level of burning and stinging associated with their instillation.

Allergic responses, if mild, can sometimes be successfully treated with mast-cell stabilizers, such as olopatadine, cromolyn, lodoxamide, or low-dose corticosteroids, such as medrysone. Preservative-free preparations are available for pilocarpine, epinephrine, timolol, and apraclonidine. Some patients with adverse reactions due to benzalkonium chloride in certain drops may be treated with other drugs using alternative preservatives. In some cases of drug intolerance, dosages below those normally prescribed can sometimes be effective; for example, latanoprost was shown similarly efficacious when given once daily or once weekly.[58] However, in many cases, the drugs tolerated are insufficient for control of the glaucoma, and laser or surgical intervention becomes necessary.

ACKNOWLEDGMENT

This work was supported by the Joseph Cohen Research Fund of the New York Glaucoma Research Institute, New York.

REFERENCES

1. Ritch R, Liebmann JM, Tello C. A construct for understanding angle-closure glaucoma: the role of ultrasound biomicroscopy. *Ophthalmol Clin North Am.* 1995;8:281–293.
2. Feitl ME, Krupin T. Hyperosmotic agents. In: Ritch R, Shields MB, Krupin T, eds. *The Glaucomas.* St Louis, MO: CV Mosby; 1996.
3. Drance SM. Effect of oral glycerol on intraocular pressure in normal and glaucomatous eyes. *Arch Ophthalmol.* 1964;72:491.
4. Oakley DE, Ellis PP. Glycerol and hyperosmolar nonketotic coma. *Am J Ophthalmol.* 1976;81:469.
5. Almog Y, Geyer O, Laser M. Pulmonary edema as a complication of oral glycerol administration. *Ann Ophthalmol.* 1986;18:38.
6. Ritch R. The pilocarpine paradox. *J Glaucoma.* 1996;5:225–227.
7. Ganias F, Mapstone R. Miotics in closed-angle glaucoma. *Br J Ophthalmol.* 1975; 59:205.
8. Airaksinen PJ, Saari KM, Tiainen TJ, et al. Management of acute closed-angle glaucoma with miotics and timolol. *Br J Ophthalmol.* 1979;63:822.
9. Kramer P, Ritch R. The treatment of angle-closure glaucoma revisited [editorial]. *Ann Ophthalmol.* 1984;16:1101–1103.
10. Ritch R. Argon laser treatment for medically unresponsive attacks of angle-closure glaucoma. *Am J Ophthalmol.* 1982;94:197.
11. Ritch R, Liebmann JM. Argon laser peripheral iridoplasty: a review. *Ophthalmic Surg Lasers.* 1996;27:289–300.
12. Tham CCY, Lai JSM, Poon ASY, et al. Immediate argon laser peripheral iridoplasty (ALPI) as initial treatment for acute phacomorphic angle-closure (phacomorphic glaucoma) before cataract extraction: a preliminary study. *Eye.* 2005;19:778–783.
13. Lai JSM, Tham CCY, Chua JKH, et al. Laser peripheral iridoplasty as initial treatment of acute attack of primary angle-closure: a long-term follow-up study. *J Glaucoma.* 2002;11:484–487.
14. Lam DSC, Lai JSM, Tham CCY. Immediate argon laser peripheral iridoplasty as treatment for acute attack of primary angle-closure glaucoma. A preliminary study. *Ophthalmology.* 1998;105:2231–2236.
15. Yip PPW, Leung WY, Hon CY, Ho CK. Argon laser peripheral iridoplasty in the management of phacomorphic glaucoma. *Ophthalmic Surg Lasers Imaging.* 2005;36: 286–291.
16. Chew PT, Aung T, Aquino MV, Rojanapongpun P; EXACT Study Group. Intraocular pressure-reducing effects and safety of latanoprost versus timolol in patients with chronic angle-closure glaucoma. *Ophthalmology.* 2004;111:427–434.

17. Aung T, Chan YH, Chew PT; EXACT Study Group. Degree of angle closure and intraocular pressure-lowering effect of latanoprost in subjects with chronic angle-closure glaucoma. *Ophthalmology*. 2005;112:267–271.

18. Sihota R, Saxena R, Agarwal HC, Gulati V. Cross-over comparison of timolol and latanoprost in chronic primary angle-closure glaucoma. *Arch Ophthalmol*. 2004;122: 185–189.

19. Kook MS, Cho HS, Yang SJ, et al. Efficacy of latanoprost in patients with chronic angle-closure glaucoma and no visible ciliary-body face: a preliminary study. *J Ocul Pharmacol Ther*. 2005;21:75–84.

20. Shirakashi M, Iwata K, Nakayama T. Argon laser trabeculoplasty for chronic angle-closure glaucoma uncontrolled by iridotomy. *Acta Ophthalmol*. 1989;67:265–270.

21. Wishart PK, Nagasubramanian S, Hitchings RA. Argon laser trabeculoplasty in narrow angle glaucoma. *Eye*. 1987;1:567.

22. Eltz H, Gloor B. Trabeculectomy in cases of angle-closure glaucoma—successes and failures. *Klin Monatsbl Augenheilkd*. 1980;177:556–561.

23. Shields MD, Ritch R, Krupin TK. Classifications and mechanisms of the glaucomas. In: Ritch R, Shields MB, Krupin T, eds. *The Glaucomas*. St Louis, MO: CV Mosby; 1996.

24. Liebmann JM, Tello C, Chew S-J, Cohen H, Ritch R. Prevention of blinking alters iris configuration in pigment dispersion syndrome and in normal eyes. *Ophthalmology*. 1995;102:446–455.

25. Karickhoff JR. Reverse pupillary block in pigmentary glaucoma: follow up and new developments. *Ophthalmic Surg*. 1993;24:562–563.

26. Adam RS, Pavlin CJ, Ulanski LJ. Ultrasound biomicroscopic analysis of iris profile changes with accommodation in pigmentary glaucoma and relationship to age. *Am J Ophthalmol*. 2004;138:652–654.

27. Heys JJ, Barocas VH. Computational evaluation of the role of accommodation in pigmentary glaucoma. *Invest Ophthalmol Vis Sci*. 2002;43:700–708.

28. Ritch R, Liebmann J, Tello C, Chew SJ. Ultrasound biomicroscopic findings in pigment dispersion syndrome. In: Krieglstein GK, ed. *Glaucoma Update V*. Heidelberg: Kaden Verlag; 1995.

29. Scheie HG, Cameron JD. Pigment dispersion syndrome: a clinical study. *Br J Ophthalmol*. 1981;65:264–269.

30. Weseley P, Liebmann J, Walsh JB, Ritch R. Lattice degeneration of the retina and the pigment dispersion syndrome. *Am J Ophthalmol*. 1992;114:539–543.

31. Becker B. Does hyposecretion of aqueous humor damage the trabecular meshwork? [editorial]. *J Glaucoma*. 1995;4:303–305.

32. Mastropasqua L, Carpineto P, Ciancaglini M, Gallenga PE. A 12-month, randomized, double-masked study comparing latanoprost with timolol in pigmentary glaucoma. *Ophthalmology*. 1999;106:550–555.

33. Becker B, Shin DH, Cooper DG, Kass MA. The pigment dispersion syndrome. *Am J Ophthalmol*. 1977;83:161–166.

34. Ritch R. A unification hypothesis of pigment dispersion syndrome. *Trans Am Ophthalmol Soc*. 1996;94:381–409.

35. Haynes WL, Alward WLM, Tello C, Liebmann JM, Ritch R. Incomplete elimination of exercise-induced pigment dispersion by laser iridotomy in pigment dispersion syndrome. *Ophthalmic Surg Lasers*. 1995;26:484–486.

36. Haynes WL, Johnson AT, Alward WLM. Incomplete elimination of exercise-induced pigment dispersion in a patient with the pigment dispersion syndrome. *Am J Ophthalmol*. 1990;109:599–601.

37. Reistad E, Shields MB, Campbell DG, et al. The influence of peripheral iridotomy on the intraocular pressure course in patients with pigmentary glaucoma. *J Glaucoma.* 2005;14:255–259.

38. Ritch R, Schlötzer-Schrehardt U. Exfoliation syndrome. *Surv Ophthalmol.* 2001;45: 265–315.

39. Grødum K, Heijl A, Bengtsson B. Risk of glaucoma in ocular hypertension with and without pseudoexfoliation. *Ophthalmology.* 2005;112:386–390.

40. Konstas AG, Mylopoulos N, Karabatsas CH. Diurnal intraocular pressure reduction with latanoprost 0.005% compared to timolol maleate 0.5% as monotherapy in subjects with exfoliation glaucoma. *Eye.* 2004;18:893–899.

41. Konstas AGP, Kozobolis VP, Tersis I, Leech J, Stewart WC. The efficacy and safety of the timolol/dorzolamide fixed combination vs latanoprost in exfoliation glaucoma. *Eye.* 2003;17:41–46.

42. Mapstone R. Pigment release. *Br J Ophthalmol.* 1981;65:258–263.

43. Shaw BR, Lewis RA. Intraocular pressure elevation after pupillary dilation in open angle glaucoma. *Arch Ophthalmol.* 1986;104:1185–1188.

44. Zugerman C, Saunders D, Levit F. Glaucoma from topically applied steroids. *Arch Dermatol.* 1976;112:1326.

45. Cubey RB. Glaucoma following the application of corticosteroid to the skin of the eyelid. *Br J Dermatol.* 1976;95;207.

46. Garbe E, LeLorier J, Bolvin J-F, Suissa S. Inhaled and nasal glucocorticoids and the risks of ocular hypertension or open-angle glaucoma. *JAMA.* 1997;277:722–727.

47. Haas JS, Nootens RH. Glaucoma secondary to benign adrenal adenoma. *Am J Ophthalmol.* 1974;78:497.

48. Kass MA, Johnson T. Corticosteroid-induced glaucoma. In: Ritch R, Shields MB, Krupin T, eds. *The Glaucomas.* St Louis, MO: CV Mosby Co; 1989.

49. Weinreb RN, et al. Acute effects of dexamethesone on intraocular pressure in glaucoma. *Invest Ophthalmol Vis Sci.* 1985;26:170.

50. Kass MA, Kolker AE, Becker B. Chronic topical corticosteroid use simulating congenital glaucoma. *J Pediatr.* 1972;81:1175.

51. Jonas JB, Degenring RF, Kreissig I, et al. Intraocular pressure elevation after intravitreal triamcinolone acetonide injection. *Ophthalmology.* 2005;112:593–598.

52. Diabetes Control, Complications Trial Research Group. The effect of intensive treatment of diabetes on the development and progression of long-term complications in insulin-dependent diabetes mellitus. *N Engl J Med.* 1993;329:977–986.

53. Goldberg MF. The diagnosis and treatment of sickled erythrocytes in human hyphemas. *Trans Am Ophthalmol Soc.* 1978;76:481.

54. Herschler J. Trabecular damage due to blunt anterior segment injury and its relationship to traumatic glaucoma. *Trans Am Acad Ophthalmol Otol.* 1977;83:OP239.

55. Mermoud A, et al. Surgical management of post-traumatic angle recession glaucoma. *Ophthalmology.* 1993;100:634.

56. Rosenbaum JT, Tammaro J, Robertson JE Jr. Uveitis precipitated by nonpenetrating ocular trauma. *Am J Ophthalmol.* 1991;112:392.

57. Bowman RJC, Cope J, Nischal KK. Ocular and systemic side effects of brimonidine 0.2% eye drops (Alphagan) in children. *Eye.* 2004;18:24–26.

58. Kurtz S, Shemesh G. The efficacy and safety of once-daily versus once-weekly latanoprost treatment for increased intraocular pressure. *J Ocul Pharmacol Ther.* 2004; 20:321–327.

13

Pregnancy and Pediatric Patients

ELLIOTT M. KANNER AND PETER A. NETLAND

Glaucoma in younger individuals is less common and is managed differently compared with adults. In young adults, pregnancy and lactation can be considerations in medical management decisions. Pediatric glaucoma is treated primarily surgically, and medications are usually in a supportive role, often to bridge the gap to surgery and clear the cornea prior to surgery. Although long-term response to medical therapy can be achieved in children, glaucoma medications are often used as adjunctive therapy after surgical treatments. The effectiveness and side effect profiles for some medications are significantly different in very young patients, which can influence management decisions. In this chapter, we review glaucoma medical therapy considerations in pregnancy, lactation, and pediatric patients.

13.1 GLAUCOMA MEDICAL THERAPY IN PREGNANCY

13.1.1 *General Considerations.* Although glaucoma is infrequently diagnosed in pregnant patients, occasionally patients with preexisting glaucoma become pregnant. Whenever medications are prescribed for glaucoma, the clinician considers the potential for systemic effects on the patient. In pregnant women, this concern extends to the developing child, as well. One major advantage to the use of topical medications for glaucoma is the reduced systemic absorption and coincident decrease in systemic symptoms. There is little literature demonstrating adverse events of topical medications during pregnancy.[1,2]

13.1.2 *Natural History of Intraocular Pressure During Pregnancy.* Metabolic and physiologic changes during pregnancy cause a mild decrease in the intraocular pressure (IOP) compared to the pressure before pregnancy. This has been proposed to occur by several mechanisms. The episcleral venous pressure decreases due to changes in the mother's hemodynamics. A metabolic acidosis occurs, which affects aqueous production and decreases IOP. Comparisons of prepregnancy and pregnancy IOP show an average decrease of 1.5 mm Hg during pregnancy.[3–5] In one study, the majority of eyes required treatment with glaucoma medications and maintained stable visual fields.[6] However, the course of glaucoma was variable, with 18% developing visual field loss and another 18% developing increased IOP without visual field loss.[6]

13.1.3 *Teratogenicity.* There are no direct studies that show teratogenicity of glaucoma medicines, and few human studies have addressed topical medications. Most data are extrapolated from similar studies of the class of medications. In one study of systemic anticholinergic medications, there were no reported gestational or congenital anomalies.[7] Adrenergic compounds interfere with contractions of the uterus (by interfering with the oxytocin pathway), and so may delay labor and cause uterine hypotony (which can prolong postpartum bleeding).[7] Prostaglandin analogs for ophthalmic use are in the same class of prostaglandins that may cause abortion when administered as a periuterine injection. The dosage used to stimulate abortion is the equivalent of 400 cc of latanoprost as formulated for ocular use;[8] however, caution is advised for use in pregnancy.

13.1.4 *FDA Safety Categories.* The Food and Drug Administration classifies drugs into several categories of safety levels for use in pregnancy. Class A drugs have an established safety record, with human testing data proving safety. Class B drugs have animal safety data but no human data to confirm. Class C drugs have either animal studies with adverse effects or no human or animal data. Class D drugs have clear risks, although use can be justified under certain conditions. Class X drugs are known to cause birth defects and should never be used during pregnancy. FDA category classifications for glaucoma medications are shown in table 13.1.

Despite the extensive classification of mediations, and high awareness among physicians regarding the importance of the cautious use of medications in women of reproductive age, a retrospective study of 152,531 deliveries from 1996 through 2000 showed that almost half of them received a drug from FDA safety category B, C, D, or X.[9]

13.2 GLAUCOMA MEDICAL THERAPY DURING LACTATION

There are few studies in the literature regarding the safety of glaucoma mediations during breast-feeding. Any medication with any degree of systemic absorption must be assumed to have a measurable level in breast milk. Due to the extreme reluctance to used any medications in pregnant and lactating women, these data are difficult to

Table 13.1 FDA Category Classifications for Glaucoma Medications

Drug Class	Pregnancy Category
Prostaglandin analogs	Class C
Beta blockers	Class C
Alpha-adrenergic agonists	
Brimonidine	Class B
Apraclonidine	Class C
Carbonate anhydrase inhibitors	Class C
Nonspecific adrenergic agonist[a]	Class B
Fixed-combination timolol-dorzolamide	Class C
Cholinergic drugs	Class C

[a]Dipivefrin.

obtain. In one study, timolol 0.5% and betaxolol were found in breast milk.[10] In fact, breast milk had higher timolol levels than did serum measured simultaneously (5.6 ng/mL vs. 0.93 ng/mL).[10] The authors concluded that this level of timolol was not of concern if the infant has normal renal and hepatic function; however, if treatment is absolutely necessary, the infant must be monitored carefully for any possible side effects. Punctal occlusion or other methods of reducing systemic uptake of any topically applied medicine are beneficial in this scenario.

13.3 GLAUCOMA MEDICAL THERAPY IN PEDIATRIC PATIENTS

13.3.1 *General Considerations.* Children are more vulnerable to side effects, due to reduced body mass and blood volume for drug distribution (resulting in higher concentrations from the same absorbed dose). Also, they may be unable to verbally describe side effects caused by medications. Thus, children on chronic medical therapy need to be carefully monitored. The medical regimen must be frequently reevaluated in an effort to use the minimum medical regimen that will result in acceptable IOP control. Glaucoma medications commonly used in children are shown in table 13.2.

13.3.2 *Specific Drug Classes*

13.3.2.1 *Prostaglandin analogs.* In pediatric patients, latanoprost has been evaluated in a variety of diagnoses including Sturge-Weber syndrome.[11–14] In one study of 31 eyes, 19% had a 34% reduction in IOP.[15] The majority of the eyes did not respond to the therapy (figure 13.1).[15] Juvenile-onset open-angle glaucoma was more likely to respond, most likely due to the anatomy of the angle more closely approximating that in the adult.[16] In this study, while the response rate was low, latanoprost was well tolerated. In glaucoma associated with Sturge-Weber, between 17% and 28% of eyes responded with a decrease in IOP.[11,12] The, majority of side effects were due to local hyperemia, with only 6% cessation of therapy from side

Table 13.2 Glaucoma Medications Commonly Used in Pediatric
Patients

Beta Blockers

Betaxolol 0.25% (qd, bid)
Levobunolol 0.25% (qd, bid)
Timolol solution 0.25% (qd, bid)
Timolol gel-forming solution 0.25% (qd)

Carbonic Anhydrase Inhibitors

Acetazolamide elixir, 5 to 15 mg/kg/day in divided doses
   (bid, tid)
Brinzolamide 1% (bid, tid)
Dorzolamide 2% (bid, tid)

Cholinergic drugs

Pilocarpine 1%, 2% (tid, qid)

Prostaglandin-Related Drugs

Bimatoprost 0.03% (qd)
Latanoprost 0.005% (qd)
Travoprost 0.004% (qd)

effects.[12] As an adjunctive therapy, latanoprost was well tolerated for a year with good IOP response.[13] Although the response rate is low in the pediatric population, in those that do respond it is very effective and offers good 24-hour control.[14] The once-daily dosing is convenient for parents, and the local systemic effects are manageable, although parents do need to be warned because they will likely note iris pigment changes, eyelash growth, and hyperemia. If used only to manage IOP prior to a definitive surgical procedure, then local side effects are seldom a problem. The frequency of these side effects in children on long-term therapy is not known.

13.3.2.2 *Beta blockers*. Prior to the commercial release of timolol, it was tested as an additional medication in uncontrolled pediatric glaucoma: 29% had a definitive improvement, 32% had a modest or equivocal improvement, while 39% demonstrated no improvement.[16] In another study of pediatric glaucoma, timolol adjunctive therapy controlled 37% of patients to below 22 mm Hg.[17] Only 7% had to discontinue timolol due to adverse events.[17] However, in another study of 89 eyes, only 20% of eyes showed any effect of timolol on IOP.[18] In another study of pediatric glaucoma, 45% of eyes had a significant drop in IOP after treatment with timolol alone (figure 13.2).[19]

As in adults, systemic levels of timolol can be found in pediatric patients after topical dosing, but at much higher levels.[20] Much of the plasma level increase can be explained by the much smaller volume of distribution in children compared to adults, especially compared the relatively small change in ocular volume. Thus, the

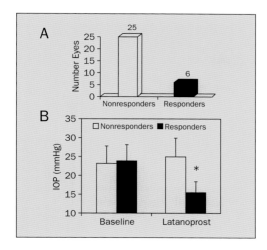

Figure 13.1. Latanoprost lowers IOP effectively in a minority of pediatric glaucomas. (A) Of 31 eyes in a series, most failed to respond (defined as < 15% decrease in IOP). (B) IOP was reduced significantly in those that did respond to latanoprost. The average IOP reduction in latanoprost responders was 8.5 ± 3.6 mm Hg (34.0% ± 10.9%; *P = 0.002). Error bars indicate standard deviation. Adapted with permission from Enyedi LB, Freeman SF, Buckley EG. The effectiveness of latanoprost for the treatment of pediatric glaucoma. *J AAPOS.* 1999;3:33–39.

small amount of systemically absorbed timolol is diluted far less and is more concentrated. Lower levels of metabolic enzymes may also prolong the half-life of medications in children by a factor of 2 to 6.[21]

Children older than 5 years of age had an average decrease of 6 beats per minute in their resting pulse rate, while there was no observed change in those younger than 5.[16] Various studies have shown rates of 4% to 13% in children,[16,17] requiring cessation of therapy in 3% to 7%.[17,18] Case reports of severe side effects have been reported in the literature, such as apnea.[22–24] While asthma provocation has been reported with timolol, there are no data comparable to those in adults on betaxolol (selective beta-1 antagonist) showing decreased pulmonary effects. The above studies are all short term, with no long-term study data currently available.

Due to the much higher level of systemic absorption in children, lower concentration 0.25% timolol rather than the 0.5% is preferred in younger children, and these children still should be thoroughly evaluated for systemic abnormalities such as cardiac disease and asthma. Systemic absorption can be reduced in the pediatric population by simple methods such as punctal occlusion, eyelid closure, or blotting the excess drops away during administration.[20]

13.3.2.3 *Carbonic anhydrase inhibitors.* In children, oral carbonic anhydrase inhibitor (CAI) administration can cause growth retardation and metabolic acidosis.[25,26] At doses of 5 to 15 mg/kg per day (divided twice or three times daily), oral acetazolamide is well tolerated, and reduces IOP and improves corneal edema presurgically.[27,28] A study of children 3 to 12 years of age comparing the effect of systemic administration of acetazolamide and topical dorzolamide showed that both were effective at lowering IOP (36% vs. 27%) in pediatric glaucoma (figure 13.3).[29]

Since the rate of side effects is lower, topical treatment is preferred, unless systemic administration is found to be more effective in the patient. In another study of children younger than age 6, the rate of discontinuation of topical dorzolamide was

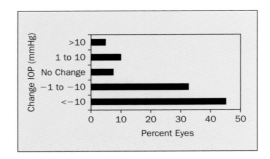

Figure 13.2. Timolol is effective in the majority of pediatric glaucomas: change from baseline IOP in 40 eyes receiving timolol therapy without additional surgery or medications. Thirty-one eyes (78%) demonstrated reduced IOP after timolol treatment. Adapted with permission from Hoskins HD Jr, Hetherington J Jr, Magee SD, Naykhin R, Migliazzo CV. Clinical experience with timolol in childhood glaucoma. *Arch Ophthalmol.* 1985;103:1163–1165.

only 1.8% in those younger than 2 and 3.0% in those between 2 and 6 years of age due to adverse reactions.[30]

13.3.2.4 *Fixed combinations.* Cosopt is a fixed-combination medication composed of dorzolamide 2% and timolol 0.5%. There is very little information in the literature about the use of the fixed combination in children. However, one study that compared dorzolamide to timolol in children used a combination if either alone was not sufficient. In this study, treatment was with 2% dorzolamide three times daily and 0.25% timolol gel-forming solution once daily in children younger than 2, and fixed combination (2%/0.5%) twice daily in older children.[30] One patient (1.8%) younger than 2 who was on 2% dorzolamide and 0.25% timolol discontinued due to bradycardia, while none of the patients on 0.25% timolol alone had such side effect.[30] Of the older patients (ages 2 to 6 years), one patient (2.9%) discontinued timolol secondary to hyperemia.[30]

13.3.2.5 *Cholinergic drugs.* Cholinergic agonists were the first medical treatment for glaucoma but are now seldom used for pediatric patients. Topical use of both pilocarpine and carbachol can be associated with cholinergic side effects, including gastrointestinal cramping, diarrhea, vomiting, headaches, hypotension, sweating, salivation, and syncope. The degree to which side effects are experienced is highly dependent on systemic absorption, which can be greater in pediatric patients.

Since the majority of pediatric glaucomas result from structural and developmental abnormalities of the angle and associated structures, these drugs may be less effective in lowering IOP. Pilocarpine (2% applied three or four times daily) has been used to a limited degree in pediatric patients.[27] This drug may be used for induction of miosis pre- and postoperatively for surgical goniotomy. The induction of myopia can significantly affect vision in pediatric patients. However, pseudophakic or aphakic

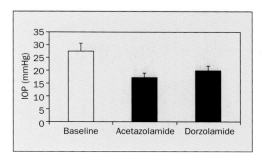

Figure 13.3. Carbonic anhydrase inhibitors in pediatric patients are additive with beta blockers. Both oral and topical medicines significantly reduced IOP from baseline (beta blocker alone). Acetazolamide decreased the IOP by 35.7% ± 15.6%, and dorzolamide by 27.4% ± 17.1%. *P < 0.01 compared with baseline. Adapted with permission from Portellos M, Buckley EG, Freedman SF. Topical versus oral carbonic anhydrase inhibitor therapy for pediatric glaucoma. *J AAPOS.* 1998;2:43–47.

patients have fewer side effects. Ocusert, a slow-release pilocarpine system, resulted in less myopic spasm from burst release but is not currently available commercially.[31]

Long-acting anticholinesterases, such as echothiophate iodide (Phospholine Iodide), are used mostly for the treatment of accommodative esotropia. Since the agents are of poor availability, with no advantages over pilocarpine and with more serious side effects, they are seldom used for glaucoma therapy. Reported side effects in children include ciliary spasms and angle closure.[32] In addition, systemic inhibition of cholinesterase activity and pseudocholinesterase in serum can cause signs of excessive parasympathetic stimulation, such as generalized weakness, nausea, diarrhea, vomiting, decreased heart rate, and salivation. When systemic levels of cholinesterase and pseudocholinesterase are reduced, the risks of anesthesia are significantly increased, due to the interaction with succinylcholine (a commonly used paralytic), which is degraded by this pathway. With low metabolism, prolonged apnea can result after surgery.

13.3.2.6 *Adrenergic agonists.* Epinephrine and dipivefrin, nonspecific adrenergic agonists, are rarely used in pediatric patients. When considered for medical therapy, systemic side effects may limit their use in this population.

Brimonidine, an alpha-2–selective agonist, has been studied in pediatric populations. One study of 30 patients (mean age, 10 years) showed a small (7%) decrease in IOP, but had a high rate of central nervous system depression (two became transiently unarousable and five others experienced fatigue).[33] In another study of 23 children (mean age, 8 years), the side effects were sufficient to merit discontinuation of therapy in 18%.[34] Other published reports include somnolence in four children, and multiple "coma" episodes, with hypotension, hypothermia, hypotonia, and bradycardia.[35,36] In one large study of 83 patients, brimonidine had only a modest effect on IOP (5 mm Hg) and a high rate (84%) of side effects, including lethargy (76%). There was an association between patient age and weight and the incidence of fatigue and lethargy. The researchers suggested caution in children younger than 6 years of age or weighing less than 20 kg.[37]

13.3.2.7 *Osmotic agents.* Glycerol (0.75 to 1.5 g/kg) in a 50% solution can be administered orally mixed with other fluids or over ice to partially mask the excessively sweet flavor. Glycerol is seldom used for the treatment of developmental glaucoma, but can be used in older children where an acute decrease in IOP is needed. Mannitol can be given intravenously (0.5 to 1.5 g/kg) and has the maximum effect within 20 to 30 minutes and lasting 4 to 10 hours. This can be useful for clearing the cornea prior to surgery. Patients must be carefully monitored during intravenous infusions of mannitol for cardiovascular and volume overload problems.

13.4 CONCLUSION

The management of glaucoma in reproductive-age women includes consideration of a second patient that does not need the medication (fetus). Proper treatment of the mother includes the consideration that therapy should not harm the unborn or breast-feeding child.

The management of pediatric glaucoma is different from that of adult glaucoma in several aspects. Pediatric glaucoma is mostly managed surgically, with medical therapy serving mostly to control the IOP during surgical planning. In addition, medical therapy can temporarily decrease the IOP to facilitate surgery by clearing the cornea, permitting certain operations. If long-term therapy is required, it is often the more severe disease that cannot be adequately managed surgically. In this situation, medication can be a useful adjunct to surgery.

The medications used in glaucoma for the most part were developed and tested primarily in adults. Future studies of the effects of glaucoma medications in pediatric patients will improve our knowledge of dosing, effectiveness, and side effect profile. As noted above, the side effects can be very different for small children, although they tend to approximate the adult level as the child grows in size and metabolic maturity. The management of pediatric glaucoma is a long-term effort, and any potential for vision loss needs to be treated aggressively, including the use of medical therapy when needed.

REFERENCES

1. Maris PJG Jr, Mandal AK, Netland PA. Medical therapy of pediatric glaucoma and glaucoma in pregnancy. *Ophthalmol Clin North Am.* 2005;18:461–468.
2. Chung CY, Kwok AK, Chung KL. Use of ophthalmic medications during pregnancy. *Hong Kong Med J.* 2004;10:191–195.
3. Becker B, Friedenwald JS. Clinical aqueous outflow. *AMA Arch Ophthalmol.* 1953;50:557–571.
4. Kass MA, Sears ML. Hormonal regulation of intraocular pressure. *Surv Ophthalmol.* 1977;22:153–176.
5. Sunness JS. The pregnant woman's eye. *Surv Ophthalmol.* 1988;32:219–238.

6. Brauner SC, Chen TC, Hutchinson BT, Chang MA, Pasquale LR, Grosskreutz CL. The course of glaucoma during pregnancy: a retrospective case series. *Arch Ophthalmol.* 2006;124:1089–1094.

7. Kooner KS, Zimmerman TJ. Antiglaucoma therapy during pregnancy—part II. *Ann Ophthalmol.* 1988;20:208–211.

8. Salamalekis E, Kassanos D, Hassiakos D, Chrelias C, Ghristodoulakos G. Intra/extra-amniotic administration of prostaglandin F2a in fetal death, missed and therapeutic abortions. *Clin Exp Obstet Gynecol.* 1990;17:17–21.

9. Andrade SE, et al. Prescription drug use in pregnancy. *Am J Obstet Gynecol.* 2004; 191:398–407.

10. Lustgarten JS, Podos SM. Topical timolol and the nursing mother. *Arch Ophthalmol.* 1983;101:1381–1382.

11. Yang CB, et al. Use of latanoprost in the treatment of glaucoma associated with Sturge-Weber syndrome. *Am J Ophthalmol.* 1998;126:600–602.

12. Altuna JC, et al. Latanoprost in glaucoma associated with Sturge-Weber syndrome: benefits and side-effects. *J. Glaucoma.* 1999;8:199–203.

13. Ong T, Chia A, Nischal KK. Latanoprost in port wine stain related paediatric glaucoma. *Br J Ophthalmol.* 2003;87:1091–1093.

14. Enyedi LB, Freedman SF. Latanoprost for the treatment of pediatric glaucoma. *Surv Ophthalmol.* 2002;47(suppl 1):S129–S132.

15. Enyedi LB, Freedman SF, Buckley EG. The effectiveness of latanoprost for the treatment of pediatric glaucoma. *J AAPOS.* 1999;3:33–39.

16. Boger WP III, Walton DS. Timolol in uncontrolled childhood glaucomas. *Ophthalmology.* 1981;88:253–258.

17. McMahon CD, Hetherington J Jr, Hoskins HD Jr, Shaffer RN. Timolol and pediatric glaucomas. *Ophthalmology.* 1981;88:249–252.

18. Zimmerman TJ, Kooner KS, Morgan KS. Safety and efficacy of timolol in pediatric glaucoma. *Surv Ophthalmol.* 1983;28(suppl):262–264.

19. Hoskins HD Jr, Hetherington J Jr, Magee SD, Naykhin R, Migliazzo CV. Clinical experience with timolol in childhood glaucoma. *Arch Ophthalmol.* 1985;103:1163–1165.

20. Passo MS, Palmer EA, Van Buskirk EM. Plasma timolol in glaucoma patients. *Ophthalmology.* 1984;91:1361–1363.

21. Harte VJ, Timoney RF. Drug prescribing in paediatric medicine. *Ir Med J.* 1980;73: 157–161.

22. Burnstine RA, Felton JL, Ginther WH. Cardiorespiratory reaction to timolol maleate in a pediatric patient: a case report. *Ann Ophthalmol.* 1982;14:905–906.

23. Bailey PL. Timolol and postoperative apnea in neonates and young infants. *Anesthesiology.* 1984;61:622.

24. Olson RJ, Bromberg BB, Zimmerman TJ. Apneic spells associated with timolol therapy in a neonate. *Am J Ophthalmol.* 1979;88:120–122.

25. Futagi Y, Otani K, Abe J. Growth suppression in children receiving acetazolamide with antiepileptic drugs. *Pediatr Neurol.* 1996;15:323–326.

26. Ritch R. Special Therapeutic Situations. In: Netland PA, Allen RC, eds. *Glaucoma Medical Therapy: Principles and Management.* San Francisco, CA: American Academy of Ophthalmology; 1999:193–201.

27. Haas J. Principles and problems of therapy in congenital glaucoma. *Invest Ophthalmol.* 1968;7:140–146.

28. Shaffer RN. New concepts in infantile glaucoma. *Trans Ophthalmol Soc U K.* 1967; 87:581–590.

14.1 CLINICAL FEATURES OF NONCOMPLIANCE

There are several ways in which patients can fail to adhere to prescribed medical regimens for glaucoma; these may include the following:

1. Failure to take the medication is the most common form of noncompliance and manifests in a variety of ways. Some patients may never intend to take a medication and thus fail to fill the initial prescription.[1] Patients can also miss doses of medications[2–6] or discontinue a medication prematurely.[7] Well-intentioned patients may be unable to deliver doses of medication to their eyes because of physical disabilities.[8,9]
2. Improper timing of medication can lead patients to space their medications too close together, leaving large stretches of time when they are undertreated (table 14.1).[3,10] Patients may also administer two different medications within too short an interval, causing the second drug to wash the first drug from the conjunctival cul-de-sac before it has the opportunity to fully penetrate the eye.
3. Overuse of a medication can be seen in patients who hope to increase a therapeutic effect[11] or who are confused with respect to their treatment regimen.
4. Use of the wrong medication may occur in patients whose regimens are complicated or whose regimens have undergone recent change.[12]

14.2 PREVALENCE OF NONCOMPLIANCE

It is difficult to estimate what percentage of patients with glaucoma fail to take their medications as prescribed, primarily because we lack a foolproof method of detecting noncompliance. Published studies report noncompliance rates of 28% to 59% among glaucoma patients.[2–7,13–15] The large range can be attributed to differences in the definitions of compliance used and in the measurement techniques employed. Rather than classifying patients as either compliant or noncompliant using an arbitrary criterion, it may be more informative to measure the level of compliance (adherence). One study used an electronic monitor to measure compliance to a treatment regimen of pilocarpine taken four times daily.[10] Monitor data indicated that patients administered a mean $\pm$ standard deviation of 76% $\pm$ 24.3% of prescribed doses. The same patients reported taking a mean $\pm$ standard deviation of 97.1% $\pm$ 5.9% of their doses. These data indicate that noncompliance is common and support the belief that patients who admit noncompliance are truthful, while patients who report good compliance may or may not be truthful.

In recent years, researchers have utilized large databases from Medicare, health plans, or insurance companies to study persistence with medication. A retrospective cohort study using health insurance claims data of 5,300 newly treated glaucoma or glaucoma-suspect patients found that persistence decreased over time and was affected by the type of glaucoma medication used.[16] Within 6 months of initiating therapy, nearly half of the patients who filled a prescription discontinued all topical ocular hypotensive medication. In addition, only 37% of these individuals continued to fill the prescription during the subsequent 3 years. Other studies report

Table 14.1 Improper Spacing of Dosing Interval[a]

Hour	02	03	04	05	06	07	08	09	10	11	12	13	14	15	16	17	18	19	20	21	22	23	24	00	01
Week 1					x				x					x				x							
					x					x				x				x							
					x					x				x				x							
					x	x				x				x				x							
						x				x				x				x							
Week 2					x													x							
					x					x				x				x							
						x				x					x										
							x			x				x				x							
						x				x				x				x							
Week 3						x				x				x				x							
						x				x					x			x							
						x				x				x				x							
						x				x				x				x							
						x					x				x										
Week 4						x				x				x				x							
						x				x				x				x							
						x				x				x				x							
						x				x				x				x							
				x																					

[a]One patient's administration of pilocarpine as measured by medication monitor.

Source: Reprinted from Kass MA, Meltzer DW, Gordon M, et al. Compliance with topical pilocarpine treatment. *Am J Ophthalmol.* 1986;101:515–523. Copyright 1986, with permission from Elsevier Science.

persistence rates as low as 20% at 18 months[17] and as high as 64% at 12 months.[18] It is important to emphasize that employing large databases to study persistence is useful but has some limitations. The data consist of prescription-refill counts gathered retrospectively. Such data cannot fully account for medication prescribed to one eye only, for medication purchased outside the health system (e.g., in Mexico or Canada), or for medication prescribed for temporary conditions. Nonetheless, these data reinforce the conclusion that defaulting is a common and serious problem in glaucoma therapy.

14.3 REASONS FOR NONCOMPLIANCE

Each mentally and physically competent patient has ultimate responsibility for compliance, but how a patient arrives at the decision to comply or not to comply with medical treatment is based on many factors. A patient's beliefs about health and disease, influenced by personal, societal, cultural, and financial factors, as well as the amount of information he or she has about the disease, play a significant role in this decision. In addition, other factors, such as the nature of the disease, the nature of the medical regimen, the patient–physician relationship, and the clinical environment, all play a role in the decision to adhere to treatment. Using hierarchical cluster analysis, Tsai et al.[19] identified 71 distinct barriers to medication compliance among patients with glaucoma. These obstacles were then grouped into four distinct categories: situational/environmental factors (e.g., lack of social support, difficulty with travel away from home, competing activities, major life events), regimen factors (e.g., side effects, cost, complexity, recent change), patient factors (e.g., knowledge, memory, motivation, comorbidity), and provider factors (e.g., dissatisfaction with physician, communication). Situational and environmental factors were thought to account for nearly half of these compliance obstacles, while the medical regimen was thought to account for one-third of the problems. Patient and provider factors were responsible for the remaining obstacles.[19] Some of these factors are addressed below.

14.3.1 *Patient Factors.* The large literature on compliance with medical regimens has shown limited correlation between noncompliance and age, sex, socioeconomic status, marital status, level of schooling, and race.[20,21] In general, studies addressing patients with glaucoma confirm these observations.[1,2,8,14,22–24] Despite some conflicting data, most studies indicate that gender is not an important indicator of compliance.[1,3,8,10,14] Likewise, a patient's age, marital status, educational level, and socioeconomic status have not been reliably linked to noncompliance with eye drops for glaucoma.[1,2,8,23,24]

While age as an independent variable is not significantly related to the level of compliance, age is often accompanied by diseases that may influence adherence. Elderly patients are more likely to suffer from multiple chronic diseases, and approximately 20% to 30% take three or more medications.[25] Polypharmacy is associated with increased risk of adverse drug reactions, drug interactions, and poor compliance.[25] Forgetfulness, poor visual acuity, parkinsonism, tremor, and hemiplegia have all been cited as reasons for noncompliance.[14] Falling asleep prior to bedtime medications or being unable to walk independently to the kitchen to use refrigerated drops can interfere with drug administration. Other physical hindrances to compliance with eye drops include difficulties with positioning the head, aiming the dropper bottle, and squeezing the bottle. Kass et al.[23] found that 20% of patients relied on another person to administer their eye drops. Winfield et al.[9] evaluated 200 patients who were prescribed eye drops for various reasons, including glaucoma; 57% of these patients admitted difficulty administering their drops, and when directly observed, only 20% instilled a drop correctly on the first try. In another study, 27% of patients were unable to put drops into each eye on the initial attempt; Uniform teaching of drop administration was correlated with an increase in the patients' ability to instill eye drops properly.[8] These studies reinforce the idea that proper eye drop instillation needs to be taught and, equally important, observed in all patients starting glaucoma therapy. Teaching alone, however, may not be enough for some patients with physical disabilities. In such cases, patients should be made aware of commercially available aids to instill medication, including Auto-squeeze, Autodrop, and Opticare.[26,27]

Patients with poor reading skills face particular difficulty accessing the health care system, understanding treatment regimens and consent forms, and following physician instructions.[28–32] Printed materials are frequently given to patients without first assessing the patient's ability to read or to read English-language materials.[33] Many materials require a higher level of literacy than that of the general population.[31,34] Physicians should evaluate the written documents they distribute and revise them to meet the reading level of their patients. They should also consider alternatives, such as photoessays, audiotapes, and videotapes for nonreaders or the visually impaired. Many patient materials are available in multiple languages.

Personal health beliefs play an important role in compliance with therapy. These beliefs include the patient's perceived vulnerability to the disease, the perceived benefit of treatment, and the perceived burden of treatment.

Patients who perceive themselves as having a serious medical problem are more compliant with the prescribed therapy.[35,36] That is, the patient must be willing and capable of accepting the illness before accepting the treatment.[37] This is especially relevant to glaucoma, given its typically asymptomatic nature. In a study of patients with ocular hypertension, better compliance with follow-up appointments was seen in the group who were prescribed treatment with eye drops than in those who were to be monitored without medication.[22] This study suggests that those who were not treated did not perceive a potential health problem and were more likely to be lost to follow-up. In addition, adherence to glaucoma therapy among patients with the diagnosis of glaucoma may be higher than in patients followed as glaucoma suspects.[16]

A study by Bloch et al.[2] found that patients were more likely to comply with glaucoma therapy if they had another chronic medical problem in addition to glaucoma.[2] These researchers suggest that this finding may be a result of the more clearly defined "sick role" of those patients who require more medical therapy; however, there is some evidence that patients must also perceive glaucoma to be a serious disease before being compliant with therapy.[2] Patients with multiple medical problems were more likely to be compliant with glaucoma therapy if they rated their glaucoma as their most troubling illness, while the noncompliers rated their other illnesses as more troubling.

The perception of the severity of glaucoma was also important in determining compliance in patients who were newly diagnosed with the disease.[1] Patients who were already taking a number of medications for other ailments were less likely to fill their prescriptions for glaucoma medications, perhaps because they thought glaucoma was "the least of their problems." On the other hand, if patients were started on multiple glaucoma medications at the initial diagnosis, they were more likely to be compliant than patients treated with a single agent. It is postulated that these patients perceived their glaucoma to be severe enough to warrant aggressive therapy.

It has been shown that a patient's knowledge of glaucoma is positively correlated with compliance. Compliant patients are more likely than noncompliers to know that intraocular pressure (IOP) plays a role in glaucoma,[6] to know the name of their eye disease and the possible effect of no treatment,[14] and to appreciate the connection between glaucoma and blindness.[2]

Another important determinant of compliance is the patient's social support system. Relatives and friends can provide transportation to appointments, remind patients to refill prescriptions and take medication, and may actually instill eye drops for some individuals.

14.3.2 *Disease Factors.* Characteristics of a particular disease are generally poor indicators of compliance; increasing severity of the disease, escalating symptoms, and increasing disability do not necessarily result in better compliance and, in fact, may sometimes lower compliance with therapy.[38] In patients with glaucoma, neither the duration of treatment[2,8,14,23] nor the severity of the disease[2,4,8,14] is significantly related to compliance with therapy. A retrospective cohort study in a group-model health maintenance organization found that glaucoma severity, measured by higher IOP and visual field loss, did not correlate with compliance.[39] A clinician's view of the severity of glaucoma may be very different from the patient's perception of the severity of his or her disease.

14.3.3 *Treatment Factors.* The tolerability, safety, dosing, and stigma of a treatment regimen have substantial impact on patient compliance. One of the major factors influencing compliance is daily dose frequency and the overall complexity of the therapeutic regimen. Numerous studies have documented a decrease in compliance with increased prescribed daily frequency of eye drops[14,24,40–42] or medications in general[43] (table 14.2). When Patel and Spaeth[24] classified glaucoma patients into three groups, those who had been prescribed one medication once or twice daily, one medication more than twice daily, and more than one medication daily, they found that the percentage of patients reporting missed doses was 51.2%, 60.7%, and 67.7%, respectively. Using an unobtrusive electronic monitor, Kass et al.[44] found that patients administered a mean of 82.7% of timolol doses prescribed twice daily versus 77.7% of pilocarpine doses prescribed four times daily.

Inconvenient dosing regimens are associated with defaulting. Patients may miss doses while at work or when they are away from home (and away from the

Table 14.2 Compliance Rate by Dosage Schedule

Dosage Schedule	Compliance Range (%)	Mean ± SEM
qd	42–93	70 ± 6
bid	50–94	70 ± 5
tid	18–89	52 ± 7
qid	11–66	42 ± 5

Note: $P < 0.05$ when comparing compliance of once- and twice-daily groups with that of either three- or four-times-daily groups.

Source: Modified by permission of the publisher from Greenberg RN. Overview of patient compliance with medication dosing: a literature review. *Clin Ther.* 1984;6:591–599. Copyright 1984 by Excerpta Medica, Inc.

medication), and are more likely to miss doses in the middle of the day for this reason.[3,14,24]

The health care claims data reported by Nordstrom et al.[16] demonstrated significantly higher persistence and adherence to glaucoma therapy with the use of prostaglandins (administered once daily), compared with topical beta blockers, carbonic anhydrase inhibitors, and alpha agonists (administered twice daily).

The cost of the medication can be an additional obstacle to compliance for many patients.[24,45] Patients may be unable to afford the medications or even the copayments for the medication prescribed.

Side effects or perceived side effects of a medication may negatively influence compliance. One study using willingness-to-pay surveys found that patients placed a higher value on eye drop medications that did not produce blurring of vision, drowsiness, or inhibition of sexual performance than they did on once-a-day use or the use of combination products.[46] In fact, 85% of patients were willing to pay, on average, 40% more for a medication that did not cause visual blurring. Uncomfortable side effects were the cause cited for stopping medication in 64% of glaucoma patients in one study.[2] In contrast, another study[24] found no correlation between side effects and noncompliance. It is possible that the patients' attitudes toward the disease and the side effects played a greater role than the actual side effects.[3] It is imperative to educate patients regarding the potential side effects of medication to avoid alarm or self-discontinuation when they are encountered.

14.3.4 *Patient–Physician Relationship.* In long-term patient–physician relationships, compliance is improved if the patient is satisfied with the doctor and believes that the physician is warm, concerned, thorough, accessible, and provides useful information about the disease and its treatment.[5,36,47] It is clear, however, that factors other than patient satisfaction affect compliance. In a study by Patel and Spaeth,[24] 98% of patients reported that their doctors were helpful and friendly, but 59% of patients were still noncompliant with their medications. It has been suggested that a combination of knowledge about the disease and its treatment and faith in the doctor motivates patients to use medications as prescribed.[37]

14.3.5 *Clinical Environment.* Continuity of care and short waiting periods in the office are associated with higher compliance in patients being treated for hypertension,[36,48] and it seems logical that this should also apply to patients being monitored for other chronic conditions, such as glaucoma. Missed visits by glaucoma patients have been associated with being a glaucoma suspect, being dissatisfied with extended clinic waiting time, and not being prescribed ocular hypotensive drops.[49,50] One study found fewer visits with an ophthalmologist to be the strongest risk factor for medication noncompliance.[39] Continuity of care not only facilitates the development of a good patient–physician relationship but also allows for reinforcement of education about glaucoma and glaucoma therapy. Brown et al.[8] found that uniform teaching by one doctor in a private practice resulted in an improved ability of patients to administer their medications, compared to patients who received variable information from different doctors at each visit in a clinic setting. This obstacle particularly affects underprivileged patients who may have reduced access to office-based physicians and may be more likely to obtain care from other sources, such as hospital outpatient departments or emergency departments.[51–54] The office and clinic staff should play a major role in providing information to glaucoma patients and instructing them about proper technique of eye drop administration.

14.4 DETECTION OF NONCOMPLIANCE

There is no gold-standard technique for detecting poor compliance; thus, in the day-to-day office practice of glaucoma, detection of noncompliance is exceedingly difficult. Methods used to detect noncompliance in clinical studies, such as electronic medication monitors, pill counts, and blood tests for drug or metabolite levels,[10,13,55–57] are expensive and may not be applicable to ophthalmic medications. Physicians are usually unable to accurately gauge the level of compliance in their own patients, even those who have been under their care for years.[3,10,55,58] The value of asking a patient about compliance is relatively low because most patients will tell their doctor "what the doctor wants to hear" instead of accurately reporting their adherence.[3,7,10,15,56,57,59–61] If a patient admits to poor compliance, he or she is likely to be telling the truth. Questionnaires have been developed to determine compliance with medical regimens.[62] It is possible that these will be useful in glaucoma management, but further research is required to prove their value (table 14.3).

Table 14.3 Self-Reported Medication-Taking Scale: A Four-Item Questionnaire

1. Do you ever forget to take your medicine?
2. Are you careless at times about taking your medicine?
3. When you feel better, do you sometimes stop taking your medicine?
4. Sometimes if you feel worse when you take the medicine, do you stop taking it?

Source: Modified with permission from Morisky DE, Green LW, Levine DM. Concurrent and predictive validity of a self-reported measure of medication adherence. *Med Care.* 1986;24:67–74.

It is often recommended that patients bring their eye drop bottles to each office visit. This is an indirect measure of adherence but may be useful in detecting gross noncompliance. In some medical systems, it may be possible to monitor the frequency of prescription refills, which, again, is an indirect measure of adherence but does provide information to the physician.

14.5 STRATEGIES TO IMPROVE COMPLIANCE

Numerous strategies have been employed to improve patient compliance. Some of these are listed in table 14.4.

14.5.1 *Simplification of Regimen.* As described above, compliance diminishes as the frequency and complexity of dosing increases. One of the most effective approaches a physician can have toward glaucoma therapy is to keep the regimen as simple as possible. One way is to prescribe daily dosing of medications instead of twice daily when possible. Using the lowest number of medications to achieve the desired therapeutic effect is also helpful, and this is aided by combination eye drops such as

Table 14.4 Improvement of Compliance

Educate

1. Explain glaucoma and rationale for treatment.
2. Anticipate and explain possible side effects.
3. Demonstrate drop administration.

Simplify

1. Prescribe least number of medications and lowest number of
   daily doses for desired therapeutic effect.
2. Tailor dosing schedule to daily events.
3. When changing regimen, change only one medication at a time.

Communicate

1. Reemphasize information about glaucoma on return visits.
2. Use printed information and videotapes.
3. Consider use of questionnaire to elicit difficulties with compliance.

Use Memory Aids

1. Have printed templates for medication schedules available.
2. Offer medications with compliance caps for appropriate patients.
3. Make patients aware of aids, such as eye drop instillation frames.

Gather Direct Information

1. Ask patients to use medication monitors.
2. Ask patients to share pharmacy records of refills.

dorzolamide–timolol (Cosopt). Finally, tailoring the dosing times to daily events, such as meals and bedtime, helps to cue the patient to take medications on schedule.[3,41,63]

14.5.2 *Improvement of Patient–Physician Relationship.* Sackett[64] has pointed out that "the easiest way to begin helping patients with low compliance is to pay more attention to them." This can be accomplished by inquiring at each visit if any problems were encountered with medications. Time can be taken to explicitly review instructions for drop use. The use of a short questionnaire may be helpful, allowing the physician to give feedback and reinforce instructions. These two aspects of physician behavior, showing concern and giving explanations, correlate positively with compliance.[65–67]

14.5.3 *Patient Education.* Too frequently, physicians assume that, because they have explained the disease process of glaucoma at the initial diagnosis, the patients will retain the information. In fact, most patients do not recall instructions given during any one outpatient visit[68] and may be especially prone to forget instructions given at an initial visit because of nervousness, shock at the diagnosis, or the large amount of information given in a short period of time. Because patients are more compliant with treatment if they understand their disease,[3,14,56,69] it is important that they understand glaucoma, the use of eye drops, the goals of treatment, and the consequences of defaulting. A rudimentary understanding of the pharmacology of the medications is also required to help avoid irregular spacing of doses or overuse of medications. Instruction in proper eye drop administration, including hand washing, sterile technique, drop separation in time, and punctal occlusion or eyelid closure, should be demonstrated by the physician or another health worker at the outset of therapy and should be reinforced periodically during follow-up visits. Patients should also be warned about potential side effects so they do not automatically discontinue a medication when a side effect occurs. They should be advised of serious side effects and instructed to call the office if they experience an alarming symptom.

It is beneficial to have a team approach to compliance so the patient receives reinforcement from different personnel in the office. Technicians and nurses can question patients about their medication schedules, check bottles, clarify instructions, and observe eye drop administration during office visits. Family members, friends, and coworkers can be enlisted to increase compliance. The pharmaceutical industry and national foundations provide literature and videotapes with information about glaucoma, treatment, and instructions for eye drop use and, in some cases, will sponsor support and discussion groups for patients. It is important to utilize resources such as these in combination with other strategies mentioned previously to help in the ongoing process of enhancing patient compliance.

14.5.4 *Memory Aids.* Printed medication timetable cards or sheets are an important method to aid patient compliance (see also Figure 11.2). These are most helpful if they list the drug name, eye to be given the dose, and the time of dose. The memory sheets can also include general information about drop-instillation technique, such as leaving 5-minute intervals between different eye drops and the use of eyelid closure and punctal occlusion.[70] The sheets can be made with colored dots that correspond to the color-coded bottle caps of different medications.[71] Large-print labels can be affixed to medication bottles[72] to aid patients with poor visual acuity.

Refill reminders, in the form of postcards or telephone calls from the pharmacist, have been shown to improve compliance.[73] However, such reminder systems are not in extensive use in the United States[74] and may cause confusion if the physician has changed a medication or the patient receives an inappropriate refill reminder.[59]

The C Cap ("C" for "compliance") is a memory aid designed to help patients remember to use their glaucoma medications at prescribed intervals. A window in the cap displays a number corresponding to the next scheduled dose; for example, a 1 or 2 appears in the window on medications prescribed twice daily. Each time a dose is taken and the cap is replaced on the bottle, the display number advances to the next scheduled dose.[75] In one study, this device helped significantly more patients achieve compliance with their regimens (67% vs. 41% prior to using the C Cap) and resulted in an IOP drop of 1.7 mm Hg.[76]

14.6 LOOKING FORWARD

In a recent editorial, Friedman et al.[77] make a strong case for a more dynamic approach to the care of glaucoma patients. They point out the importance of identifying all patients with glaucoma, retaining these patients under active care, and facilitating adherence with treatment. It seems likely that electronic compliance monitors will be commercially available in the near future. Physicians and patients could agree to use these devices and to share the information on compliance to improve patient care. Similarly, physicians and patients could agree to share information about prescription refills. With this information, physicians could actively monitor patient adherence and persistence with therapy. The information would allow physicians to make rational recommendations about changing medical therapy, enlisting help from friends and relatives, or performing surgery. Data from electronic monitors and prescription refill records could also be used to assess the value of medication questionnaires, educational programs, and behavioral interventions. Data would allow physicians to determine the most effective approaches for different groups of patients.[77]

REFERENCES

1. Gurwitz JH, Glynn RJ, Monane M, et al. Treatment for glaucoma: adherence by the elderly. *Am J Public Health*. 1993;83:711–716.
2. Bloch S, Rosenthal AR, Friedman L, Caldarolla P. Patient compliance in glaucoma. *Br J Ophthalmol*. 1977;61:531–534.
3. Granstrom PA. Glaucoma patients not compliant with their drug therapy: clinical and behavioural aspects. *Br J Ophthalmol*. 1982;66:464–470.
4. Granstrom PA, Norell SE. Visual ability and drug regimen: relation to compliance with glaucoma therapy. *Acta Ophthalmol*. 1983;61:206–219.
5. Spaeth GL. Visual loss in a glaucoma clinic, I: sociological considerations. *Invest Ophthalmol*. 1970;9:73–82.

6. Vincent P. Factors influencing patient non-compliance: a theoretical approach. *Nurs Res.* 1971;20:509–516.

7. Norell SE, Granstrom PA. Self-medication with pilocarpine among outpatients in a glaucoma clinic. *Br J Ophthalmol.* 1980;64:137–141.

8. Brown MM, Brown GC, Spaeth GL. Improper topical self-administration of ocular medication among patients with glaucoma. *Can J Ophthalmol.* 1984;19:2–5.

9. Winfield AJ, Jessiman D, Williams A, Esakowitz L. A study of the causes of non-compliance by patients prescribed eyedrops. *Br J Ophthalmol.* 1990;74:477–480.

10. Kass MA, Meltzer DW, Gordon M, et al. Compliance with topical pilocarpine treatment. *Am J Ophthalmol.* 1986;101:515–523.

11. Solomon DK, Baumgartner RP, Glascock LM, et al. Use of medication profiles to detect potential therapeutic problems in ambulatory patients. *Am J Hosp Pharm.* 1974;31:348–354.

12. Geletko SM, Rana KZ. Improving adherence with complicated medication regimens. *Med Health R I.* 1998;81:54–57.

13. Alward PD, Wilensky JT. Determination of acetazolamide compliance in patients with glaucoma. *Arch Ophthalmol.* 1981;99:1973–1976.

14. MacKean JM, Elkington AR. Compliance with treatment of patients with chronic open-angle glaucoma. *Br J Ophthalmol.* 1983;67:46–49.

15. Norell SE, Granstrom PA, Wassen R. A medication monitor and fluorescein technique designed to study medication behaviour. *Acta Ophthalmol.* 1980;58:459–467.

16. Nordstrom BL, Friedman DS, Mozafari E, et al. Persistence and adherence with topical glaucoma therapy. *Am J Ophthalmol.* 2005;140:598–606

17. Spooner JJ, Bullano MF, Ikeda LI, et al. Rates of discontinuation and change of glaucoma therapy in a managed care setting. *Am J Manag Care.* 2002;8(suppl):S262–S270.

18. Dasgupta S, Oates V, Bookhart BK, et al. Population-based persistency rates for topical glaucoma medications measured with pharmacy claims data. *Am J Manag Care.* 2002;8(suppl):S255–S261.

19. Tsai JC, McClure CA, Ramos SE, et al. Compliance barriers in glaucoma: a systematic classification. *J Glaucoma.* 2003;12:393–398.

20. Marston MV. Compliance with medical regimens: a review of the literature. *Nurs Res.* 1970;19:312–323.

21. Mitchell JH. Compliance with medical regimens: an annotated bibliography. *Health Educ Monogr.* 1974;2:75–87.

22. Bigger JF. A comparison of patient compliance in treated vs untreated ocular hypertension. *Trans Am Acad Ophthalmol Otolaryngol.* 1976;81:277–285.

23. Kass MA, Hodapp E, Gordon M, et al. Part 1. Patient administration of eyedrops: interview. *Ann Ophthalmol.* 1982;14:775–779.

24. Patel SC, Spaeth GL. Compliance in patients prescribed eyedrops for glaucoma. *Ophthalmic Surg.* 1995;26:233–236.

25. Corlett AJ. Caring for older people: aids to compliance with medication. *BMJ.* 1996;313:926–929.

26. Walker R. Aids for eye drop administration. *Pharm J.* 1992;249:608.

27. Morrison J. Eye drop aids and counseling sessions for glaucoma patients. *Hosp Pharm Prac.* 1993;3:413–418.

28. French KS, Larrabee JH. Relationship among education material readability, client literacy, perceived beneficence, and perceived quality. *J Nurs Care Qual.* 1999;13:68–82.

29. Weiss BD, Reed RL, Kligman EW. Literacy skills and communication methods of low-income older persons. *Pat Educ Counsel.* 1995;25:109–119.

30. Baker DW, Parker RM, Williams MV, et al. The health care experience of patients with low literacy. *Arch Fam Med.* 1996;5:329–334.

31. Davis TC, Jackson TH, George RB, et al. Reading ability in patients in substance misuse treatment centers. *Intl J Addict.* 1993;28:571–582.

32. Meade CD, Howser DM. Consent forms: how to determine and improve their readability. *Oncol Nurs Forum.* 1992;19:1523–1528.

33. Stephens NS. Patient education materials: are they readable? *Oncol Nurs Forum.* 1992;19:83–85.

34. Merritt SL, Gates MA, Skiba K. Readability levels of selected hypercholesteremia patient education literature. *Heart Lung.* 1993;22:415–420.

35. Becker MH. The health belief model and sick role behavior. *Health Educ Monogr.* 1974;2:409–419.

36. Dunbar JM, Stunkard AJ. Adherence to diet and drug regimen. In: Rifkind B, Levy R, Dennis B, Ernst N, eds. *Nutrition, Lipids, and Coronary Heart Disease.* New York: Raven Press; 1979:391–423.

37. Dowell J, Hudson H. A qualitative study of medication-taking behaviour in primary care. *Fam Pract.* 1997;14:369–375.

38. Haynes RB. Determinants of compliance: the disease and mechanics of treatment. In: Haynes RB, Taylor DW, Sackett DL, eds. *Compliance in Health Care.* Baltimore, MD: Johns Hopkins University Press; 1979:49–62.

39. Gurwitz JH, Yeomans SM, Glynn RJ, et al. Patient demographics in the managed care setting: the case of medical therapy for glaucoma. *Med Care.* 1998;36:357–369.

40. Akafo SK, Thompson JR, Rosenthal AR. A cross-over trial comparing once daily levobunolol with once and twice daily timolol. *Eur J Ophthalmol.* 1995;5:172–176.

41. Eisen SA, Miller DK, Woodward RS, et al. The effect of prescribed daily dose frequency on patient medication compliance. *Arch Intern Med.* 1990;150:1881–1884.

42. Greenberg RN. Overview of patient compliance with medication dosing: a literature review. *Clin Ther.* 1984;6:592–599.

43. Monane M, Bohn RL, Gurwitz JH, et al. The effects of initial drug choice and co-morbidity on antihypertensive therapy compliance: results from a population-based study in the elderly. *Am J Hypertens.* 1997;10:697–704.

44. Kass MA, Gordon M, Mosley RE Jr, et al. Compliance with topical timolol treatment. *Am J Ophthalmol.* 1987;103:188–193.

45. Stewart WC, Sine C, Cate E, et al. Daily cost of b-adrenergic blocker therapy. *Arch Ophthalmol.* 1997;115:853–856.

46. Jampel HD, Schwartz GF, Robin AL, et al. Patient preference for eye drop characteristics. A willingness-to-pay analysis. *Arch Ophthalmol.* 2003;121:540–546.

47. Stunkard AJ. Adherence to medical treatment: overview and lessons from behavioral weight control. *J Psychosom Res.* 1981;25:187–197.

48. Finnerty FA Jr. The problem of noncompliance in hypertension. *Bull NY Acad Med.* 1982;58:195–202.

49. Kosoko O, Quigley HA, Vitale S, et al. Risk factors for noncompliance with glaucoma follow-up visits in a residents' eye clinic. *Ophthalmology.* 1998;105:2105–2111.

50. Schwartz GF. Compliance and persistency in glaucoma follow-up treatment. *Curr Opin Ophthalmol.* 2005;16:114–121.

51. Ayanian JZ, Kohler BA, Abe T, et al. The relationship between health insurance coverage and clinical outcomes among women with breast cancer. *N Engl J Med.* 1993;329:326–331.

52. Cohen JW. Medicaid policy and the substitution of hospital outpatient care for physician care. *Health Serv Res.* 1989;24:33–66.

53. The Medicaid Access Study Group. Access of Medicaid recipients to outpatient care. *N Engl J Med.* 1994;330:1426–1430.

54. Long SH, Settle R, Stuart B. Reimbursement and access to physicians' services under Medicaid. *J Health Econ.* 1986;5:235–251.

55. Kass MA, Gordon M, Meltzer DW. Can ophthalmologists correctly identify patients defaulting from pilocarpine therapy? *Am J Ophthalmol.* 1986;101:524–530.

56. Norell SE. Improving medication compliance: a randomised clinical trial. *BMJ.* 1979; 2:1031–1033.

57. Yee RD, Hahn PM, Christensen RE. Medication monitor for ophthalmology. *Am J Ophthalmol.* 1974;78:774–778.

58. Blowey DL, Hebert D, Arbus GS, et al. Compliance with cyclosporine in adolescent renal transplant recipients. *Pediatr Nephrol.* 1997;11:547–551.

59. Cramer JA. Overview of methods to measure and enhance patient compliance. In: Cramer JA, Spilker B, eds. *Patient Compliance in Medical Practice and Clinical Trials.* New York: Raven Press; 1991:3–10.

60. Norell SE. Monitoring compliance with pilocarpine therapy. *Am J Ophthalmol.* 1981; 92:727–731.

61. Straka RJ, Fish JT, Benson SR, Suh JT. Patient self-reporting of compliance does not correspond with electronic monitoring: an evaluation using isosorbide dinitrate as a model drug. *Pharmacotherapy.* 1997;17:126–132.

62. Morisky DE, Green LW, Levine DM. Concurrent and predictive validity of a self-reported measure of medication adherence. *Med Care.* 1986;24:67–74.

63. Rudd P. Clinicians and patients with hypertension: unsettled issues about compliance. *Am Heart J.* 1995;130:572–579.

64. Sackett DL. A compliance practicum for the busy practitioner. In: Haynes RB, Taylor DW, Sackett DL, eds. *Compliance in Health Care.* Baltimore, MD: Johns Hopkins University Press; 1979:286–294.

65. Bartlett EE, Grayson M, Barker R, et al. The effects of physician communications skills on patient satisfaction, recall, and adherence. *J Chronic Dis.* 1984;37:755–764.

66. Cramer JA. Feedback on medication dosing enhances patient compliance. *Chest.* 1993;104:333–334.

67. Waitzkin H. Doctor–patient communication: clinical implications of social scientific research. *JAMA.* 1984;252:2441–2446.

68. Higbee M, Dukes G, Bosso J. Patient recall of physician's prescription instructions. *Hosp Formulary.* 1982;17(4):553–556.

69. Morisky DE, Malotte CK, Choi P, et al. A patient education program to improve adherence rates with antituberculosis drug regimens. *Health Educ Q.* 1990;17:253–267.

70. Kooner KS, Zimmerman TJ. A glaucoma medication time-table card. *Ann Ophthalmol.* 1987;19:43–44.

71. Faucher D, Gunn M, Morris M, et al. Why some eye surgery patients are seeing dots. *Nursing.* 1993;23:41.

72. Ritch R, Liebmann J, Steinberger D. A labelling method for eyedrops to improve compliance. *Ophthalmic Surg.* 1993;24:861.

73. Simkins CV, Wenzloff NJ. Evaluation of a computerized reminder system in the enhancement of patient medication refill compliance. *Drug Intell Clin Pharm.* 1986;20:799–802.

74. Robbins J. *The Forgetful Patient: The High Cost of Improper Patient Compliance.* Schering Report IX. Kenilworth, NJ: Schering Laboratories; 1987.
75. Sclar DA, Skaer TL, Chin A, et al. Effectiveness of the C Cap in promoting prescription refill compliance among patients with glaucoma. *Clin Ther.* 1991;13:396–400.
76. Chang JS Jr, Lee DA, Peturrsson G, et al. The effect of a glaucoma medication reminder cap on patient compliance and intraocular pressure. *J Ocul Pharmacol.* 1991;7:117–124.
77. Friedman DS, Cramer J, Quigley H. A more proactive approach is needed in glaucoma care. *Arch Ophthalmol.* 2005;123:1134–1135.

15

From Medical
to Surgical Therapy

ROBERT N. WEINREB AND FELIPE A. MEDEIROS

*F*or both the patient and the clinician, the decision to advance from medical therapy to surgery in glaucoma is an important one. Thoughtful consideration and assessment of the benefits and risks are essential. Although a lower intraocular pressure (IOP) following glaucoma surgery is generally considered beneficial to the eye, the risk of vision loss without surgery must outweigh the risk of vision loss with surgery. For this reason, medical therapy is the preferred initial treatment in most circumstances. With medical therapy, one or more drugs in the form of eye drops are prescribed to achieve a target IOP—the level below which the optic nerve function is stable and not expected to worsen. However, some clinicians have advocated early surgical intervention when glaucoma is first diagnosed.

Proponents of early surgery, and particularly those who advocate the benefits and success of glaucoma surgery as the initial therapeutic measure for primary open-angle glaucoma, cite the limitations of medical treatment. These include ocular and systemic side effects of medical treatment, cost of medication, poor compliance, and loss of visual function despite presumed adequate medical treatment. Under these conditions, early surgical intervention clearly is warranted in some patients. In particular, early surgery should be considered in those patients who are unlikely to comply with medical therapy, who require an unusually low target IOP, and in whom adequate IOP control is unlikely to be achieved with medical treatment.

In addition to these indications for early surgery, it has been suggested that patients not treated previously with a medical regimen have a better chance of success with trabeculectomy than do those who have received medical therapy. In this regard, some topical medications have been associated with an adverse effect on subsequent trabeculectomy because of deleterious effects, particularly of their preservatives, on the conjunctiva or Tenon's capsule. Without definitive data, however, most ophthalmologists view the potential complications of glaucoma surgery as serious enough that other therapeutic modalities should be employed first. Therefore, for most patients, surgery should be performed only when medical therapy has failed or is likely to fail. In other words, surgery to lower IOP is generally indicated for glaucoma patients on maximum tolerable medical therapy who have had maximal laser benefit and whose target IOP is exceeded.

15.1 MAXIMUM MEDICAL THERAPY

With six available classes of topical medications to use for IOP lowering, there is a seemingly bewildering array of treatment choices.[1] The large number of these choices has contributed to the ambiguity of the term "maximum medical therapy." The added benefit of a third or fourth topical agent is often minimal for most patients, and certainly the use of six classes of drugs is not feasible. Further, in clinical practice, combinations of each available medical agent at their highest concentrations are not indicated before a surgical approach is considered.

A medical treatment regimen needs to be customized to each individual patient to optimize the benefits and avoid the risks of the administered drugs. Clinicians should generally measure IOP more than once and preferably at different times of the day when establishing baseline IOP prior to surgery. Assuming topical agents have been administered appropriately, a single determination of IOP may be sufficient when it is markedly elevated. Certainly, drugs that have intolerable side effects should be excluded from consideration when assessing whether medical control of IOP can be achieved satisfactorily. An ineffective drug should be discontinued and similarly excluded. Medical contraindications may preclude the use of various agents.

Poor adherence or persistence with a prescribed medical regimen also needs to be considered when assessing maximum tolerable medical therapy. Patients who continue to worsen despite apparent IOP control should be questioned about their use of prescribed medications. Patients who are administering their medication only prior to a scheduled visit to the ophthalmologist, and not during the interval between visits, most likely will benefit little from long-term medical treatment. Patients who have well-controlled IOP when under the surveillance of their ophthalmologist, but who cannot remember to use their eye drops or are poorly persistent for a multitude of other reasons, ought to be considered for surgical treatment. With any patient on maximum tolerable medical therapy, poor adherence or persistence should be suspected because of the greater probability of side effects when numerous drugs are prescribed, as well as the difficult dosing schedules. In the latter situation, patients may have had prescribed six different eye drops with schedules varying from one to four times daily. Therefore, the term "maximum medical therapy" is used to indicate that no further escalation of medical treatment is available, appropriate, or likely to provide a clinically significant lowering of IOP.

15.2 THE OPTIC NERVE AND TARGET INTRAOCULAR PRESSURE

In the absence of structural of functional findings on examination of the optic nerve, the clinician certainly must refrain from rapidly advancing therapy to an intolerable or unacceptable level. Nevertheless, advancing optic disk or retinal nerve fiber layer damage even without observable visual field loss is progression and under certain circumstances can be an indication for surgery. Efforts should be directed at estimating the rate or risk of progression. Glaucoma patients who are at highest risk for progression should be identified and the threshold for surgery lowered. Conversely, those glaucoma patients who are at lowest risk should be followed with structural and functional testing of the optic nerve to identify early progression.[2] The risk of progression needs to be weighed against the risks and benefits of surgery and the life expectancy of the patient.

Regardless of whether there is an apparently adequate IOP with medical treatment, surgery is indicated if there is progressive worsening of the visual field, progressive optic disk damage, or thinning of the retinal nerve fiber layer. IOP that consistently exceeds the target suggests the possibility of progression even if the visual field, the optic disk appearance, and retinal nerve fiber layer are unchanged. The extent and location of damage may alter the threshold for surgery. Patients with advanced damage or damage threatening central vision should have lower IOP than those with early disease. One also should keep in mind that elderly patients with slow progression may have no change in quality of life during their lifetime and often can be observed on medical treatment. In addition, patients who have become blind from glaucoma in one eye despite good medical management and those with a strong family history of blindness from glaucoma are candidates for earlier surgical intervention. With so many classes of medication available, it is essential that the ophthalmologist set an appropriate IOP target and not wait for progressive visual field or optic disk changes before escalating therapy.

15.3 NEUROPROTECTION

Neuroprotection is a therapeutic paradigm for slowing or preventing death of neurons, including retinal ganglion cells and their axons (optic nerve fibers), to maintain their physiological function.[3] The underlying theoretical basis for a neuroprotective strategy in glaucoma appears sound. Moreover, considerable data from retinal ganglion cell culture and animal models of optic nerve injury support a neuroprotective strategy. Randomized controlled trials are evaluating neuroprotective strategies in patients with glaucoma. For neuroprotection to become an integral part of our therapy for glaucoma, it is necessary that clinical research complement and extend available basic research. If neuroprotection does become a viable therapy for glaucoma, it is likely that it will be complementary, and not replace, IOP-lowering medical therapy.

15.4 LASER SURGERY

Many types of open-angle glaucoma are amenable to treatment with laser trabeculoplasty. In contrast, only some types of closed-angle glaucoma, particularly (but not exclusively) those with a component of pupillary block, are amenable to treatment with laser iridotomy. Laser trabeculoplasty is usually performed over 360° of the anterior chamber angle during one or two sessions using appropriate treatment parameters. Except in situations where it has not performed correctly or in the presence of pseudoexfoliative glaucoma, retreatment is seldom effective. Although retreatment with selective laser trabeculoplasty has been touted as more effective than argon laser trabeculoplasty, studies to prove this have not yet been reported. Retreatment with either laser can be attempted, however, before proceeding to trabeculectomy if the clinician and the patient are willing to incur certain risks: possible deterioration of the condition during the additional delay, a reduced level of expectation for success, and temporary or sustained elevation of IOP.

Certain types of patients tend to respond poorly to laser surgery; therefore, laser surgery should not be offered routinely to patients with childhood glaucoma, inflammatory glaucoma, angle-recession glaucoma, iridocorneal endothelial syndrome, corticosteroid-induced glaucoma, and chronic angle-closure glaucoma. Laser surgery is difficult, if not impossible, to perform in certain other patients, such as those who cannot cooperate or hold a steady position at the laser, whose cornea is edematous, or whose angle cannot be adequately visualized.

15.5 SURGICAL CONSIDERATIONS

15.5.1 *Nonpenetrating Drainage Surgery.* For some surgeons, nonpenetrating glaucoma surgery (NPGS) provides an alternate surgical approach to trabeculectomy for moderate lowering of IOP in glaucoma patients. Lower IOP can be achieved with trabeculectomy than with NPGS, but short-term complications are fewer with NPGS. Further, NPGS is technically more challenging with a longer operative time. Despite potential advantages, there is still need for further evaluation of the technical details and standardization of the technique to improve the learning curve and efficiency of the procedure before NPGS is adopted widely.

15.5.2 *Sequence of Laser Surgery and Trabeculectomy.* The appropriate sequence of surgical therapy in patients whose IOP is uncontrolled by maximum tolerable and effective medical treatment is debatable. After follow-up of 4 to 7 years, the Advanced Glaucoma Intervention Study,[4] a randomized, controlled trial sponsored by the National Eye Institute and initiated in 1988 to compare visual outcomes of two sequences of surgical therapy, has suggested that initial trabeculectomy, rather than laser trabeculoplasty, may be preferable in white patients. In contrast, laser trabeculoplasty may be preferable for a first surgical intervention in African American patients. Longer follow-up and confirmatory data from other studies will be essential for determining whether the race-related differences in treatment outcome persist over the long term.

15.6 SURGICAL CONTRAINDICATIONS

A blind, painful eye is an absolute contraindication to glaucoma surgery. Because there is no visual benefit to be gained, pain control can be more safely and effectively achieved through other means. Surgery also is contraindicated for a blind, painless eye. In addition to being unable to improve vision, the clinician would be incurring a small risk of inducing sympathetic ophthalmia. Eyes with ocular neoplasms and individuals with poor hygiene should be considered poor risks for trabeculectomy; instead, noninvasive surgical therapy, such as cyclodestructive surgery, should be considered. Patients with iris neovascularization or neovascular glaucoma should be treated first with retinal ablation by panretinal photocoagulation and/or peripheral cryotherapy to induce regression of neovascularization.

15.7 CONCLUDING COMMENT

The clinician needs to keep in mind that the goal of glaucoma therapy is to sustain the vision-related quality of life and to maintain both the visual field and the structural integrity of the optic nerve. When the clinician is considering whether or when to advance from medical to surgical therapy, individual patient variations need to be taken into account. Selection of a target IOP for each individual eye is important, and surgical intervention should be considered if this target is not achieved with the appropriate medical therapy. Although these indications represent a prevailing view, they should be considered only as guidelines,[5,6] and not as a substitute for the experience and judgment of an individual ophthalmologist. Ophthalmic practice is continually evolving, and indications are likely to change as new knowledge is acquired.

REFERENCES

1. Zimmerman TJ, Fechtner RD. Maximal medical therapy for glaucoma. *Arch Ophthalmol.* 1997;115:1579–1580.
2. Weinreb RN, Friedman DS, Fechtner RD, et al. Risk assessment in the management of patients with ocular hypertension. *Am J Ophthalmol.* 2004;138:458–467.
3. Weinreb RN, Levin LA. Is neuroprotection a viable therapy for glaucoma? *Arch Ophthalmol.* 1999;117:1540–1544.
4. AGIS Investigators. The Advanced Glaucoma Intervention Study (AGIS), 4: comparison of treatment outcomes within race—seven-year results. *Ophthalmology.* 1998;105: 1146–1164.
5. Weinreb RN, Crowston JG, eds. *Glaucoma Surgery.* Amsterdam: Kugler Publications; 2005.
6. Weinreb RN, Mills RP, eds. *Glaucoma Surgery: Principles and Techniques.* 2nd ed. New York: Oxford University Press; 1998. *American Academy of Ophthalmology Monograph Series*; No 4.

Self-Study Examination

The self-study examination is intended for use after completion of the monograph. The examination for *Glaucoma Medical Therapy: Principles and Management* consists of 46 multiple-choice questions followed by the answers to the questions and a discussion for each answer. The Academy recommends that you not consult the answers until you have completed the entire examination.

Questions

The questions are constructed so that there is one "best" answer, unless indicated otherwise. Despite the attempt to avoid ambiguous selections, disagreement may occur about which selection constitutes the optimal answer. After reading a question, record your initial impression on the answer sheet (facing page).

Answers and Discussions

The "best" answer(s) to each question is provided after the examination. The discussion that accompanies the answer is intended to help you confirm that the reasoning you used in determining the most appropriate answer was correct. If you missed a question, the discussion may help you decide whether your "error" was due to poor wording of the question or to your misinterpretation. If, instead, you missed the question because of miscalculation or failure to recall relevant information, the discussion may help fix the principle in your memory.

Self-Study Examination Answer Sheet

Glaucoma Medical Therapy: Principles and Management

Circle the letter of the response option that you regard as the "best" answer to the question.

Question	Answer	Question	Answer
1	a b c d	24	a b c d
2	a b c d	25	a b c d
3	a b c d	26	a b c d
4	a b c d	27	a b c d
5	a b c d	28	a b c d
6	a b c d	29	a b c d
7	a b c d	30	a b c d
8	a b c d	31	a b c d
9	a b c d	32	a b c d
10	a b c d	33	a b c d
11	a b c d	34	a b c d
12	a b c d	35	a b c d
13	a b c d	36	a b c d
14	a b c d	37	a b c d
15	a b c d	38	a b c d
16	a b c d	39	a b c d
17	a b c d	40	a b c d
18	a b c d	41	a b c d
19	a b c d	42	a b c d
20	a b c d	43	a b c d
21	a b c d	44	a b c d
22	a b c d	45	a b c d
23	a b c d	46	a b c d

Questions

Chapter 1

1. The main route of topical ocular drug delivery into the anterior chamber of the eye is through the
   a. Conjunctiva
   b. Cornea
   c. Eyelids
   d. Sclera

2. The blood–ocular barrier includes tight junctions between the
   a. Capillary endothelial cells in the retina and iris
   b. Nonpigmented ciliary epithelial cells
   c. Retinal pigment epithelial cells
   d. All of the above

3. Iris color can interfere with ocular drug effects.
   a. True
   b. False
   c. Unknown
   d. Maybe

4. The conjunctival cul-de-sac compartment has a volume of
   a. 1 µL
   b. 7 µL
   c. 50 µL
   d. 100 µL

5. Nasolacrimal occlusion may
   a. Decrease systemic absorption of topically applied drugs
   b. Increase the ocular penetration of topically applied drugs
   c. Improve the therapeutic index of topically applied drugs
   d. All of the above

Chapter 2

6. Prostaglandin analogs reduce intraocular pressure by
   a. Reducing aqueous production
   b. Reducing outflow facility
   c. Reducing episcleral venous pressure
   d. Increasing uveoscleral outflow

7. A documented side effect associated with latanoprost use is
   a. Darkening of iris color
   b. Lowering of blood pressure
   c. Lowering of heart rate
   d. Impotence

8. The recommended dosing regimen for latanoprost is
   a. Daily in the morning
   b. Daily in the evening
   c. Twice daily
   d. Three times daily

9. Latanoprost has an additive ocular hypotensive effect with
   a. Timolol
   b. Acetazolamide
   c. Pilocarpine
   d. All of the above

Chapter 3

10. All the following are nonselective ocular beta blockers *except*
    a. Levobunolol
    b. Timolol in gellan gum
    c. Betaxolol
    d. Carteolol

11. A patient with a hypersensitivity to benzalkonium chloride might best tolerate which of the following beta blockers?
    a. Levobunolol
    b. Timolol in gellan gum
    c. Betaxolol
    d. Carteolol

12. Which of the following beta blockers does not exacerbate reactive airway disease?
    a. Timolol maleate
    b. Betaxolol
    c. Carteolol
    d. None of the above

Chapter 4

13. The most common systemic side effect of topical clonidine is
    a. Tachycardia
    b. Bronchospasm
    c. Hypotension
    d. Headache

14. Brimonidine is an
    a. Alpha-2 agonist
    b. Alpha-1 and alpha-2 agonist
    c. Alpha-2 antagonist
    d. Alpha-1 agonist

15. The most common ocular side effect of apraclonidine is
    a. Cataract
    b. Allergy
    c. Corneal edema
    d. Iritis

Chapter 5

16. The major mechanism by which cholinergic drugs reduce intraocular pressure is enhancement of
    a. Unconventional or uveoscleral outflow
    b. Trabecular outflow by a direct effect on the trabecular meshwork
    c. Trabecular outflow as a result of ciliary muscle contraction, which expands the trabecular meshwork
    d. Trabecular outflow as a result of iris contraction

17. Indirect cholinomimetics initiate their effect by
    a. Binding directly to muscarinic receptors
    b. Suppressing enzymes that inactivate acetylcholine
    c. Suppressing acetylcholine release from nerve terminals
    d. Increasing the sensitivity of postsynaptic nerve terminals to acetylcholine

18. High doses of cholinomimetics are not indicated for
    a. Acute angle-closure glaucoma
    b. Open-angle glaucoma
    c. Dark-eyed individuals
    d. Light-eyed individuals

Chapter 6

19. (For this question, more than one answer may be selected.) Which of the following are available as topical ophthalmic formulations?
    a. Acetazolamide
    b. Brinzolamide
    c. Methazolamide
    d. Dorzolamide

20. Side effects associated with systemic administration of carbonic anhydrase inhibitors include
    a. Anorexia
    b. Malaise
    c. Depression
    d. All of the above

21. (For this question, more than one answer may be selected.) Patients with which of the following conditions may be at risk for severe adverse effects following therapy with systemic carbonic anhydrase inhibitors?

a. Diabetes
b. Hepatic insufficiency
c. Chronic obstructive pulmonary disease
d. Pseudotumor cerebri

Chapter 7

22. Advantage(s) of fixed combination drugs include
    a. Reduced number of drops per day
    b. Reduced "washout" effect
    c. Reduced amount of preservative dose
    d. All of the above

23. Compared with concomitant dosing with the individual components, fixed combination drugs are likely to
    a. Have reduced side effects and similar efficacy
    b. Have similar efficacy and side effects
    c. Have increased efficacy and similar side effects
    d. Have reduced side effects and efficacy

24. Compared with either individual component, fixed combination products should be associated with
    a. Less reduction of intraocular pressure
    b. The same reduction of intraocular pressure
    c. Greater reduction of intraocular pressure
    d. Varying effects on intraocular pressure

Chapter 8

25. The most commonly used intravenous osmotic drug is
    a. Urea
    b. Sodium ascorbate
    c. Mannitol
    d. Glycerol

26. (For this question, more than one answer may be selected.) In diabetic patients, the preferred osmotic drugs are
    a. Glycerol
    b. Isosorbide
    c. Ethyl alcohol
    d. Mannitol

27. Osmotic drugs may be useful in all of the following situations *except*
    a. Angle-closure glaucoma
    b. Secondary glaucoma with acute and highly elevated intraocular pressure
    c. Chronic primary open-angle glaucoma
    d. Perioperative treatment

Chapter 9

28. Which of the following medications can lower intraocular pressure when administered systemically?
    a. Beta blockers
    b. Calcium channel blockers
    c. Central sympatholytics
    d. All of the above

29. Consumption of beverages containing which of the following may lead to unexpectedly low measurements of intraocular pressure?
    a. Tea
    b. Coffee
    c. Alcohol
    d. Orange juice

30. Which of the following psychoactive substances can lower intraocular pressure?
    a. Lysergic acid diethylamide (LSD)
    b. Amphetamines
    c. Heroin
    d. Marijuana

Chapter 10

31. All of the following are major risk factors associated with the development and progression of glaucoma *except*
    a. Elevated intraocular pressure
    b. Migraine headache
    c. Family history of glaucoma
    d. Age

32. All of the following statements regarding the Collaborative Normal-Tension Glaucoma Study are true *except*
    a. It was a randomized treatment of patients with normal-tension glaucoma.
    b. Target intraocular pressure was defined as 20% reduction from the baseline intraocular pressure.
    c. Cataract formation was significantly less than in the control group.
    d. Visual field loss was significantly reduced in the treated group.

33. The condition least likely to be of concern when selecting a medical regimen for a patient beginning medical therapy is
    a. A childhood history of asthma
    b. Elevated serum high-density lipoprotein (HDL)
    c. A clinical history of depression
    d. High myopia

Chapter 11

34. When considering the addition of a beta-blocking topical agent to a patient's medical regimen, the clinician should take into account the patient's
    a. Pulmonary history
    b. Cardiac history
    c. Current systemic medications
    d. All of the above

35. Maximum medical therapy is
    a. The therapy that the patient can tolerate, even if only one or no drug
    b. At least three glaucoma medications
    c. A level of medical therapy best determined by the physician
    d. Not considered when deciding to perform laser trabeculoplasty

36. The classes of topical medications that are additive are
    a. Prostaglandins
    b. Alpha agonists
    c. Beta blockers
    d. All of the above

37. The decision to advance medical therapy is best based on
    a. A change in intraocular pressure
    b. A single visual field
    c. The appearance of the optic nerve
    d. Change or expected change over time in optic nerve structure or function

Chapter 12

38. The differential diagnosis of pigmentation on the trabecular meshwork includes all of the following *except*
    a. Pigment dispersion syndrome
    b. Exfoliation syndrome
    c. Steroid-induced glaucoma
    d. Angle recession

39. Which of the following conditions can respond paradoxically to pilocarpine with worsening of angle-closure glaucoma?
    a. Pupillary block
    b. Plateau iris syndrome
    c. Aqueous misdirection
    d. Pupillary block and aqueous misdirection

40. Miotic treatment may prevent progression of the process leading to glaucoma by interfering with the mechanism leading to trabecular damage in all of the following conditions *except*
    a. Pigment dispersion syndrome
    b. Creeping angle closure

    c. Neovascular glaucoma

    d. Exfoliation syndrome

41. The appropriate initial therapy for congenital glaucoma is

    a. Trabeculectomy

    b. Goniotomy

    c. Trabeculotomy

    d. Either goniotomy or trabeculotomy

Chapter 13

42. According to the Food and Drug Administration, drugs with an established safety record with human testing done proving safety are classified as

    a. Class A

    b. Class B

    c. Class C

    d. Class X

43. In lactating women, the concentration of timolol in breast milk may be

    a. Lower than serum level

    b. The same as serum level

    c. Higher than serum level

    d. Not detectable

44. In pediatric patients treated with glaucoma medications, responder rates are typically

    a. Zero (no patients respond)

    b. Higher compared with adults

    c. The same compared with adults

    d. Lower compared with adults

Chapter 14

45. Compliance is best correlated with patients'

    a. Socioeconomic status

    b. Age

    c. Perception of their disease

    d. Sex

46. All of the following factors are associated with increased compliance with glaucoma medications *except*

    a. Simplification of the regimen

    b. Knowledge of the pathophysiology of glaucoma

    c. Severity of glaucoma

    d. Enhancement of the patient–physician relationship

Answers and Discussions

Chapter 1

1. *Answer—b.* The main route of topical ocular drug delivery into the anterior chamber of the eye is through the cornea. Drugs may also be absorbed from the cul-de-sac across the conjunctiva and enter the eye through the sclera, but this is a minor route of drug delivery into the anterior chamber.

2. *Answer—d.* The eye is relatively isolated from the systemic circulation by the blood–retina, blood–vitreous, and blood–aqueous barriers. These types of junctions prevent large molecules, such as plasma proteins, from entering the eye through the blood circulation.

3. *Answer—a.* Iris color is determined by the amount of melanin in the iris stroma. The onset and duration of the drug action after topical application are correlated with the retention of the drug in the melanin-containing iris. Many liposoluble drugs are bound by the melanin and slowly released later.

4. *Answer—b.* The human cul-de-sac has a volume of about 7 μL, which can expand momentarily and variably to 30 μL. A normal blink eliminates about 2 μL of excess fluid from the cul-de-sac.

5. *Answer—d.* Nasolacrimal occlusion may allow a reduction in the dosage and frequency of administration of various topically applied drugs. The benefit of nasolacrimal occlusion should be determined individually for each patient. It is important to train the patient on the proper performance of punctal occlusion for its benefit to be fully realized. Simple eyelid closure may also reduce nasolacrimal drainage of topically applied drugs.

Chapter 2

6. *Answer—d.* Prostaglandins primarily act by increasing uveoscleral outflow and outflow facility. They have not been shown to reduce aqueous production or episcleral venous pressure.

7. *Answer—a.* Latanoprost can cause darkening of iris color and increased pigmentation of eyelashes in some patients. There have been reports of uveitis and cystoid macular edema in some patients using latanoprost. These patients generally have had other risk factors for these conditions, and latanoprost itself has not been proven to cause either of these conditions. Latanoprost is not known to cause any systemic side effects.

8. *Answer—b.* Although latanoprost may be used once daily at any time of day, there is conflicting evidence that evening dosing is most effective.

9. *Answer—d.* Latanoprost has been shown to have an additive effect on the reduction of intraocular pressure when used in combination with any of the various classes of hypotensive medications.

Chapter 3

10. *Answer—c.* Betaxolol is a relatively selective beta-1 adrenergic antagonist. The other drugs are nonselective.

11. *Answer—b.* The preservative for the timolol in gellan gum is benzododecinium bromide. The preservative in the other preparations is benzalkonium chloride. Timolol maleate is available in a preservative-free preparation.

12. *Answer—d.* No ocular beta blocker is without risk for exacerbating reactive airway disease. The selectivity of betaxolol is only relative.

Chapter 4

13. *Answer—c.* Topical clonidine may cause significant systemic hypotension. For this reason, topical clonidine is not available for clinical use in the United States.

14. *Answer—a.* Brimonidine is a highly selective lipophilic alpha-2 agonist. Apraclonidine is more hydrophilic and has alpha-1 and alpha-2 agonist activity.

15. *Answer—b.* Hyperemia and allergy are commonly encountered ocular side effects associated with the use of apraclonidine. The allergic reaction may be delayed and may produce a follicular conjunctivitis.

Chapter 5

16. *Answer—c.* Although there is some evidence in organ culture systems for enhancement of trabecular outflow by an effect directly on the trabecular meshwork, the main mechanism is via ciliary muscle contraction. When the muscle contracts, tendons and connecting fibrils inserting into the trabecular meshwork and the inner wall of Schlemm's canal cause an unfolding of the meshwork and a widening of the canal to facilitate aqueous flow. Ciliary muscle contraction decreases uveoscleral outflow.

17. *Answer—b.* Indirect cholinomimetics act by suppressing cholinesterase activity, thereby decreasing acetylcholine inactivation, so that the neurotransmitter can act at muscarinic receptors to initiate a response.

18. *Answer—a.* High doses of cholinomimetics can create or increase pupillary block, further complicating angle-closure glaucoma. Moderate doses, such as pilocarpine 2%, induce adequate miosis, in most instances, to help reverse acute angle-closure glaucoma.

Chapter 6

19. *Answer—b,d.* Brinzolamide (Azopt) and dorzolamide (Trusopt) are available in the United States as topical ophthalmic formulations. Acetazolamide is available in oral and intravenous preparations. Methazolamide is an orally administered carbonic anhydrase inhibitor.

20. *Answer—d.* The side effects of systemic carbonic anhydrase inhibitors are legion and troublesome for patients. Anorexia, malaise, and depression are frequently encountered. In addition, aplastic anemia is a rare idiosyncratic adverse effect.

21. *Answer—a,b,c.* The metabolic acidosis associated with systemic administration of carbonic anhydrase inhibitors may cause serious problems in diabetic patients susceptible to ketoacidosis; in patients with hepatic insufficiency, because they are unable to tolerate the obligatory increase in serum ammonia; and in patients with respiratory acidosis and chronic obstructive pulmonary disease. Patients with pseudotumor cerebri may benefit from systemic administration of carbonic anhydrase inhibitors.

Chapter 7

22. *Answer—d.* Fixed combination drugs may reduce the total number of drops administered per day, reduce the amount of preservative instilled in the eye. In addition, they may reduce the "washout" effect by avoiding the rapid-sequence administration of the components when given separately. Cost savings is a potential advantage.

23. *Answer—b.* A useful fixed combination drug should have similar efficacy and side effects compared with the individual components administered in separate bottles. Other advantages of fixed combination products are attractive to patients and clinicians, including convenience and avoidance of "washout" effect.

24. *Answer—c.* Useful fixed combination products should have greater efficacy compared with any individual component. If the efficacy is the same as a single component administered as monotherapy, it would be preferable to treat with the single drug.

Chapter 8

25. *Answer—c.* Urea and sodium ascorbate are distributed in total body water and have a less pronounced osmotic effect compared with mannitol. Also, there are significant practical problems in the preparation and administration of urea and sodium ascorbate. Glycerol is an oral osmotic agent.

26. *Answer—b,d.* Glycerol and ethyl alcohol are metabolized and cause increased caloric load after ingestion, which may be a problem, particularly in diabetic patients.

27. *Answer—c.* Osmotic drugs are not useful in the long-term medical management of chronic glaucoma. They are, however, useful in the therapy of acutely elevated intraocular pressure and in the perioperative treatment of certain glaucoma patients.

Chapter 9

28. *Answer—d.* Medications prescribed by physicians for systemic disorders may affect intraocular pressure. Clinical measurement of intraocular pressure

should be interpreted after considering the patient's topical and systemic medications.

29. *Answer—c.* Alcohol has an osmotic effect, which can cause reduction of intraocular pressure. Patients who ingest alcohol-containing beverages prior to their appointments may temporarily lower their intraocular pressure.

30. *Answer—d.* Marijuana has an ocular hypotensive effect. Ophthalmologists who care for glaucoma patients can better interpret intraocular pressure measurements when they are aware of recent marijuana use by their patients.

Chapter 10

31. *Answer—b.* All are major risk factors for the development of glaucoma except migraine headache. Although not included as a requirement in the definition of glaucoma, elevated intraocular pressure is one of the greatest single risk factors in the development of glaucoma. Intraocular pressure affects risk in a dose-dependent manner. The risk of developing glaucoma is 10 times greater for the individual with intraocular pressure greater than 23 mm Hg compared to one with intraocular pressure less than 16 mm Hg. A positive family history of glaucoma is present in approximately 50% of patients with primary open-angle glaucoma, which is the cause of most glaucoma in the United States. A positive family history increases the risk of developing primary open-angle glaucoma by 4- to 7-fold in first-degree relatives. Glaucoma is uncommon before the age of 40 years, but increases dramatically after the age of 50. In some studies, the prevalence of glaucoma is greater than 10% of individuals older than 70 to 80. Migraine headaches may be a risk factor for normal-tension glaucoma. However, the role of vasospastic disease in the development of most other types of glaucoma is uncertain. Race is another major risk factor, which is not listed in the question. African Americans have a significantly greater risk of developing glaucoma than do whites.

32. *Answer—b.* The target intraocular pressure in the treated group in this well-executed clinical trial was defined as a 30% reduction in intraocular pressure from the baseline value. A significant number of patients developed cataracts after filtration surgery. When this fact was taken into account, progression of visual field loss was significantly reduced in the treated group (80% survival vs. 40% in the control group).

33. *Answer—b.* Low serum high-density lipoprotein (HDL) is a risk factor for atherosclerotic vascular disease. Carteolol is a beta blocker that is less likely to reduce serum HDLs than are nonselected beta blockers. A history of childhood asthma suggests the possibility of latent reactive airway disease. Patients with a history of asthma or chronic obstructive pulmonary disease are at significantly increased risk of developing reactive airway disease. Beta blockers can aggravate or induce clinical depression in susceptible individuals. Knowledge of a history of clinically treated depression should be obtained prior to initiating beta-blocker therapy. High myopia is a risk factor for retinal

detachment; these patients are at increased risk of retinal detachment with the use of miotics.

Chapter 11

34. *Answer—d.* The use of topical beta blockers is dependent on the patient's systemic health. Topical beta blockers are relatively contraindicated in individuals with asthma, heart block, or a history of congestive heart failure. Topical beta blockers may give less than the expected intraocular pressure–lowering effect if used in the presence of a systemic beta blocker.

35. *Answer—a.* Maximum medical therapy must be a level of medical treatment that is tolerable to the patient; the level is arrived at through consultation between physician and patient. It is not based on a set number of medications. The choice to perform surgery should always involve consideration of medical therapy.

36. *Answer—d.* Each of these medications, as well as carbonic anhydrase inhibitors, is additive to the others.

37. *Answer—d.* The level of intraocular pressure is important only in its relationship to the optic nerve. Certain individuals can tolerate higher intraocular pressures than can other individuals. Some normal-tension glaucoma patients may not tolerate intraocular pressure higher than 10 mm Hg. A change in intraocular pressure alone is not indicative of the need to intervene. A single visual field should not be relied on as an accurate indicator of function; rather, a series of at least two fields should be examined whenever possible. This is a subjective test, with limited reproducibility. The optic nerve appearance alone may sometimes indicate the need for treatment, but a better indicator is change or expected change over time in the structure or function of the optic nerve.

Chapter 12

38. *Answer—c.* Pigment dispersion syndrome leads initially to deposition of dense, often black, pigmentation over 360° of the trabecular meshwork. In the regression phase of the disease, the pigment is more prominent in the superior angle than in the inferior angle (pigment reversal sign). In exfoliation syndrome, the pigment is usually denser in the inferior angle, is usually of varying shades of brown, and is often accompanied by Sampaolesi's line. Trauma causing angle recession often leads to pigment deposition on the meshwork, particularly inferiorly. The meshwork in steroid-induced glaucoma is usually unpigmented or shows no more than age-related pigment changes. It should be noted, however, that patients with pigment dispersion syndrome tend to be steroid responders, whereas those with exfoliation syndrome respond similarly to the general population.

39. *Answer—c.* Pilocarpine constricts the pupil, but also increases lens axial thickness and shallows the anterior chamber. In pupillary block and plateau

iris syndrome, the effect on the pupil is significantly greater than that on the lens. In aqueous misdirection, pilocarpine worsens the block.

40. *Answer—c.* By eliminating pupillary movement, pilocarpine eliminates iridozonular contact in pigment dispersion syndrome and reduces or eliminates friction between the lens and the iris in exfoliation syndrome. By keeping the angle open, progressive formation of peripheral anterior synechiae can be prevented in creeping angle closure. Pilocarpine does not help to prevent progression of neovascular glaucoma.

41. *Answer—d.* Goniotomy and trabeculotomy are equally successful in treating congenital glaucoma. Trabeculectomy is recommended only after failure of these procedures to lower intraocular pressure sufficiently.

Chapter 13

42. *Answer—a.* No glaucoma medication is classified as Class A. All glaucoma medications are FDA Class B and C, with no human data to confirm safety in pregnancy.

43. *Answer—c.* The concentration of timolol in breast milk is higher than serum level, indicating that the drug is concentrated in breast milk during lactation.

44. *Answer—d.* In pediatric patients treated with glaucoma medications, responder rates are usually lower compared with responder rates in adults. In children, responder rates to glaucoma medications vary by age and type of glaucoma.

Chapter 14

45. *Answer—c.* No studies have found a clear correlation between common demographic variables, such as age, race, sex, or education, and compliance. The best correlation is seen when patients perceive their disease to be serious.

46. *Answer—c.* Increasing severity of glaucoma, escalating symptoms, or increasing disability does not necessarily result in better compliance and may actually decrease compliance.

Index